Diagnosis of Endometrial Biopsies and Curettings

Michael T. Mazur   Robert J. Kurman

Diagnosis of Endometrial Biopsies and Curettings

A Practical Approach

With 209 Illustrations

Springer-Verlag
New York Berlin Heidelberg London Paris
Tokyo Hong Kong Barcelona Budapest

Michael T. Mazur, M.D.
Crouse Irving Memorial Hospital
State University of New York
Health Science Center
Syracuse, NY 13210
USA

Robert J. Kurman, M.D.
Departments of Gynecology and
  Obstetrics and Pathology
The Johns Hopkins Hospital
and
The Johns Hopkins University
  School of Medicine
Baltimore, MD 21287
USA

Library of Congress Cataloging-in-Publication Data
Mazur, Michael T.
    Diagnosis of endometrial biopsies and curettings : a practical
approach / Michael T. Mazur, Robert J. Kurman.
        p.   cm.
    Includes bibliographical references and index.
    ISBN 0-387-94230-0. — ISBN 3-540-94230-0: DM158.00
    1. Endometrium—Histopathology. I. Kurman, Robert J. II. Title.
    [DNLM: 1. Endometrium—pathology. 2. Uterine Diseases—pathology.
WP 400 M476d 1994]
RG318.M39 1994
618.1'407—dc20
DNLM/DLC
for Library of Congress   94-10428
                                                             CIP

Printed on acid-free paper.

Production coordinated by Chernow Editorial Services, Inc. and managed by Theresa
Kornak; manufacturing supervised by Gail Simon.
Typeset by Asco Trade Typesetting Ltd., Hong Kong.
Printed and bound by Maple-Vail, York, PA.
Printed in the United States of America.

9 8 7 6 5 4 3 2 1

ISBN 0-387-94230-0 Springer-Verlag New York Berlin Heidelberg
ISBN 3-540-94230-0 Springer-Verlag Berlin Heidelberg New York

Preface

The incentive for writing this book came from a short course, "Endometrial Biopsy Interpretation," that we presented for five years at the United States and Canadian Academy of Pathology. The enthusiastic response we received from this endeavor prompted us to consider writing a practical text on the histologic interpretation of these specimens, which are commonly encountered in the surgical pathology laboratory but are given short shrift in standard texts. Several gynecologic pathology textbooks, such as *Blaustein's Pathology of the Female Genital Tract*, 4th ed. (1994), describe the morphologic features and classification of benign and malignant endometrial lesions, but little attention is given to the subtle differences between physiologic changes and pathologic conditions and the artifacts of biopsy and processing. In addition, microscopic findings that can be safely ignored because they have no clinical bearing are generally not discussed in standard texts. It is our impression that it is precisely these areas that present most of the difficulties in daily practice, more so, in fact, than the diagnosis of a malignant tumor.

This text is not a reference or atlas that describes pathologic curiosities that one might never encounter in a lifetime of practice. Instead, we attempt to provide a logical approach to formulating a pathologic diagnosis from the diverse array of fragmented, often scant pieces of tissue and blood received in the laboratory. As such, the material is presented in a less traditional fashion. Conventional histopathologic classifications remain an integral part of the text, but the various chapters focus on a clinically oriented approach to the microscopic diagnosis of common problems. For example, the individual chapters address the clinical questions and specifics of reporting the findings, aspects that vary according to the patient's age and the clinical circumstances.

One important subject is that of changes in the endometrium induced by breakdown and bleeding, independently of the underlying pathology. These alterations are highly prevalent in endometrial biopsies and are often misinterpreted, so they are described in detail. The updated World Health Organization classification of endometrial hyperplasia is based on the distinction of atypical and non-atypical hyperplasia. This topic is especially important, since cytologic atypia is the critical prognostic feature in their behavior, yet the characteristics of what constitutes atypia are not well appreciated. Metaplasia and other benign changes can mimic hyperplasia and carcinoma, so the text focuses on these lesions in detail. Clinical management of endometrial carcinoma is greatly influenced by the histologic evaluation of the curettings. Accordingly, the discussion of endometrial carcinoma considers not only the differential diagnosis, but also the grading of carcinoma and the distinction of endometrial from endocervical primary tumors.

Trophoblast presents unique problems in diagnosis. This is largely because the pathologist lacks experience with the diverse morphologic array of trophoblastic changes in benign and malignant lesions. Gestational trophoblastic disease is rare in routine practice. Furthermore, trophoblast of abortion specimens, including the trophoblast of the implantation site, usually receives little scrutiny. Two chapters have been included to cover this complex subject, one devoted to physiologic and one to neoplastic conditons.

Almost all the illustrations used in this text are from biopsies, and some show artifact and distortion, as occurs in routine specimens. We intentionally use this less-than-perfect material, since it better illustrates the problems that the pathologist faces in the interpretation of these specimens.

Since this monograph is not a reference text or atlas, we suggest reading it in its entirety in order to appreciate the clinically oriented problem-solving approach that we advocate. We hope that the reader finds this approach informative, useful, and enjoyable.

Michael T. Mazur
Robert J. Kurman

Contents

1
Introduction

Endometrial biopsies and curettings are among the most common tissue specimens received in the pathology laboratory. In several ways these specimens present a unique challenge for the surgical pathologist. Normal endometrium undergoes a variety of morphologic changes, especially during the reproductive years when cyclical hormonal influences and pregnancy affect uterine growth. Biopsy-induced artifacts confound this heterogeneous group of morphologic changes. Whether the biopsy is limited or a thorough curettage, the procedure usually is "blind," with no visualization of the tissue sampled. The final specimen contains multiple, irregularly oriented tissue fragments mixed with blood and contaminating cervical tissue and mucus.

Interpreting the biopsy material demands a logical approach that considers many factors. These include patient history, the specific needs of the clinician performing the biopsy, and an appreciation of the limitations, potential pitfalls, and complex array of patterns encountered in the microscopic sections. As with any pathologic specimen, proper interpretation requires careful fixation, processing, and sectioning of the tissue.

Indications for Biopsy

There are four main indications for endometrial biopsy or curettage[1-7]:

1. Determination of the cause of abnormal uterine bleeding.
2. Evaluation of the status of the endometrium in infertile patients, including histologic dating.
3. Evacuation of products of conception, either spontaneous abortions or termination of pregnancy.
4. Assessment of the response of the endometrium to hormonal therapy, especially estrogen replacement in perimenopausal and postmenopausal women.

Other indications for biopsy may arise. An occasional patient will have atypical or abnormal glandular cells in a cervical–vaginal cytologic specimen that requires endometrial sampling to exclude hyperplasia or carcinoma. Some clinicians sample the endometrium prior to hysterectomy to exclude significant pathology, although this procedure yields little pathology in the absence of a history of abnormal bleeding.[8] Likewise, endometrial biopsy as a screening device for perimenopausal and postmenopausal patients has a very low yield of significant abnormalities.[9]

At times these indications for endometrial sampling overlap. For example, some complications of pregnancy, such as a missed abortion or trophoblastic disease, are accompanied by abnormal uterine bleeding. Nonetheless, these broad categories provide a clinicopathologic framework for approaching the microscopic analysis of endometrial biopsy specimens. The text has therefore been divided into chapters that correspond to these clinical indications.

Clinical History and Biopsy Interpretation

In addition to considering the indication for the biopsy, interpretation requires appropriate clinical data. Important information for all biopsies includes patient age, menstrual status (last menstrual period), and hormone therapy. Other parts of the clinical history vary in their importance depending on the indication for biopsy.

Abnormal Uterine Bleeding

The most common reason for performing an endometrial biopsy is abnormal uterine bleeding, a term that refers to any nonphysiologic uterine bleeding. Age and menstrual/menopausal status are especially important data, since causes of abnormal uterine bleeding vary significantly according to the age and menstrual status, as discussed below. Abnormal uterine bleeding is a common sentinel of a number of different uterine disorders ranging from dysfunctional (nonorganic) abnormalities or complications of pregnancy to organic lesions such as hyperplasia or carcinoma.[5,6,10-12] There are several clinical terms used to describe different patterns of bleeding (Table 1.1).

The prevalence of the various abnormalities that lead to abnormal bleeding is difficult to determine precisely, varying with the patient population and the terms used by investigators.[2-4] A practical approach to the diagnostic possibilities of abnormal bleeding takes age into account (Tables 1.2 to 1.5). Pregnancy-related and dysfunctional (ovulatory) disorders are more common in younger patients, whereas atrophy and organic lesions become more frequent at older ages.[6] Among studies of patients of the same age there is a wide variation in the prevalence of some abnormalities. Polyps in perimenopausal and postmenopausal patients have been found in from 2% to 24% of patients.[13-19] Hyperplasia is found in up to 16% of postmenopausal patients undergoing biopsy, and endometrial carcinoma

TABLE 1.1. Clinical terms.

Amenorrhea	Absence of menstruation
Hypermenorrhea	Uterine bleeding occurring at regular intervals but increased in amount. The period of flow is normal
Hypomenorrhea	Uterine bleeding occurring at regular intervals but decreased in amount. The period of flow is the same as or less than the usual duration
Menorrhagia	Excessive uterine bleeding in both amount and duration of flow occurring at regular intervals
Metrorrhagia	Uterine bleeding, usually not heavy, occurring at irregular intervals
Menometrorrhagia	Excessive uterine bleeding, usually with prolonged period of flow, occurring at frequent and irregular intervals
Oligomenorrhea	Infrequent or scanty menstruation. Usually at intervals greater than 40 days
Abnormal uterine bleeding (AUB)	A term that describes any form of pathologic bleeding pattern from the uterus. Menorrhagia, metrorrhagia, menometrorrhagia, and postmenopausal bleeding are all forms of AUB
Dysfunctional uterine bleeding (DUB)	Abnormal uterine bleeding with no organic cause. The term implies bleeding due to abnormalities in ovulation or follicle development
Postmenopausal bleeding (PMB)	Abnormal uterine bleeding that occurs at least one year after menopause (the cessation of menses)

in less than 10% of patients.[13] One consistent observation in studies of postmenopausal patients is the finding that atropy is a common cause of abnormal bleeding, being found in 25% or more of cases.[13,14,16,19-21]

TABLE 1.2. Causes of abnormal uterine bleeding in adolescence.

Common	Uncommon
Dysfunctional bleeding	Endometritis
Anovulatory cycles	Clotting disorders
Complications of pregnancy[a]	

[a]See Chapter 3, Table 3.1 (Complications of pregnancy).

TABLE 1.3. Causes of abnormal uterine bleeding in the reproductive years.

Common	Uncommon
Complications of pregnancy[a]	Hyperplasia
Endometritis	Neoplasia
Dysfunctional bleeding	Endometrial carcinoma
Anovulatory cycles	Cervical carcinoma
Inadequate luteal phase	Clotting disorders
Irregular shedding	
Organic lesions	
Leiomyomas	
Polyps (endometrial, endocervical)	
Adenomyosis	
Exogenous hormones	
Birth control	
Progestin therapy	

[a]See Chapter 3, Table 3.1 (Complications of pregnancy).

TABLE 1.4. Causes of abnormal uterine bleeding in perimenopausal years.

Common	Uncommon
Dysfunctional bleeding	Complications of pregnancy[a]
Anovulatory cycles	Endometritis
Organic lesions	Adenomyosis
Hyperplasia	Neoplasia
Polyps (endometrial, endocervical)	Cervical carcinoma
	Endometrial carcinoma
Exogenous hormones	Sarcoma
Estrogen replacement	Clotting disorders
Progestin therapy	

[a]See Chapter 3, Table 3.1 (Complications of pregnancy).

TABLE 1.5. Causes of abnormal uterine bleeding in postmenopausal years.

Common	Uncommon
Atrophy	Endometritis
Organic lesions	Sarcoma
Hyperplasia	Clotting disorders
Polyps (endometrial)	
Neoplasia	
Endometrial carcinoma	
Exogenous hormones	
Estrogen replacement	
Progestin therapy (e.g., therapy of breast carcinoma)	

Even among perimenopausal and postmenopausal patients, the proportion of cases due to any of these conditions is age dependent. Atrophy and carcinoma occur more frequently in patients over 60 years of age, whereas polyps and hyperplasia are more common in patients who are perimenopausal or more recently postmenopausal. In addition to these uterine causes of bleeding, other abnormalities, such as atrophic vaginitis, can cause vaginal bleeding, and this bleeding may be difficult to distinguish from uterine bleeding until the patient undergoes a thorough clinical evaluation.

Ideally, the clinical history that accompanies an endometrial sample should include some description of the pattern and amount of bleeding. Often in the reproductive-age or perimenopausal patient the history is simply dysfunctional uterine bleeding (DUB). Clinically, this term suggests no other causes for bleeding except ovarian dysfunction. Nonetheless, a history of DUB commonly presupposes the etiology and, therefore, implicitly asks that organic lesions be excluded.

A history of risk factors for hyperplasia and adenocarcinoma, including anovulation, obesity, hypertension, diabetes, and exogenous estrogen use, serves to alert the pathologist that the patient is at increased risk for these disorders. This information, however, is rarely included on the requisition. Typically, there is little accompanying clinical information except the patient's age and a short history of abnormal bleeding. Consequently, hyperplasia and adenocarcinoma must be diagnostic considerations for most endometrial specimens received in the laboratory. On rare occasions, one can encounter hyperplasia or even adenocarcinoma in biopsies undertaken during an infertility workup where the clinical question was histologic dating rather than suspicion of these disorders.

Infertility Biopsy

When a patient undergoes biopsy for infertility, the clinical information often is limited, but here, too, the history should include the date of the last menstrual period (LMP) to give an approximate time in the menstrual cycle. This information is useful but not precise for determining the actual day of the cycle, since ovulatory frequency and follicular phase length are highly variable among patients. Usually the main concern in biopsies for infertility is whether there is morphologic evidence of ovulation and, if so, the histologic date (Chapter 3). The gynecologist may seek other specific information, such as response to hormone therapy, so it is important that the pathologist be given ay additional history that may be necessary for the interpretation.

Products of Conception

When endometrial sampling is done to remove products of conception, clinical information often is sparse, since the main goal of the procedure is simply to remove the placental and fetal tissue. Significant pathologic changes are rare. Nonetheless, it is helpful to know if pregnancy is suspected, and, if so, the approximate gestational age of the pregnancy. If there is a suspicion of trophoblastic disease, this should be stated. In such instances the human chorionic gonadotropin (hCG) titer is relevant. If an ectopic pregnancy is suspected, alerting the pathologist can ensure rapid processing and interpretation of the specimen.

Hormone Therapy

Since the endometrium is hormonally responsive tissue, the history of hormone use is important information. Clinical uses of steroid hormones (estrogens, progestins, or both) include oral contraceptives, postmenopausal replacement therapy, and therapy for endometriosis, hyperplasia, DUB, infertility, and breast carcinoma. As with other facets of the clinical data, this information may be absent or, if present, unreadable on the requisition. Consequently, the pathologist must be prepared to encounter hormonal effects in the absence of history indicating use of hormones.

Other Considerations

Pregnancy history is useful, especially in premenopausal patients, regardless of the indication for biopsy, since recent and remote effects of pregnancy, such as a placental site nodule or gestational trophoblastic disease, may be encountered in biopsy material. The history of recent or remote pregnancies is expressed as gravidity and parity. The letter G (gravidity) followed by a number (G1, G2, etc.) indicates the number of pregnancies, and the letter P (parity) followed by a number indicates the number of deliveries. For example, G4, P2 indicates that a woman has had four pregnancies and two deliveries. Further information on parity often is designated by four numbers indicating full-term pregnancies, premature pregnancies (> 20 but < 37 weeks gestation), abortions (< 20 weeks gestation), and living children. Thus a patient who is G5, P3013 is currently pregnant and has had three previous full-term pregnancies and one abortion, and the three children from the term pregnancies are alive.

The type of procedure, i.e., biopsy versus curettage, can be another important consideration in the interpretation of some cases. This information can be critical for deciding whether focal changes represent significant abnormalities and for determining whether or not small specimens are adequate. Although office-based biopsies generally provide a representative sample, they may not contain sufficient tissue to ensure the best diagnosis of some changes. For example, the irregular glands of hyperplasia may resemble patterns seen in some polyps, low-grade adenocarcinomas, and even artifactually distorted normal endometrium. Therefore, at times it can be difficult to be certain whether changes truly represent a hyperplastic proliferation in small biopsy samples. Furthermore, atypia can be focal in hyperplasia, and limited sampling may not be sufficient to exclude this type of focal abnormality, thus affecting the degree of confidence the pathologist may have in excluding atypia. With limited sampling, the full diagnosis is not always possible, although even scant specimens usually yield some useful information. On occasion a more thorough sample is necessary to permit the best diagnosis.

These basic clinical data are not excessive, but requisition forms are notorious for their lack of clinical information, so the pathologist must be prepared to address many endometrial specimens with a minimum of information. When the information supplied is not sufficient for accurate histologic assessment, the pathologist and gynecologist must communicate verbally.

Clinical Queries and Reporting

Selecting the best diagnostic term can be as challenging as the interpretation of the specimen. In general, it is best to avoid diagnostic terms such as "no pathologic diagnosis" or "no significant pathologic findings," since there is a wide range of normal histology. When the tissue lacks abnormalities, stating the normal phase of the endometrium, e.g., proliferative or secretory, provides more useful information for the clinician.

In biopsies for abnormal uterine bleeding, the pathologic information sought varies with the patient's age and clinical history. The gynecologist wishes to know the following:

1. Is there an organic lesion, such as a complication of pregnancy, inflammation, or a polyp?
2. Is there evidence of active or old breakdown and bleeding?
3. Is there evidence to suggest dysfunctional bleeding?
4. Is there evidence of hyperplasia or carcinoma?

For example, in the premenopausal patient the possibility of pregnancy and related bleeding is a frequent question. In a perimenopausal patient the concern shifts to hyperplasia and carcinoma, and in postmenopausal patients the importance of ruling out carcinoma becomes paramount. In any of these conditions, glandular and stromal breakdown may be present either focally or diffusely. It is the underlying disorder that is most important to report. The changes of breakdown and bleeding are secondary and do not indicate a primary disorder by themselves. Nonetheless, when there is a history of abnormal bleeding, it can be helpful to note whether or not there is histologic evidence of glandular and stromal breakdown (Chapter 5), especially if the tissue lacks evidence of an organic process such as hyperplasia or carcinoma. This information serves to document to the gynecologist that bleeding is, in fact, endometrial in origin. Even when there is no evidence of active bleeding,

foci of stromal foam cells or hemosiderin, sometimes with fibrosis, indicate that abnormal bleeding has taken place and deserve comment.

Besides reporting the morphologic changes present, noting significant negative findings can be helpful to the clinican. As an example, the diagnosis of chronic endometritis is more helpful if it includes a comment regarding the presence or absence of specific etiologic factors such as evidence of a recent pregnancy. Likewise, if an organic lesion such as a polyp is present, it is helpful to indicate whether noninvolved tissue is present and, if so, its appearance. In perimenopausal and postmenopausal patients, if the gynecologist indicates a specific concern regarding the presence of hyperplasia, atypia, or carcinoma, then a statement noting the absence of these lesions is reassuring.

For all cases, specimen adequacy is a consideration, but this only needs to be specifically addressed in limited samples where the diagnosis is not clear-cut. Scant tissue obtained by an office-based biopsy may be insufficient to allow thorough assessment of the status of the endometrium. In these cases the pathologist should indicate in the report that the specimen is scant. For instance, small samples may reveal hyperplastic glands, but it may be difficult to determine whether the abnormality represents a localized hyperplastic polyp or a diffuse hyperplasia. Some assessment of the endometrium can be done even on very limited specimens. For example, histologic dating is possible on small samples. Atrophic endometrium typically yields a very small amount of tissue, yet these specimens should not be regarded as inadequate (Chapter 5). The subsequent chapters consider in greater detail the queries likely to arise in different circumstances and the information that the pathologist should incorporate in the final report.

References

1. Noyes RW, Hertig AT, Rock J: Dating the endometrial biopsy. Fertil Steril 1950;1:3–25.
2. Baitlon O, Hadley JO: Endometrial biopsy. Pathologic findings in 3,600 biopsies from selected patients. Am J Clin pathol 1975;63:9–15.
3. Nickelsen C: Diagnostic and curative value of

uterine curettage. Acta Obstet Gynecol Scand 1980;65:693–697.

4. Van Bogaert L-J, Maldague P, Staquet J-P: Endometrial biopsy interpretation. Shortcomings and problems in current gynecologic practice. Obstet Gynecol 1978;51:25–28.

5. Galle PC, McRae MA: Abnormal uterine bleeding. Finding and treating the cause. Postgrad Med 1993;93:73–81.

6. Speroff L, Glass RH, Kase NG: Clinical Gynecologic Endocrinology and Infertility. 4th ed. Baltimore: Williams & Wilkins, 1989.

7. Merrill JA: The interpretation of endometrial biopsies. Clin Obstet Gynecol 1991;34:211–221.

8. Stovall TG, Solomon SK, Ling FW: Endometrial sampling prior to hysterectomy. Obstet Gynecol 1989;73:405–409.

9. Archer DF, McIntyre-Seltman K, Wilborn WW, Dowling EA, Cone F, et al: Endometrial morphology in asymptomatic postmenopausal women. Am J Obstet Gynecol 1991;165:317–322.

10. Goldfarb JM, Little AB: Abnormal vaginal bleeding. N Engl J Med 1980;302:666–669.

11. Povey WG: Abnormal uterine bleeding at puberty and climacteric. Clin Obstet Gynecol 1970;13: 474–488.

12. Stenchever MA: Significant symptoms and signs in different age groups. In: Comprehensive Gynecology. Herbst AL, Mishell DR, Jr, Stenchever MA, Droegemueller W, eds. St. Louis: Mosby, 1992; 161–183.

13. Rubin SC: Postmenopausal bleeding: Etiology, evaluation, and management. Med Clin N Am 1987;71:59–69.

14. Schindler AE, Schmidt G: Post-menopausal bleeding: A study of more than 1000 cases. Maturitas 1980;2:269–274.

15. Van Bogaert L-J: Clinicopathologic findings in endometrial polyps. Obstet Gynecol 1988;71: 771–773.

16. Choo YC, Mak KC, Hsu C, Wong TS, Ma HK: Postmenopausal uterine bleeding of nonorganic cause. Obstet Gynecol 1985;66:225–228.

17. Mencaglia L, Perino A, Hamou J: Hysteroscopy in perimenopausal and postmenopausal women with abnormal uterine bleeding. J Reprod Med 1987; 32:577–582.

18. Pacheco JC, Kempers RD: Etiology of postmenopausal bleeding. Obstet Gynecol 1968;32:40–46.

19. Lidor A, Ismajovich B, Confino E, David MP: Histopathological findings in 226 women with post-menopausal uterine bleeding. Acta Obstet Gynecol Scand 1983;65:41–43.

20. Meyer WC, Malkasian GD, Dockerty MB, Decker DG: Postmenopausal bleeding from atrophic endometrium. Obstet Gynecol 1971; 38:731–738.

21. Gambrell RD: Postmenopausal bleeding. J Am Geriatr Soc 1974;22:337–343.

2
Normal Endometrium and Infertility Evaluation

The histologic features of what constitutes "normal" endometrium change with a woman's age, through the premenarchal, reproductive, perimenopausal, and postmenopausal years.[1-3] During the reproductive years, the cyclical hormonal changes of the menstrual cycle provide a continuously changing morphologic phenotype which is "normal." The combination of these changes with artifacts and sampling limitations can make normal patterns difficult to interpret. During the reproductive years, deviations from normal, either in histologic pattern or in temporal relationship to ovulation, often indicate underlying abnormalities that may cause female infertility.

The endometrial biopsy is an important part of the evaluation of the female with infertility.[4,5] Biopsies for the evaluation of infertility often are performed in the office using a small curette or a Pipelle aspirator and therefore tend to be small.[6] Occasionally, biopsy or curettage is part of a comprehensive workup of the patient in the operating room that includes laparoscopy, hysteroscopy, or hysterosalpingography to assess the presence or absence of uterine or tubal lesions that contribute to infertility. In these cases, the endometrial sampling may not be timed as precisely for the mid to late luteal phase. Nonetheless, histologic evaluation provides the gynecologist with information regarding the response of the endometrium to hormonal stimulation, including indirect evidence of ovulatory function. The secretory phase is constant in the normal cycle, lasting 14 days from the time of ovulation to the onset of menstruation.[1] Variations in cycle length occur because of variations in the proliferative phase of cycle. The duration of the proliferative phase varies between cycles and between women. Accordingly, the gynecologist correlates the cycle date by histology with the woman's cycle date based on the time of onset of the upcoming menstrual period, not the last menstrual period.

The findings in the biopsy help confirm that ovulation occurred, and indicate whether there was sufficient secretory effect, mediated by progesterone, during the luteal phase. To fully utilize the morphologic interpretation, the gynecologist compares the histologic date to the date obtained from clinical data, including the date of the rise in the basal body temperature, the time of the serum luteinizing hormone (LH) surge, transvaginal ultrasound evaluation of follicular or corpus luteum development, serum progesterone level, or subtraction of 14 days from the onset of menses.[4,7-9] Consequently, the biopsy typically is timed to coincide with the luteal (secretory) phase of the cycle. In addition to obtaining the precise histologic date, an endometrial biopsy is performed as part of the infertility workup to exclude other organic uterine abnormalities.

This chapter reviews the morphologic variations due to ovarian hormonal stimulation as a background for the interpretation of endometrial biopsies in infertility patients. These patterns include changes due to normal hormonal fluctuations during the menstrual cycle and variations in normal development that are due to abnormalities in the endogenous ovarian hormonal levels during the reproductive years. The latter represent the so-called dysfunctional abnormalities that are, for the most part, due to abnormalities in ovarian follicular development or in hormone production by the corpus luteum. Ovarian dysfunction also can result in abnormal bleeding, and Chapter 5 reviews dysfunctional uterine bleeding due to ovulatory abnormalities. During gestation the endometrium undergoes other "normal," i.e., physiologic, alterations discussed in Chapter 3.

General Considerations in Histologic Evaluation

Histologic evaluation begins with identification of surface epithelium, a prerequisite for orienting the underlying glands and stroma. The surface epithelium is less responsive to sex steroid hormones than the underlying glands, but it often shows alteration in pathologic conditions, especially when the abnormalities are subtle or focal. For example, during the proliferative phase, estrogenic stimulation induces development of ciliated cells along the surface.[10] In contrast, ciliated surface epithelial cells are far more frequent in pathologic conditions, particularly those associated with unopposed estrogen simulation, such as hyperplasia and metaplasia.[2,3,11–13]

The subsurface endometrium is divided into two regions, the functionalis (stratum spongiosum) and the basalis (stratum basale) (Fig. 2.1). The functionalis, situated between the surface epithelium and the basalis, is important to evaluate, since it shows the greatest degree of hormonal responsiveness. The size and distribution of glands as well as the cytologic features of the glandular epithelial cells are important features

in the histologic evaluation. Under normal conditions, the glands should be regularly spaced and have a perpendicular arrangement from the basalis to the surface epithelium. In the secretory phase, the endometrium also shows a stratum compactum, a thin region beneath the surface epithelium. In the stratum compactum the stroma is dense and the glands are straight and narrow, even when the glands in the functionalis are tortuous. The basalis adjoins the myometrium and regenerates the functionalis and surface epithelium following shedding of the upper layers during menses. The endometrium of the basalis is less responsive to steroid hormones, and typically shows irregularly shaped, inactive-appearing glands, dense stroma, and aggregates of spiral arteries. The spiral arteries of the basalis have thicker muscular walls than those in the functionalis. In biopsies, tissue fragments that contain basalis often do not have surface epithelium. The glands and stroma of the basalis cannot be dated, since they are unresponsive to steroid hormones. A specimen consisting solely of endometrium from the basalis is therefore inadequate for dating.

Endometrial tissue from the lower uterine segment or isthmus is from another region of the endometrium that is less responsive to steroid hormones. Tissue from this region has shorter, poorly developed, inactive glands dispersed in a distinctive stroma (Fig. 2.2). The columnar cells lining the glands resemble those found in the glands of the corpus. Some glands show a transition to mucinous endocervical-type epithelium, however, and the latter represent glands near the junction with the endocervix. The stromal cells in the lower uterine segment are elongate and resemble fibroblasts with more abundant eosinophilic cytoplasm, in contrast to the oval to rounded stromal cells with minimum cytoplasm of the corpus.

The tangential orientation of the functionalis in biopsies and the tortuosity of the glands, particularly in the late proliferative phase, often lead to irregular cross sections of the tissue. In these areas gland development can be difficult to assess. Furthermore, not all fragments of tissue in a biopsy or curettage include surface epithelium to help with orientation of the glands. Nonetheless, at least focally, portions of better-oriented glands usu-

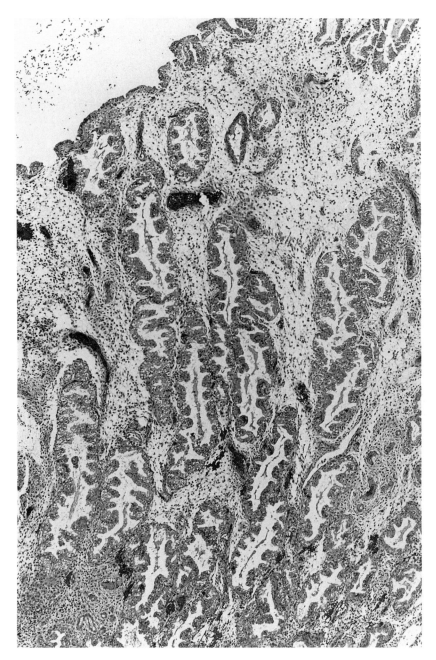

FIGURE 2.1. Normal secretory phase endometrium. Surface epithelium orients the tissue. The midportion of the tissue consists of the functionalis where glands, stroma, and blood vessels demonstrate the typical patterns of maturation through the menstrual cycle. The basalis in the lower portion of the illustration consists of irregular, closely spaced glands, dense stroma, and aggregates of arteries. The stratum compactum is composed of the surface epithelium and a subjacent thin layer of dense stroma.

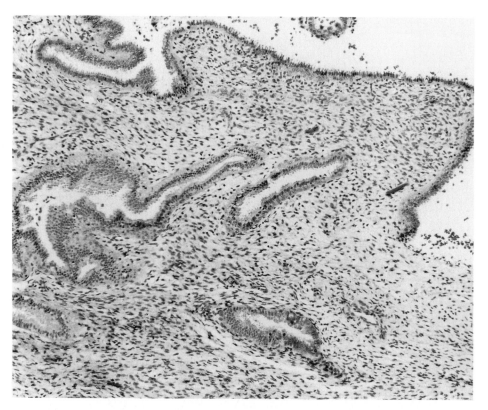

FIGURE 2.2. Lower uterine segment. Small, poorly developed glands in nonreactive stroma that is composed of widely spaced spindle cells. Tissue from the lower uterine segment cannot be dated.

ally can be traced through the functionalis to the surface epithelium. Visual extrapolation and comparison of tissue from area to area may be necessary to determine the status of glands in the functionalis, however.

Histologic Dating of the Normal, Cycling Endometrium

In the ovulatory patient, normal endometrium has two phases. The first is the proliferative (follicular or preovulatory) phase characterized by active growth of glands, stroma, and vessels influenced by estradiol produced mainly by granulosa cells in the ovarian follicles. Following ovulation, the secretory (luteal or postovulatory) phase reflects the effect of the combined production of progesterone and estradiol by luteinized granulosa and theca cells of the corpus luteum.[4] The regular sequence of morphologic changes deter-

mined by the fluctuating levels of ovarian steroid hormones forms the basis for histologic dating.

Dating uses an arbitrarily defined "normal" cycle of 28 days, with day 1 the first day of menstrual bleeding.[1] Histologic dating is most precise in the postovulatory secretory phase, since the follicular phase can be highly variable in length. Furthermore, proliferative phase changes are not as discrete as those in the secretory phase. The date of the secretory phase is expressed either as the day in the 28-day menstrual cycle, assuming ovulation occurs on day 14, or as the postovulatory day (e.g., secretory day 21 or postovulatory [P.O.] day 7). Local custom often determines the preferred method of stating the histologic date.

There are nine histologic features of the glands and stroma that determine the phase of the cycle and the histologic date (Table 2.1).[1] Five of these features affect glands: 1) gland tortuosity, 2) gland mitoses, 3) orientation of nuclei (pseudostratified

TABLE 2.1. Morphologic features used in endometrial dating.

Glandular changes
 1. Tortuosity
 2. Mitoses
 3. Orientation of nuclei (pseudostratified or basal)*
 4. Subnuclear cytoplasmic vacuoles*
 5. Secretory exhaustion (luminal secretions)*
Stromal changes
 6. Edema*
 7. Mitoses
 8. Predecidua*
 9. Granular lymphocyte infiltrate*

*Salient features used in dating the secretory phase.

TABLE 2.2. Proliferative phase changes.[a]

Early (4–7 days)
 Thin regenerating epithelium
 Short narrow glands with epithelial mitoses
 Stroma compact with mitoses (cells stellate or spindle
  shaped)
Mid (8–10 days)
 Long, curving glands
 Columnar surface epithelium
 Stroma variably edematous, mitoses frequent
Late (11–14 days)
 Tortuous glands
 Pseudostratified nuclei
 Moderately dense, actively growing stroma

[a] These changes are subtle. They are rarely used for actual dating.

versus basal), 4) subnuclear cytoplasmic vacuoles, and 5) luminal secretions with secretory exhaustion. Four features relate to the stroma: 6) edema, 7) stromal mitoses, 8) predecidual change, and 9) infiltration of granular lymphocytes. Practically,

the most important glandular features are orientation of nuclei, subnuclear cytoplasmic vacuoles, and luminal secretions with secretory exhaustion

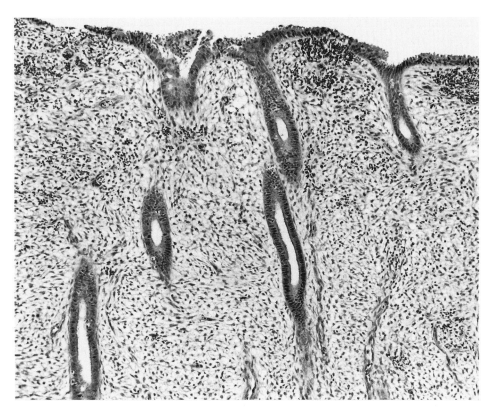

FIGURE 2.3. Proliferative endometrium. Glands are tubular and regularly spaced in abundant stroma. The stroma contains small vessels with thin walls. Both the glandular and the stromal cells show mitotic activity. Focal hemorrhage beneath the surface epithelium is a result of the biopsy and does not represent a pathologic change.

(3, 4, and 5), and the most important stromal features are edema, predecidual change, and granular lymphocytic infiltration (6, 8, and 9). These salient features are usually readily apparent when present, allowing the pathologist to apply a histologic date.

Proliferative Phase Endometrium

During the proliferative phase, the endometrium grows from about 0.5 mm up to 4.0 to 5.0 mm in thickness, so by the late proliferative phase, a biopsy obtains a moderate amount of tissue. Proliferative endometrium has three stages: early, mid, and late (Table 2.2).[2] These divisions are seldom used in biopsies, however. Usually the diagnosis of proliferative phase alone is sufficient, indicating that the endometrium is actively growing, shows a normal glandular distribution, and shows no evidence of ovulation.

Active growth of endometrium is the main characteristic of the entire proliferative phase (Figs. 2.3 and 2.4). Glands and stroma show brisk mitotic activity. In early proliferative phase endometrium, the functionalis contains small, tubular glands. The glands progressively elongate and become tortuous from the mid to the late proliferative phase because the gland growth is disproportionate to the stromal growth. Despite the tortuosity, the glands maintain a relatively regular spacing from each other. Throughout the proliferative phase, the epithelium lining the glands has pseudostratified, oval nuclei and dense basophilic cytoplasm. The pseudostratified nuclei remain oriented to the basement membrane, but some nuclei are raised above the basement membrane, giving a two-dimensional layering of the nuclei. The pseudostratification of the nuclei and the presence of mitotic activity in the glands and stroma are two constant features of the proliferative phase.

In the proliferative phase, the stromal cells are

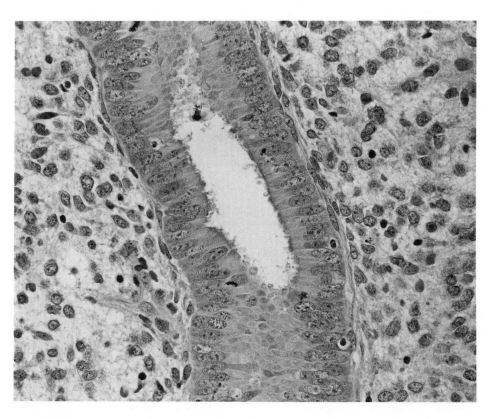

FIGURE 2.4. Proliferative endometrium. Proliferative phase gland shows pseudostratified nuclei with mitotic activity. The stromal cells have plump nuclei and indistinct cytoplasm. Scattered lymphocytes are normally present.

widely separated in the functionalis (Fig. 2.4). They are small and oval, having dense nuclei, scant wisps of cytoplasm, and ill-defined cell borders. Some stromal edema is normal at mid proliferative phase. A few lymphocytes also are scattered throughout the stroma, being most prominent around the vessels. Small spiral arteries and thin-walled venules are present.

The orientation and outline of proliferative phase glands and their relationship to intact stroma are important features for recognizing this normal pattern, since hyperplastic glands or glands in polyp can have identical cytologic features to glands in the proliferative phase. The regular spacing and uniform shape of the glands are characteristics of normal proliferative endometrium. Assessing gland orientation can be complicated, however, by biopsy-induced fragmentation, an especially common artifact in early to mid proliferative phase biopsies where the mucosa is still thin. Detached and disrupted glands may appear abnormally crowded or irregular. To separate fragmentation artifact from true abnormalities, it is therefore important to assess the integrity of the stroma as well as of the glands and to use surface epithelium to help orient the tissue fragments. Detached and poorly oriented glands that show pseudostratified nuclei and mitotic activity usually represent proliferative endometrium unless better-oriented tissue suggests another diagnosis. Proliferative phase glands also frequently show the telescoping artifact (see below).

Secretory Phase Endometrium

In the secretory phase, the glands and stroma develop, in an orderly sequence, specific histologic features of secretory activity from histologic day 16 through day 28. The endometrium attains a thickness of up to 7.0 to 8.0 mm. Unlike the proliferative phase, the changes in the glands and stroma are relatively discrete, varying sharply from one day to the next, thus permitting accurate dating. Dating of the first half of the secretory phase is based primarily on glandular changes. Dating of the second half is based mainly on stromal alterations (Table 2.3).

The morphologic changes of the secretory phase begin 36 to 48 hours after ovulation. There is an interval phase of 36 to 48 hours between

TABLE 2.3. Endometrial dating, secretory phase.[a,b]

Interval phase, 14–15 d. No datable changes for 36–48 hours after ovulation	
Early secretory phase, 16–20 d. Glandular changes predominate	
16 d	Subnuclear vacuoles (note: scattered small irregular vacuoles can be caused by estrogen alone)
17 d	Regular vacuolation—nuclei lined up with subnuclear vacuoles
18 d	Vacuoles decreased in size
	Early secretions in lumen
	Nucleus approaches base of cell
19 d	Few vacuoles remain
	Intraluminal secretion
	No pseudostratification, no mitoses
20 d	Peak of intraluminal secretions
Mid to late secretory phase, 21–27 d. Stromal changes predominate, variable secretory exhaustion	
21 d	Marked stromal edema
22 d	Peak of stromal edema—cells have "naked nuclei"
23 d	Periarteriolar predecidual change
	Spiral arteries prominent
24 d	More prominent predecidual change
	Stromal mitoses recur
25 d	Predecidual differentiation begins under surface epithelium
	Increased numbers of granular lymphocytes
26 d	Predecidua starts to become confluent
27 d	Granular lymphocytes more numerous
	Confluent sheets of predecidua
	Focal necrosis
24–27 d.	Secretory exhaustion of glands—tortuous with intraluminal tufts (saw-toothed), ragged luminal borders, variable cytoplasmic vacuolization, and luminal secretions

[a] d. = day of ideal 28-day menstrual cycle.
[b] To state as postovulatory day, subtract 14.

ovulation and the first recognizable histologic changes of the endometrium due to ovulation. During the interval phase, the glands become more tortuous and begin to show subnuclear vacuoles (Fig. 2.5). The first diagnostic evidence of ovulation, however, is the presence of abundant subnuclear glycogen vacuoles in the undulating, tortuous glands (Fig. 2.6). At this time the stroma is indistinguishable from that of the late proliferative phase. Since focal subnuclear vacuolization may occur in the proliferative phase, at least 50% of the glands should contain vacuoles to confirm ovulation. In addition, at least 50% of the cells in a

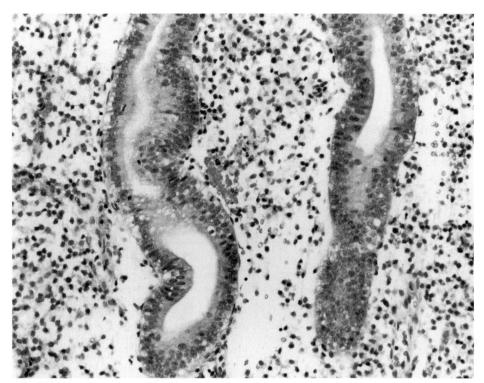

FIGURE 2.5. Interval endometrium. The glands maintain proliferative phase characteristics and show scattered subnuclear vacuoles. The extent of cytoplasmic vacuolization is not sufficient to be certain ovulation has occurred.

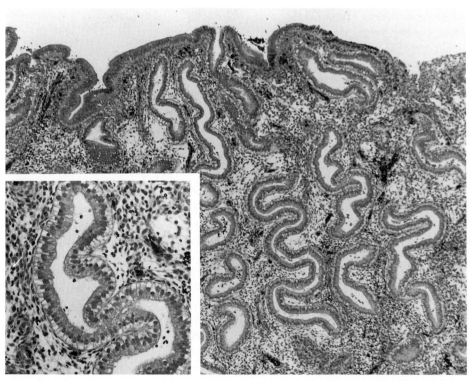

FIGURE 2.6. Early secretory endometrium, day 16–17. Postovulatory changes are clearly present with a regular distribution of subnuclear vacuoles in the serpiginous glands. The stroma shows no changes compared to the late proliferative phase. *Inset*: Every gland cell contains a vacuole, resulting in a uniform alignment of nuclei away from the basement membrane.

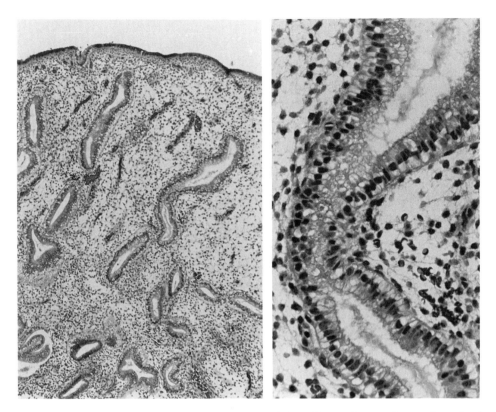

FIGURE 2.7. Early secretory endometrium, day 17–18. Glandular cell vacuoles remain prominent but begin to migrate to the supranuclear cytoplasm. A portion of the stroma shows mild edema.

gland should contain vacuoles. If the 50% rule is not fully met, but the clinical history and morphology suggest recent ovulation, the endometrium may be in the interval phase. Special stains for glycogen add little to routine histologic evaluation for establishing the presence of secretory changes.

Subnuclear vacuoles are abundant by day 17, and by day 18 the vacuoles begin to move from the basal to the supranuclear cytoplasm (Fig. 2.7). Concurrently, the nuclei become basally oriented. At this time the nuclei line up in a single layer perpendicular to the basement membrane. The cytoplasmic contents then form mucin and are expelled into the gland lumen. Luminal secretions peak at day 20 (Fig. 2.8).

After day 20, the stromal changes are more important than the glandular changes for dating. Nonetheless, the glands do continue to show increasing tortuosity, and variable amounts of luminal secretions persist until just before menses. From days 20 to 22 the glands in the functionalis begin to show secretory exhaustion, a change that becomes more prominent by days 24 to 25 (Fig. 2.9). Secretory exhaustion is characterized by the presence of a single layer of cells that lie in disarray with loss of orientation. The cytoplasmic border along the luminal surface becomes ragged, and luminal secretions are usually, though not invariably, present. By days 24 to 25 the glands often develop a serrated, "sawtoothed" luminal border (Fig. 2.10). The glandular cells may continue to show a variable degree of vacuolization throughout the remainder of the secretory phase. Cytoplasmic vacuolization is a physiologic change as long as the glands otherwise have appropriate tortuosity; the cytoplasmic changes from vacuolization to complete secretory exhaustion with no vacuoles represent a continuum of normal development. By day 27, cellular necrosis becomes evident with accumulation of nuclear dust in the basal cytoplasm of the

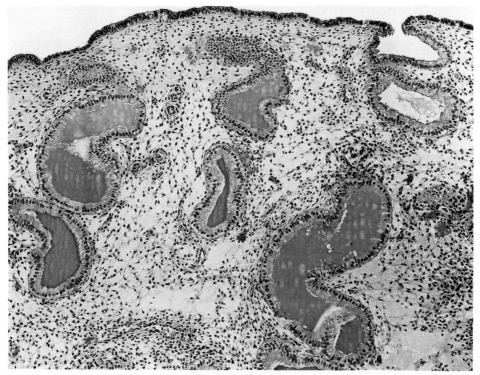

FIGURE 2.8. Mid secretory endometrium, day 20–21. Glands are distended with secretions. The stroma shows edema and there is no predecidual change.

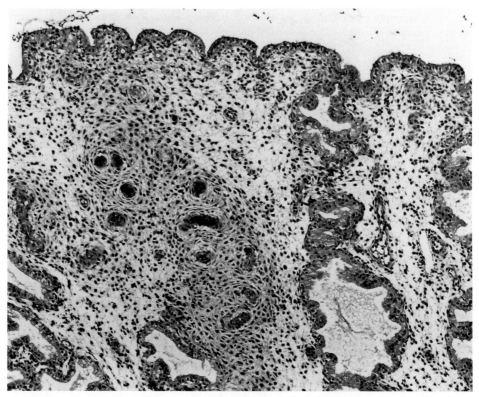

FIGURE 2.9. Late secretory endometrium, day 23–24. Predecidual stromal change is evident around spiral arteries with intervening zones showing edema. The glands are tortuous and show secretory exhaustion.

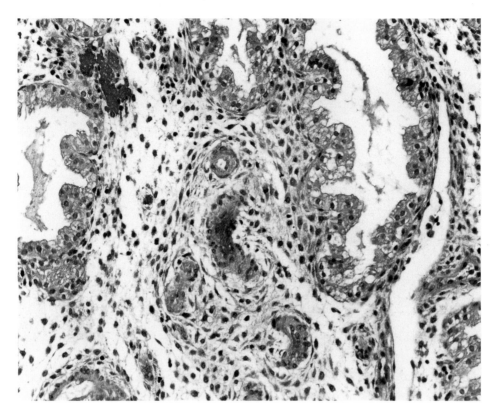

FIGURE 2.10. Late secretory endometrium. Stromal cells around spiral arteries show predecidual change with increased cytoplasm. The gland shows secretory exhaustion with disarray of the nuclei and patchy cytoplasmic vacuolization.

glandular epithelial cells. Throughout the secretory phase, the glands in the stratum compactum immediately beneath the surface epithelium remain small and tubular despite their increasing tortuosity in the functionalis.

As the glandular cells develop cytoplasmic vacuoles and produce luminal secretions, edema, the first stromal change, begins and peaks quickly at days 21 to 22 (Table 2.3). Once stromal changes begin, the glandular changes are less important for dating. Because of the edema, the stromal cells take on the so-called naked nucleus appearance at days 21 to 22. With this change the stromal cells are widely dispersed and have small nuclei with scant, imperceptible cytoplasm (Fig. 2.8). This phase of pure stromal edema is brief, and the subsequent predecidual transformation of the stroma becomes the main feature in dating the late secretory phase. Although stromal edema is maximum at days 21 to 22, edema begins in a

patchy distribution in the early secretory phase at days 17 to 18. Therefore, some edema in the earlier portion of the secretory phase does not represent an irregularity of maturation.

Predecidual change characterizes the late secretory phase (days 23 to 28). With the appearance of predecidua (not "pseudodecidua"), the cells gain identifiable cytoplasm (Fig. 2.9). These cells become oval to polygonal shaped in the functionalis and show a moderate amount of eosinophilic to amphophilic cytoplasm (Figs. 2.10 and 2.11). Just below the surface epithelium they can be spindle shaped. Cell borders of predecidual cells often are indistinct in formalin-fixed specimens. Predecidual transformation begins on day 23 around spiral arteries, making their walls appear thicker and leading to prominence of the vessels (Fig. 2.9). In the predecidua there is a resurgence of stromal mitotic activity at day 24, while the glandular epithelium lacks mitoses.

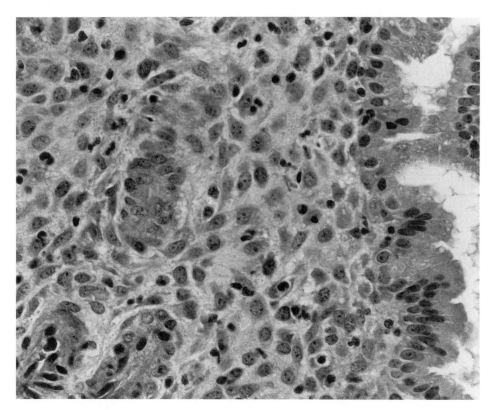

FIGURE 2.11. Predecidua and granular lymphocytes in late secretory endometrium. Predecidualized stromal cells in the late secretory phase appear oval to polygonal with a moderate amount of pale cytoplasm. At this time in the secretory phase, mitotic activity recurs in the stromal cells. Stromal granular lymphocytes are scattered throughout the stroma. These cells have dark, often lobulated nuclei.

The amount of predecidua increases, extending to the subsurface stroma on day 25. The predecidual change around vessels and beneath the surface epithelium becomes confluent, forming larger sheets by day 26 (Fig. 2.12). Predecidua is easy to recognize when advanced, but this change can be subtle when it is early and not confluent. Intervening stroma often shows some edema, and dating remains based on the most advanced changes. By day 27, predecidual change is extensive.

With predecidual transformation, the stroma shows a gradually increasing number of smaller mononuclear and bilobate cells with faintly granular cytoplasm (Fig. 2.11). Others have small round and dense nuclei. Variably termed "stromal granulocytes," "granulated lymphocytes," "K cells," "leukocytes," or "neutrophils," these cells are not polymorphonuclear leukocytes (neutrophils).[2,3,14] The latter occur normally only in menstrual endometrium. Recent immunohistochemical studies reveal that most of these cells are T lymphocytes.[15-17] We therefore prefer the designation "granular lymphocytes." They are normally present in small numbers earlier in the cycle but become prominent by the late secretory phase.

At day 27 the endometrium is premenstrual. Predecidua is present in sheets with many interspersed granular lymphocytes. The glands are highly convoluted and saw-toothed. The glands begin to show individual cell necrosis with nuclear dust at their base. On day 28 fibrin thrombi begin to form in small vessels, and hemorrhage follows with extravasation of erythrocytes into the stroma.

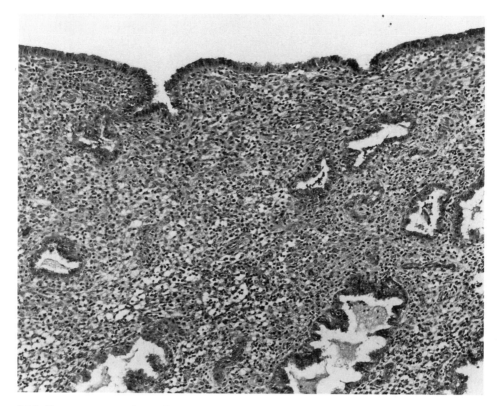

FIGURE 2.12. Late secretory endometrium, day 26–27. The stroma consists of sheets of predecidualized cells with a heavy infiltrate of granular lymphocytes. The glands in the functionalis remain tortuous and show a variable amount of intraluminal secretion. In the stratum compactum beneath the surface epithelium the glands are small and tubular.

Menstrual Endometrium

Menstrual endometrium shows glandular and stromal breakdown that rapidly affects all the functionalis by the end of day 28. This stage shows fibrin thrombi in small vessels, condensed and collapsed stroma, and necrotic debris (Fig. 2.13). With this necrosis, a true neutrophilic infiltrate becomes a part of the physiologic process.[18] When the bleeding is extensive, it may not be possible to assess the development of the glands or stroma or the "normality" of the tissue. Once breakdown starts, the stromal cells coalesce into aggregates and clusters that often show little cytoplasm. With extensive stromal collapse during menstruation, the predecidual change in the stromal cells becomes indistinct (Fig. 2.14). The extensive breakdown also can result in striking morphologic alterations with artifactual glandular crowding. As a result, menstrual endometrium can be confused with hyperplasia or even carcinoma if the background bleeding pattern is not recognized. Conversely, hyperplasia and carcinoma are proliferative processes that rarely show extensive breakdown of the type displayed by menstrual endometrium. Because of the artifacts induced by the breakdown and bleeding of the menstrual phase, this tissue is not suitable for evaluation of glandular and stromal development. Some advocate biopsy at the onset of bleeding in order to be certain that the procedure does not interrupt an early pregnancy, but this tissue is not optimal unless obtained very early in the menstrual phase before breakdown becomes extensive.[4]

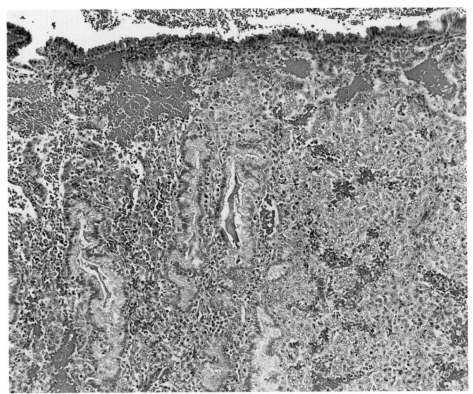

FIGURE 2.13.   Menstrual endometrium. Hemorrhage into the stroma forms lakes of erythrocytes. The hemorrhage disrupts the glands and stroma, although the tortuosity of the glands persists.

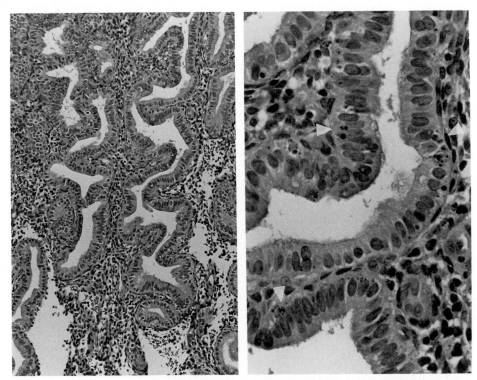

FIGURE 2.14.   Menstrual endometrium. Glands and stroma near the basalis undergo collapse as the superficial tissue sloughs. The glands retain tortuous shapes but show nuclear dust accumulating in the subnuclear cytoplasm (arrowheads). Predecidual change in the stroma has become indistinct.

Pitfalls in Dating

The preceding description summarizes the basic histologic changes of endometrial development. In addition to understanding the normal morphology in ideal situations, there are a number of practical points to consider when interpreting the endometrial biopsy. There are several caveats and potential pitfalls, knowledge of which assists in accurate diagnosis of normal endometrium and helps avoid errors in dating. The following, in our opinion, are especially important aspects to consider in evaluating this biopsy material:

1. Endometrium with surface epithelium is best for interpretation. Absence of surface epithelium compromises the interpretation.
2. Tissue from the lower uterine segment or basalis is not satisfactory for dating. Endometrium from these regions does not respond fully to hormones.
3. Straight, tubular glands beneath the surface are normal and not a sign of irregularity in maturation in the late secretory phase.
4. Scattered subnuclear vacuoles in glands are *not* sufficient evidence of ovulation. Greater than 50% of the glands must show subnuclear vacuoles to be certain that ovulation has occurred.
5. The presence of secretions in the glandular lumen does not indicate secretory endometrium. Proliferative, hyperplastic, and neoplastic glands can contain luminal secretions. It is the glandular cytoplasm and nuclear changes that are most important for determining the presence of absence of secretory changes.
6. Focal glandular crowding due to tangential sectioning can occur in proliferative or secretory endometrium (Figs. 2.15 and 2.16). This artifact can result in back-to-back glands that do not represent hyperplasia.
7. Focal cystic glands or nonreactive glands can occur in normal endometrium and have no significance by themselves.
8. Patchy stromal edema is normal by days 17 to 18 of the secretory phase and does not signify irregular maturation.

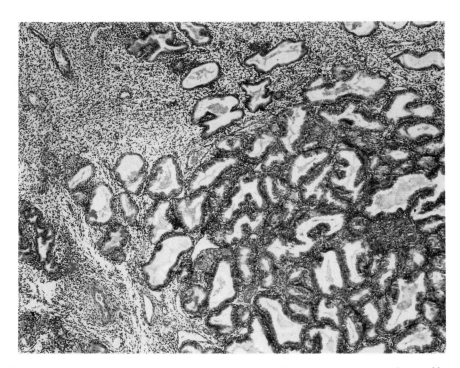

FIGURE 2.15. Artifactual crowding of late secretory endometrium. Tangential sectioning of normal late secretory endometrium near the basalis yields a pattern of focal glandular crowding. This artifact has no significance and should not be misinterpreted as hyperplasia.

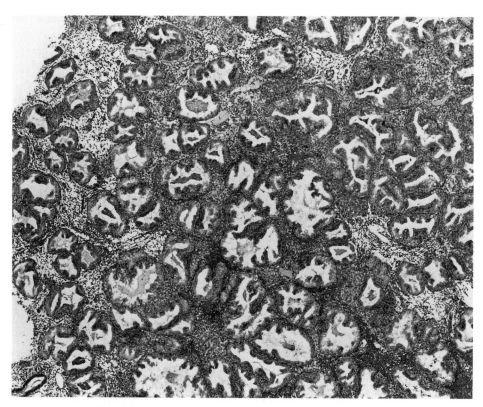

FIGURE 2.16. Artifactual crowding of late secretory endometrium. Another example of late secretory phase glands that appear crowded due to tangential sectioning. This pattern is neither hyperplastic nor "hypersecretory," however. Identifying surface epithelium elsewhere in the sections often helps to avoid misinterpretation of these normal glands.

9. Identifying very early pregnancy based on endometrial changes alone is very difficult. Apparent "hypersecretory" late secretory phase glands with vacuolated cytoplasm usually are a variation of normal development and do not, by themselves, indicate early pregnancy (see Chapter 3).

10. Compact predecidua with spindle-shaped stromal cells may not be appreciated as a true predecidual reaction. Directing attention to stromal changes around spiral arteries assists in the identification of predecidua.

11. Lymphocytes and granular lymphocytes normally become prominent in the stroma of the late secretory phase. These do not represent inflammation.

12. If the tissue is difficult to date because of apparent discordance in features, the possibility of chronic endometritis or a polyp should be considered.

13. The endometrium should not be dated when polyps, inflammation, or other abnormalities are present.

Artifacts and Contaminants

Besides variations in the normal anatomy, such as the basalis and lower uterine segment, several artifacts of the biopsy frequently complicate the histologic patterns. One artifact, tissue fragmentation caused by mechanical disruption of the tissue, is frequent in endometrial biopsies. Typically, glands are detached from the surrounding stroma, and fragmented glands become randomly oriented, often appearing closely spaced (Fig.

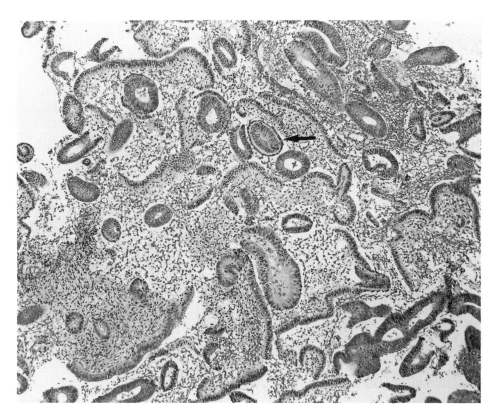

FIGURE 2.17. Artifactual fragmentation. Normal proliferative phase endometrium is fragmented as a result of the procedure. The glands have a haphazard arrangement that should not be confused with a significant abnormality. Focal "telescoping" artifact also is present (*arrow*).

2.17). Fragmentation can be mistaken for real crowding that occurs in hyperplasia or carcinoma. Fragmentation and close apposition of disparate tissues such as cervical epithelium and functionalis also leads to confusing patterns. Artifactually crowded glands lack a continuous investment of tissue and are not connected by intervening stroma. These latter features help in recognition of the artifact. Fragmentation also is a common feature of atrophy (Chapter 5).

Another frequent change is so-called telescoping of glands.[19] Telescoping may occur in either proliferative or secretory phase endometrium (Fig. 2.18), but it also complicates many nonphysiologic conditions. Telescoping results in a pattern of an apparent gland within the lumen of another gland and can mimic hyperplasia or neoplasia (Fig. 2.19). This artifact seems to be a result of mechanical disruption of the gland during curettage, since it rarely occurs in hysterectomy specimens. Tangential sectioning of tortuous glands also contributes to this phenomenon. Fortunately, telescoping rarely presents difficulty in interpretation once the observer understands the phenomenon. In questionable cases, the cytology of the glandular cells and comparison with surrounding tissue establishes this change as an artifact.

Endometrial biopsies also often contain contaminants from the cervix. Most of these contaminants are obvious. Strips of bland squamous or mucinous epithelium and irregular pools of extracelluar mucin are common (Fig. 2.20). The extracellular mucin may contain neutrophils, cell debris, macrophages, or giant cells, but all these are normal when mixed with mucin and have no pathologic significance in the absence of inflammation in the endometrial stroma. Occasionally, benign cervical contaminants become more complex and troublesome in biopsies. En-

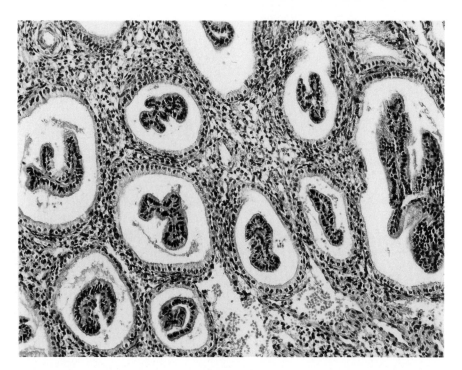

FIGURE 2.18. Telescoping artifact. Normal secretory endometrium shows telescoping artifact with a gland-in-gland appearance. This common alteration is an apparent result of the biopsy procedure and has no significance.

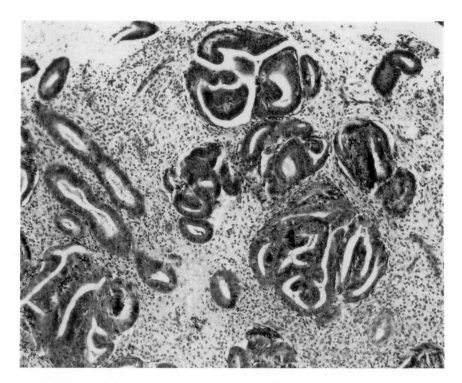

FIGURE 2.19. Telescoping with focal artifactual gland crowding. Focus of disrupted glands shows apparent gland crowding due to telescoping and fragmentation. This is a common artifact seen in normal proliferative and secretory endometrium that should not be mistaken for hyperplasia.

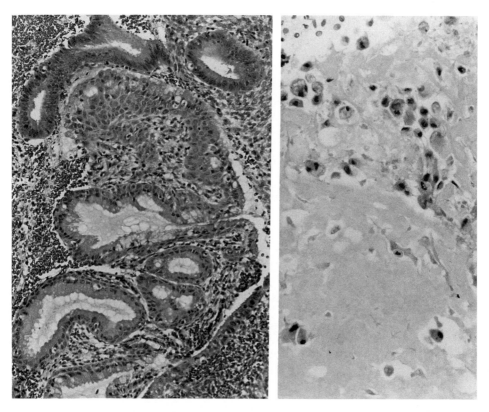

FIGURE 2.20. Cervical contaminants. *Left*. Fragmentation has resulted in a strip of mucinous glandular epithelium adjacent to detached proliferative phase glands. *Right*. Amorphous endocervical mucus with a few macrophages may be admixed with endometrial tissues. This finding has no significance.

docervical glands with squamous metaplasia or microglandular hyperplasia yield complex patterns, but these elements are cytologically bland and usually blend into more typical cervical epithelium (Fig. 2.21). In questionable cases, continuity with endometrial surface epithelium may help to establish origin in the corpus. It is also helpful to look at the surrounding stroma and see if it is of endometrial or endocervical type. Rarely, an endometrial biopsy also may reveal an admixture of fragments of tissue from cervical dysplasia, squamous carcinoma, or adenocarcinoma. Chapter 9 addresses the differential diagnosis of endocervical versus endometrial carcinoma.

Other types of cells may be admixed with endometrium, complicating the pattern. Occasionally, curettage yields sheets of histiocytes with no associated mucin or other tissue (Fig. 2.22). These histiocytes apparently reside in the endometrial cavity, and show the typical histiocyte cytology with a lobulated nucleus and amphophilic cytoplasm. We have seen them in association with hydrometra and with benign bleeding patterns. They apparently represent a response to intracavitary debris. They are benign but can mimic endometrial stromal cells or stromal cell lesions. Immunohistochemical stains for histiocyte markers, such as lysozyme, HAM 56, or KP 1, can facilitate recognition of these cells. Stromal foam cells represent stromal cells that are filled with lipid from erythrocytes in areas of chronic nonphysiologic bleeding. Separate fragments of adipose tissue with clearly identifiable fat cells in an endometrial biopsy almost always represent omentum or extrauterine pelvic soft tissue and indicate perforation of the uterus. We have also occasionally seen colonic mucosa in endometrial biopsies. In these circumstances the clinician should be notified immediately.

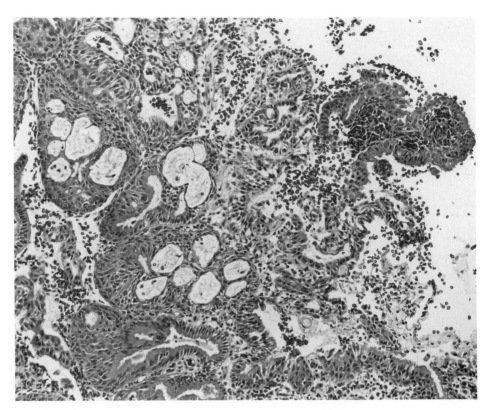

FIGURE 2.21. Cervical contaminant. Fragmented endocervical epithelium with microglandular hyperplasia lies adjacent to a fragment of endometrium showing breakdown. Other fields in the section showed proliferative endometrium.

Luteal Phase Defect and Abnormal Secretory Phase Patterns

Luteal phase defect (LPD), or inadequate luteal phase, is a recognized cause of infertility, so-called ovulatory infertility.[4,20-22] This disorder is sporadic and relatively common, but it is a significant factor in infertility in less than 5% of patients in most studies.[4,22] LPD also has been implicated as a factor in early habitual spontaneous abortion and in abnormal uterine bleeding.[23] The etiology of LPD is obscure. Usually the abnormality appears to arise due to hypothalamic or pituitary dysfunction that causes decreased levels of follicle-stimulating hormone (FSH) in the follicular phase, abnormal luteinizing hormone (LH) secretion, decreased levels of LH and FSH at the time of ovulation, or elevated prolactin levels.[4,20,24] Women with apparent LPD often have relatively low progesterone levels during the luteal phase.[7,25-29] Endometrial biopsy often is an integral component of the diagnosis and management of this disorder,[24,27,30,31] although some authors suggest that endometrial biopsy with histologic dating has limited utility in luteal phase evaluation.[9,32,33]

In LPD, ovulation occurs, but the subsequent luteal phase does not develop appropriately. There is insufficient progesterone production to support development of the endometrium to histologic day 28 of the cycle. Usually, this abnormality is recognized clinically when the histologic date lags more than 2 days from the actual postovulatory date.[20,30] In this circumstance LPD is clinically significant only if the abnormal lag in maturation occurs in at least two consecutive biopsies.[30,31,34] Using the criterion for a lag in secretory phase development by dates, there usually is no morphologic abnormality. Clinical evaluation, including the basal body temperature

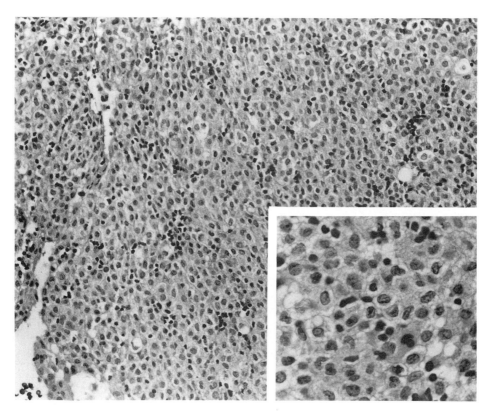

FIGURE 2.22. Histiocytes. A detached aggregate of histiocytes superficially resembles endometrial stroma. *Inset*: The cells have cytologic features of histiocytes with oval, folded unclei and faintly vacuolated cytoplasm. A lack of intrinsic vasculature helps to indicate that this is a contaminant.

or the onset of menses after biopsy, establishes the diagnosis in this situation.

Because of inadequate progesterone production, LPD may also cause abnormalities in the development of secretory endometrium.[31,35] In fact, experimental evidence shows that variations in the relative amounts of the sex steroid hormones, estradiol and progesterone, affect endometrial development.[36] In these experimental conditions, relatively low doses of estrogen and progesterone result in glandular and stromal hypoplasia. Higher doses of estrogen but low doses of progesterone result in stromal inadequacy, while high levels of progesterone and low doses of estrogen lead to glandular inadequacy. These data suggest that variations in follicle and corpus luteum development with decreases in hormone production alter the development of secretory endometrium following ovulation.

Morphologic features of LPD other than a retarded histologic date are poorly characterized. Usually, LPD is believed to cause discordance in the development of the glands and the stroma.[31,35,37] The resulting pattern is that of irregular maturation, with different areas showing a marked (greater than 4 days) variation in development. Although LPD can be reflected in endometrial morphologic abnormalities such as irregular maturation, there are no large-scale studies that have clearly indentified specific pathologic features of this condition.

On occasion, endometrial biopsies show abnormal secretory phase patterns.[31,35,37,38] In such cases the endometrium typically shows secretory changes that cannot be assigned to any day of the normal cycle (Figs. 2.23 and 2.24). The pattern may show true irregular maturation with a large variation in the pattern of endometrial development from field to field. For example, some areas may show early secretory changes characteristic

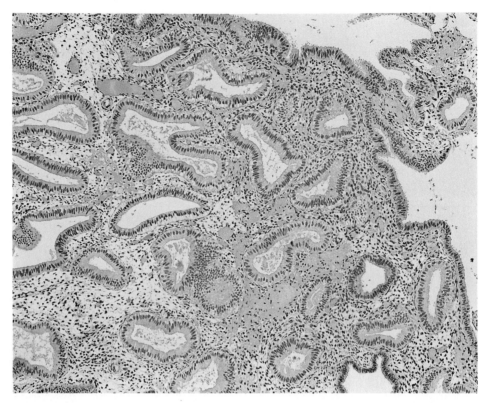

FIGURE 2.23. Abnormal secretory phase pattern. Endometrial biopsy in a premenopausal woman being evaluated for infertility shows secretory changes that cannot be assigned to a specific histologic date of the normal menstrual cycle. The glands show secretory changes but have tubular outlines and lack appropriate tortuosity. Further, some glands lack secretory vacuoles. The stroma shows edema in this field but other areas lack this stromal response (see Fig. 2.24).

of about days 18 to 19, while other areas show foci of predecidua consistent with at least day 24. Pathologic processes other than LPD can cause abnormal secretory phase development, however (Table 2.4). When abnormal secretory phase patterns are due to specific abnormalities such as inflammation or polyps, the primary abnormality may be evident. In other cases there may be no identifiable etiology for the abnormally developed secretory pattern. In this latter group of cases, the abnormality may be dysfunctional, related to abnormal development of the corpus luteum, or the aberration may be secondary to underlying pathology that is not adequately sampled. Such cases can only be classified as abnormal secretory phase pattern (see below).

Clinical Queries and Reporting

Using endometrial biopsy or curettage in the infertility workup, the gynecologist seeks the following information: 1) histologic evidence of ovulation, 2) histologic date of secretory phase specimens, and 3) presence or absence of endometrial abnormalities that may be responsible for infertility. Demonstrating the presence of secretory phase changes indicates that ovulation has occurred. Dating the secretory phase gives a general assessment of progesterone production by the corpus luteum and the ability of the endometrium to respond to progesterone.

In practice, a span of up to 3 days in date from field to field is acceptable as normal, especially in mid to late secretory endometrium where areas of

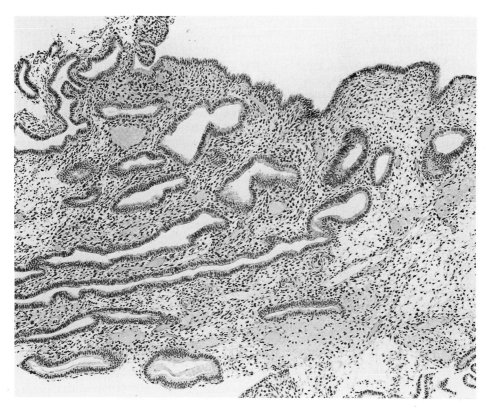

FIGURE 2.24. Abnormal secretory phase pattern. Another area from the specimen shown in Fig. 2.23 shows poorly developed secretory glands and dense stroma that lacks edema. The cause of this type of abnormality cannot be determined by morphology alone.

TABLE 2.4. Causes of undatable endometrium.

Hormonal effects
  Anovulation
  Luteal phase defect
  Persistent corpus luteum
  Exogenous hormones
  Pregnancy
Organic lesions
  Polyps
  Leiomyomas
  Chronic inflammation
  Hyperplasia
  Carcinoma
  Atrophy
  Adhesions
Sampling problems
  Fragmentation
  Lack of surface epithelium

edematous stroma alternate with areas of predecidualized stroma. Also, the glandular changes in the late secretory phase can be highly variable.

The pathologist should date the tissue on the basis of the most advanced changes using a 2-day span (e.g., days 24 to 25). Dating the secretory phase is somewhat subjective and neither completely exact nor reproducible, and therefore it is also important that everyone involved in the interpretation and clinical application of histologic dating understand the limitations of this morphologic assessment. Studies of interobserver variation show that 80% or more of endometrial biopsies for dating are within 2 days of each other when evaluated by experienced pathologists. Furthermore, 80% of the time the dates are within 2 days of the expected day compared with basal body temperature and menstruation.[39] Some investigators find that the criteria for histologic dating do not have sufficient precision to determine the degree of corpus luteum function in the late secretory phase.[40] The field-to-field variations in normal late secretory endometrium probably lead to some of the interobserver and intraobserver variations found in dating. With experience, a pathologist should be able to provide a reasonable assessment of the endometrial development in the secretory phase.

Although it is obvious that for the infertility patient every attempt should be made to provide an accurate date, there are cases where precise histologic dating is not possible. When accurate dating cannot be done, it is important, if possible, to indicate why (Table 2.4). Hormonal effects, various organic lesions, and sampling problems all can make dating difficult or impossible. Other organic factors such as inflammation, adhesions, or polyps may interfere with pregnancy (Chapter 7). These abnormalities affect fertility by altering the development of the glands and stroma, thereby preventing normal implantation or mechanically disrupting the early implanting placenta. Therefore, when present these abnormalities should be reported. If factors preclude reporting a specific date, an attempt should be made to decide whether the endometrium is proliferative or secretory, because secretory phase development generally indicates that ovulation has occurred.

On occasion the biopsy shows an abnormal secretory pattern. In such cases the abnormal pattern may be due to an LPD or to some other pathologic factor that is not identifiable in the specimen. In practice, a descriptive diagnosis of the changes (e.g., "secretory with irregular maturation" or "abnormal secretory phase pattern") with a description of the abnormality is sufficient to indicate that the secretory development is not normal. The clinician can use this information in combination with other clinical observations to determine its significance and possible cause. Descriptive diagnoses should be used carefully, however. The term "dyssynchronous endometrium" has been used to describe apparent alterations in secretory phase development. "Dyssynchronous" is not a word with a specific meaning, and therefore its use can be confusing unless there is clear communication between the pathologist and the gynecologist regarding its meaning.

Recently, morphometric analysis has been attempted to increase the accuracy of endometrial histologic dating.[41] It was found that five morphometric measurements, including mitotic rate in gland cells, amount of luminal secretion, volume fraction of gland occupied by gland cell, amount of pseudostratification of gland cells, and amount of predecidual reaction, added precision to histologic dating.[41] Furthermore, immunohistochemical analysis for specific secretory products of the endometrium may help to identify LPDs.[42,43] These data indicate that further refinements in evaluation of normal endometrium may evolve that have clinical utility. Presently, however, routine histologic evaluation remains a cost-effective method of determining the relative degree of endometrial development through the menstrual cycle.

References

1. Noyes RW, Hertig AT, Rock J: Dating the endometrial biopsy. Fertil Steril 1950;1:3–25.
2. Dallenbach-Hellweg G: Histopathology of the Endometrium. 4th ed. New York: Springer-Verlag, 1987.
3. Hendrickson MR, Kempson RL: Surgical Pathology of the Uterine Corpus (Major Problems in Pathology series). Volume 12. Philadelphia: W.B. Saunders, 1980.
4. Speroff L, Glass RH, Kase NG: Clinical Gynecologic Endocrinology and Infertility. 4th ed. Baltimore: Williams & Wilkins, 1989.
5. Merrill JA: The interpretation of endometrial biopsies. Clin Obstet Gynecol 1991;34:211–221.
6. Hill GA, Herbert CM III, Parker RA, Wentz AC: Comparison of late luteal phase endometrial biopsies using the Novak curette or Pipelle endometrial suction curette. Obstet Gynecol 1989;73: 443–446.
7. Hecht BR, Bardawil WA, Khan-Dawood FS, Dawood MY: Luteal insufficiency: Correlation between endometrial dating and integrated progesterone output in clomiphene citrate-induced cycles. Am J Obstet Gynecol 1990;163:1986–1991.
8. Shoupe D, Mishell DR, Jr, Lacarra M, Lobo RA, Horenstein J, et al: Correlation of endometrial maturation with four methods of estimating day of ovulation. Obstet Gynecol 1989;73:88–92.
9. Peters AJ, Lloyd RP, Coulam CB: Prevalence of out-of-phase endometrial biopsy specimens. Am J Obstet Gynecol 1992;166:1738–1746.
10. Masterson R, Armstrong EM, More IAR: The cyclical variation in the percentage of ciliated cells

in the normal human endometrium. J Reprod Fertil 1975;42:537–540.

11. Hendrickson MR, Kempson RL: Ciliated carcinoma—a variant of endometrial adenocarcinomal: A report of 10 cases. Int J Gynecol Pathol 1983;2:1–12.

12. Kurman RJ, Norris HJ: Endometrial hyperplasia and metaplasia. In: Blaustein's Pathology of the Female Genital Tract. 4th ed. Kurman RJ, ed. New York: Springer-Verlag, 1994;411–437.

13. Silverberg SG, Kurman RJ: Tumors of the uterine corpus and gestational trophoblastic disease. Atlas of Tumor Pathology, 3rd series, Fascicle 3. Washington, DC: Armed Forces Institute of Pathology, 1992.

14. Buckley CH, Fox H: Biopsy Pathology of the Endometrium. New York: Raven Press, 1989; 234–247.

15. Bulmer JN, Lunny DP, Hagin SV: Immunohistochemical characterization of stromal leucocytes in nonpregnant human endometrium. Am J Reprod Immmunol Microbiol 1988;17:83–90.

16. King A, Wellings V, Gardner L, Loke YW: Immunocytochemical characterization of the unusual large granular lymphocytes in human endometrium throughout the menstrual cycle. Hum Immunol 1989;24:195–205.

17. Bulmer JN, Hollings D, Ritson A: Immunocytochemical evidence that endometrial stromal granulocytes are granulated lymphocytes. J Pathol 1987;153:281–288.

18. Poropatich C, Rojas M, Silverberg SG: Polymorphonuclear leukocytes in the endometrium during the normal menstrual cycle. Int J Gynecol Pathol 1987;6:230–234.

19. Numers CV: On the traumatic effect of curettage on the endometrial biopsy, with special reference to so-called invagination pictures and the "crumbling endometrium." Acta Obstet Gynecol Scand 1942;28:305–313.

20. Jones GS: Luteal phase insufficiency. Clin Obstet Gynecol 1972;16:255-273.

21. Wentz AC: Diagnosing luteal phase inadequacy. Fertil Steril 1982;37:334.

22. Wentz AC, Kossoy LR, Parker RA: The impact of luteal phase indaequacy in an infertile population. Am J Obstet Gynecol 1990;162:937–945.

23. Kurman RJ, Mazur MT: Benign diseases of the endometrium. In: Blaustein's Pathology of the Female Genital Tract. 4th ed. Kurman RJ, ed. New York: Springer-Verlag, 1994;367–409.

24. Daly DC, Walters CA, Soto-Albors CE, Riddick DH: Endometrial biopsy during treatment of luteal phase defects is predictive of therapeutic outcome. Fertil Steril 1983;40:305–310.

25. Rosenfeld DL, Garcia C: A comparison of endometrial histology with simultaneous plasma progesterone determinations in infertile women. Fertil Steril 1976;27:1256–1266.

26. Annos T, Thompson IE, Taymor ML: Luteal phase deficiency and infertility: Difficulties encountered in diagnosis and treatment. Obstet Gynecol 1981;55:705–710.

27. Rosenfeld DL, Chudow S, Bronson RA: Diagnosis of luteal phase inadequacy. Obstet Gynecol 1980;56:193–196.

28. Cooke ID, Morgan CA, Parry TE: Correlation of endometrial biopsy and plasma progesterone levels in infertile women. J Obstet Gynaecol Br Commonw 1972;79:647–650.

29. Cumming DC, Honore LH, Scott JZ, Williams KP: The late luteal phase in infertile women: Comparison of simultaneous endometrial biopsy and progesterone levels. Fertil Steril 1985;43:715–719.

30. Wentz AC: Endometrial biopsy in the evaluation of infertility. Fertil Steril 1980;33:121-124.

31. Witten BI, Martin SA: The endometrial biopsy as a guide to the management of luteal phase defect. Fertil Steril 1985;44:460–465.

32. Balasch J, Fabregues F, Creus M, Vanrell JA: The usefulness of endometrial biopsy for luteal phase evaluation in infertility. Hum Reprod 1992;7: 973–977.

33. Scott RT, Snyder RR, Strickland DM, Tyburski CC, Bagnall JA, et al: The effect of interobserver variation in dating endometrial histology on the diagnosis of luteal phase defects. Fertil Steril 1988;50:888–892.

34. Downs KA, Gibson M: Basal body, temperature graph and the luteal phase defect. Fertil Steril 1983;40:466–468.

35. Dallenbach-Hellweg G: The endometrium of infertility. A review. Path Res Pract 1984;178:527–537.

36. Good RG, Moyer DL: Estrogen–progesterone relationships in the development of secretory endometrium. Fertil Steril 1968;19:37–45.

37. Gillam JS: Study of the inadequate secretion phase endometrium. Fertil Steril 1955;6:18–36.

38. Noyes RW: The underdeveloped secretory endometrium. Am J Obstet Gynecol 1959;77:929–945.

39. Noyes RW, Haman JO: The accuracy of endometrical dating. Fertil Steril 1953;4:504–517.

40. Li T-C, Dockery P, Rogers AW, Cooke ID: How precise is histologic dating of endometrium using the standard dating criteria? Fertil Steril 1989;51: 759–763.

41. Li TC, Rogers AW, Dockery P, Lenton EA, Cooke ID: A new method of histologic dating of human endometrium in the luteal phase. Fertil Steril 1988; 50:52–60.

42. Graham RA, Seif MW, Aplin JD, Li TC, Cooke ID, et al: An endometrial factor in unexplained infertility. Br Med J 1990;300:1428–1431.

43. Seif MW, Aplin JD, Buckley CH: Luteal phase defect: The possibility of an immunohistochemical diagnosis. Fertil Steril 1989;51:273–279.

3
Pregnancy, Abortion, and Ectopic Pregnancy

Recognition of the features of gestational endometrium, trophoblast, and villi, as well as the pathologic changes in chorionic tissues, is an important part of endometrial biopsy interpretation. Correct identification of gestational endometrium and placental tissue is important for several reasons. First, the presence of intrauterine products of conception generally excludes the diagnosis of ectopic pregnancy. Second, normal trophoblastic cells can appear atypical and even neoplastic, since they are primitive and highly proliferative. Third, identification of products of conception can help explain other pathologic states such as abnormal bleeding or chronic endometritis.

The vast majority of endometrial specimens showing apparent gestational changes are curettings from an abortion, usually before the 20th week of pregnancy. There are several types of abortion specimens. "Spontaneous abortions" are unexpected and unplanned interruptions of pregnancy that present with bleeding and passage of tissue. Approximately 15% to 20% of recognized early pregnancies end in a spontaneous abortion.[1–4] In addition, many other early pregnancies spontaneously abort before pregnancy is recognized by the woman and are occult.[5,6] Most spontaneous abortions occur before 12 weeks of pregnancy, and at least half of these are due to a genetic (karyotypic) anomaly. An "incomplete abortion" is a spontaneous abortion in which the conceptus and decidua are incompletely passed, thus requiring curettage. A "missed abortion" refers to an abortion with retained products of conception but no abnormal bleeding for 5 to 8 weeks after death of the embryo or fetus. The criteria for diagnosis of a missed abortion vary among practitioners and institutions. "Therapeutic abortions" are those in which the pregnancy is electively terminated.

Besides abortions, several other complications of pregnancy, such as retained placenta or placental implantation site, ectopic pregnancy, or gestational trophoblastic disease, lead to endometrial curettage (Table 3.1). These types of specimens show either trophoblastic tissue in the endometrium, the effects of trophoblastic tissue on the endometrium, or a combination of trophoblastic tissue and its effects.

TABLE 3.1. Complications of pregnancy.

Spontaneous abortion
Missed abortion
Retained placental tissue/implantation site
Ectopic pregnancy
Placenta accreta, increta, and percreta
Gestational trophoblastic disease

Endometrial Glands and Stroma in Pregnancy

Early Gestational Endometrium (1 to 3 Weeks Postfertilization)

This chapter first reviews the physiologic changes of the endometrium in pregnancy, especially early pregnancy. This is followed by a discussion of normal placental implantation and growth as well as benign and pathologic conditions of trophoblast. Chapter 4 reviews the closely related topic of gestational trophoblastic disease.

Fertilization occurs in the fallopian tube soon after ovulation, and implantation (nidation) of the developing blastocyst takes place on day 20 or 21 (postovulatory day 6 or 7). Implantation occurs on the surface of the endometrium, usually on the mid portion of the posterior wall. The ovulatory cycle during which fertilization and implantation take place is called the cycle of conception. Immediately after implantation, subtle changes begin to appear in the glands and stroma, although the tissue retains the overall

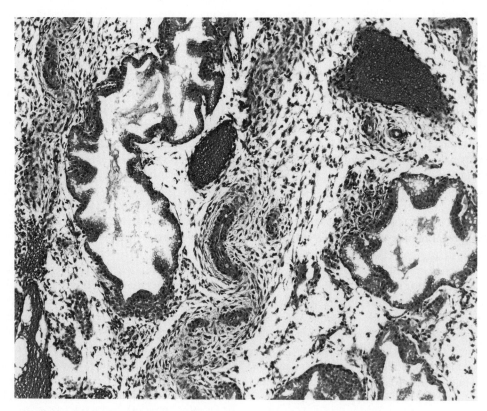

FIGURE 3.1. Early gestational endometrium, cycle of conception. Inadvertent endometrial biopsy in the cycle of conception shows distended, coiled glands and engorged vessels. Early decidual reaction is present around thickened spiral arteries. In the absence of trophoblast or chorionic villi, these features are too subtle to be diagnostic of early pregnancy until the stroma shows more advanced decidual change.

characteristics of the mid to late secretory phase for several days. An endometrial biopsy or curettage performal inadvertently at this time, usually during infertility evaluation, may not include trophoblast or disrupt the early gestation, yet will show very early pregnancy-related changes. These changes include recrudescence or accentuation of glandular secretions, distension of the glands, edema, and an extensive predecidual reaction.[7-10] The coiled glands show secretory activity and a serrated lumen, but they appear distended or wider than those in the late secretory phase of a menstrual cycle (Fig. 3.1). Vascular prominence with engorgement and dilatation of superficial veins and capillaries also occurs,[8] and the spiral arteries develop thicker walls.

Other reported changes in the cycle of conception include persistent basal cytoplasmic vacuoles in late secretory phase glands,[9] a disparity between development of the glands and stroma,[11] or a histologic date earlier than the cycle date as determined by basal body temperature or luteinizing hormone (LH) surge.[11-14] One study reported that in the cycle of conception pronounced stromal edema and vascular engorgement of capillaries and small veins correlated better with pregnancy than did the glandular changes.[7] Since menstruation does not occur, there is no substantial change in the number of true granular lymphocytes at this time.

Practically, however, the morphologic changes during the first 1 to 2 weeks after conception are subtle. It is difficult to decide whether the vacuolated cytoplasm within glandular epithelium reflects normal persistence of vacuoles in the late secretory phase or the changes of pregnancy. It usually is not possible to be certain of pregnancy-related changes until after 2 weeks when decidua, as opposed to predecidua, is fully developed (see below).

Within 10 to 15 days of fertilization, the endometrium gradually begins to show more characteristic changes of pregnancy as differentiation to decidua progresses (Table 3.2). The most striking change occurs in stromal cells that become decidualized. As compared to predecidual cells, decidual cells are larger and contain more abundant eosinophilic to amphophilic cytoplasm that may show faint vacuoles (Figs. 3.2 and 3.3). These cells become more clearly polyhedral with well-defined cell membranes. Nuclei of the decidualized stromal cells are round to oval and uniform with finely dispersed chromatin. These nuclei have smooth outlines with only slight irregularities in the nuclear membrane and small to indistinct nucleoli (compare with Fig. 3.15). Occasional decidualized stromal cells are binucleate. Stromal granular lymphocytes persist in early pregnancy and become prominent among decidual cells. The presence of granular lymphocytes may suggest a chronic inflammatory infiltrate, but the granular lymphocytes, in contrast to inflammatory cells, have characteristic lobated nuclei and plasma cells are not present.

Along with progressive decidual transformation of the stromal cells, the glands and vessels undergo pronounced alterations. Secretory changes in the glands become more prominent with further increases in the extent of cytoplasmic vacuolization and increased luminal secretions that distend the glands (Fig. 3.4). Besides hypersecretory activity, the glands become highly

TABLE 3.2. Histologic changes of the endometrium in pregnancy.[a]

Duration of pregnancy[b]	Stroma	Glands	Vessels
1–3 weeks	Edema, then progressive decidual change	Hypersecretory with cytoplasmic vacuoles, luminal secretions Saw-toothed, tortuous, distended Rare Arias-Stella reaction	Spiral arteries begin to thicken Superficial venules congested, dilated
4 or more weeks	Marked decidual change	Irregular with marked atrophy Variable Arias-Stella reaction, clear cytoplasm, optically clear nuclei	Spiral arteries thickened Superficial venules dilated

[a] Changes of endometrial glands, stroma, and vessels only.
[b] Duration from time of fertilization (day 15–16 of menstrual cycle). Add 2 weeks for time from last menstrual period.

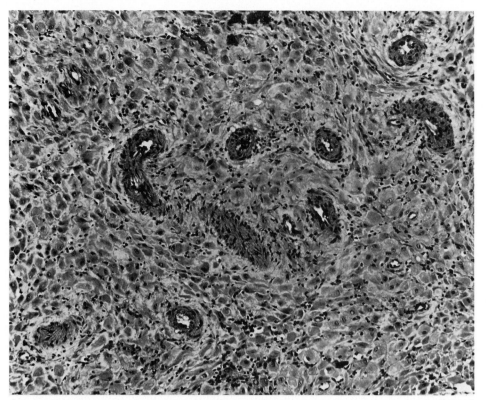

FIGURE 3.2. Early gestational endometrium with decidualized stroma. Endometrial stroma from a first-trimester abortion shows prominent decidual transformation. The decidualized cells have abundant, pale cytoplasm and uniform round to oval nuclei. Granular lymphocytes are numerous. Spiral artery walls are thicker than in nongestational endometrium.

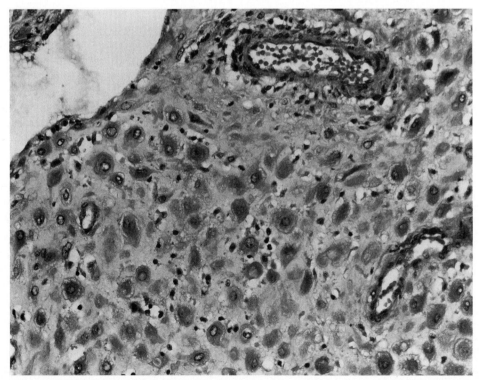

FIGURE 3.3. Decidualized stroma. Decidual cells have prominent cell borders and uniform, round to oval nuclei. Their cytoplasm has small vacuoles. A portion of atrophic gland is present in the left upper corner.

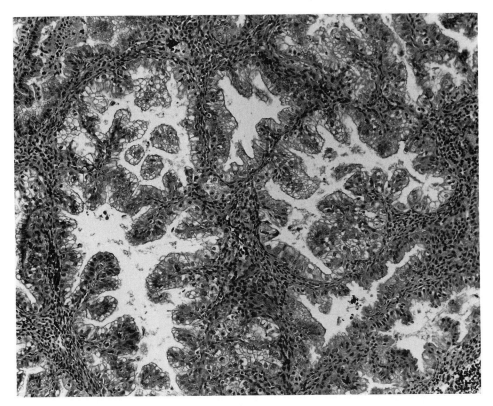

FIGURE 3.4. Gestational endometrium. Hypersecretory pattern of endometrial glands in early pregnancy with extensive cytoplasmic vacuolization. Decidualized stroma was present in other areas of the sections.

coiled with prominent serrations and papillary folds of epithelium projecting into the lumen. The epithelial cells become stratified. Concurrently, spiral arteries develop thicker walls and become more prominent (Fig. 3.2).

Endometrium in Later Pregnancy (4 or More Weeks Postfertilization)

With advancing gestational age, pregnancy-related patterns become more pronounced (Table 3.2). The decidualized stromal cells are more widespread and prominent, especially as the cell borders become better defined. They develop an epithelioid appearance and can show small cytoplasmic vacuoles. Decidual cell nuclei become somewhat larger and some appear vesicular, but they maintain their uniform contours. The decidua shows small foci of physiologic necrosis during pregnancy, as it remodels during growth of the fetus and placenta and as the decidua capsularis fuses with the decidua parietalis. These small foci of necrosis with a localized neutrophilic response are normal. They do not reflect an infectious or septic process, and they do not indicate a significant abnormality of the decidua. The stroma continues to contain a sprinkling of granular lymphocytes that remain throughout gestation.

The hypersecretory pattern of the glands begins to regress early in pregnancy, and with increasing decidual transformation of the stroma there usually is a mixture of hypersecretory and atrophic glands. The glands are most atrophic in areas of decidualization (Fig. 3.5). Conversely, in areas where the glands appear hypersecretory, the stroma is not decidualized (Fig. 3.4). By the end of the first trimester, the glands for the most part are atrophic and have lost their luminal secretions. They form irregular, dilated spaces with indistinct epithelium, making them difficult to distinguish from vascular channels.

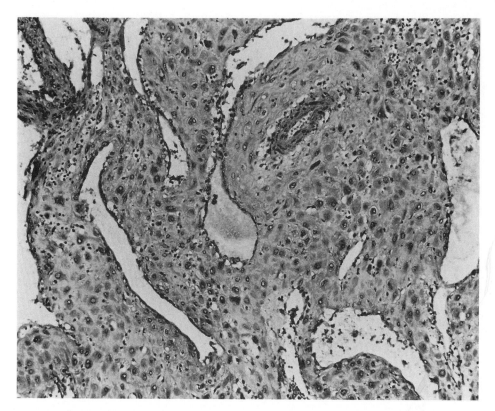

FIGURE 3.5. Gestational endometrium. Endometrium from spontaneous abortion shows diffuse decidual reaction of stroma. The glands are dilated and lined by atrophic, indistinct epithelial cells. Therapy with high-dose progestins could induce a similar pattern.

As pregnancy advances, the spiral arteries increase in thickness, a feature that persists to term and is helpful in recognizing gestational changes. Some authors suggest that in the first trimester the arteries develop a characteristic atherosclerosis-like change when an intrauterine pregnancy is present, characterized by subintimal proliferation of myofibroblasts with foam cells.[15] In addition, the venules beneath the surface epithelium dilate. Dilated superficial venules are not a specific change of pregnancy, however, since they may also be observed in progestin effect, hyperplasia, and occasionally in polyps when the endometrium grows but does not undergo cyclical shedding.

Arias-Stella Reaction

Four to eight weeks after blastocyst implantation, the endometrium often shows at least a focal Arias-Stella reaction in the glands.[16–20] This glandular change is a physiologic response to the presence of chorionic tissue either in the uterus or at an ectopic site. The morphologic features of the Arias-Stella reaction include nuclear enlargement up to three times normal size and nuclear hyperchromasia, often accompanied by abundant vacuolated cytoplasm (Figs. 3.6 and 3.7). These large nuclei may contain prominent cytoplasmic invaginations.[21] The cells typically are stratified and the nuclei hobnail-shaped, bulging into the gland lumen. Mitotic figures are rarely present.

The Arias-Stella reaction has two histologic patterns (Fig. 3.8).[18,20] One is a "hypersecretory" change characterized by highly convoluted glands lined by cells with stratified nuclei and abundant clear to foamy cytoplasm. The other pattern has been termed "regenerative," although this hypothesized etiology for the change

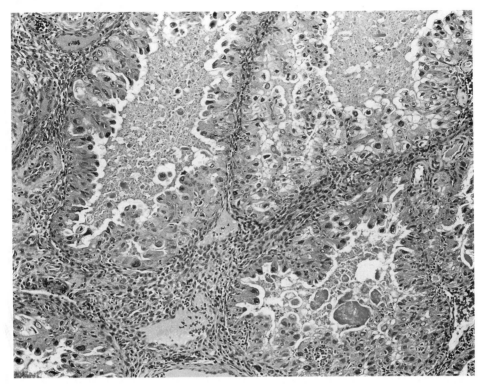

FIGURE 3.6. Arias-Stella reaction. Distended glands from an abortion specimen show prominent Arias-Stella reaction with hyperchromatic nuclei that bulge into the glandular lumen. Identical changes can be seen with an ectopic pregnancy.

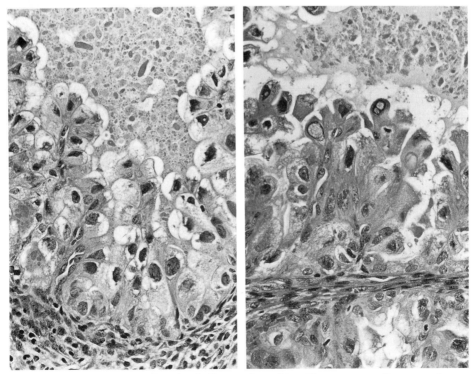

FIGURE 3.7. Arias-Stella reaction. *Left.* Arias-Stella reaction with a "hypersecretory" pattern shows stratified nuclei and vacuolated cytoplasm. *Right.* Arias-Stella reaction with "regenerative" pattern shows hobnail cells with dense cytoplasm. Several nuclei show prominent cytoplasmic invaginations.

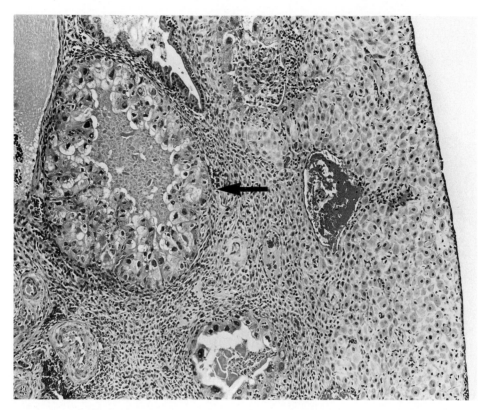

FIGURE 3.8. Gestational endometrium with Arias-Stella reaction. A dilated gland in decidualized stroma shows Arias-Stella reaction with stratified, enlarged, and hyperchromatic nuclei (*arrow*). A gland in the upper portion of the field does not show Arias-Stella change. A dilated venule is present beneath surface epithelium on the right.

remains unsubstantiated. This pattern is characterized by glands lined by enlarged hobnail cells with little cytoplasmic secretory activity. In fact, the two patterns are not very distinct and there is frequent overlap between them.

The degree and extent of the Arias-Stella reaction are highly variable in normal and abnormal intrauterine gestation and in ectopic pregnancy and gestational trophoblastic disease[18,20,22–25] This change occurs as early as 4 days after implantation,[17] although it generally is seen after about 14 days.[18] The Arias-Stella reaction persists up to at least 8 weeks following delivery. This process may be extensive, involving many glands, or the reaction can be focal, involving only a few glands (Fig. 3.8). The change can even be limited to part of a gland, leaving the remaining nuclei unaffected. There is no apparent relation between the presence and extent of

the Arias-Stella reaction and the status of the fetus. The Arias-Stella reaction is almost unique to pregnancy or gestational trophoblastic disease. Similar phenomena are rarely produced by administration of exogenous progestins.

Other Glandular Changes in Pregnancy

Besides the Arias-Stella reaction, the endometrial gland cells may undergo other specific changes in the presence of trophoblastic tissue. One such change is abundant clear cytoplasm.[16] This phenomenon overlaps with the Arias-Stella reaction yet does not show the nuclear enlargement of the latter. With this change the gland cells accumulate abundant amounts of clear, glycogen-rich cytoplasm (Fig. 3.9). The nuclei in areas of clear cell change can become stratified, and this, combined with the abundant clear cytoplasm,

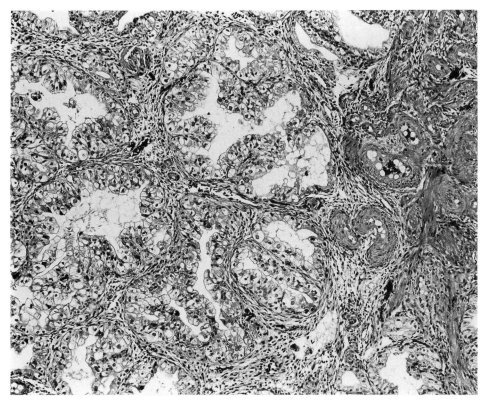

FIGURE 3.9. Gestational endometrium with clear cell change. Glands in early gestational endomtrium are lined by cells with abundant clear cytoplasm. The cells lack the nuclear enlargement of the Arias-Stella reaction.

can result in apparent obliteration of the gland lumens.

Another pregnancy-related change is optically clear nuclei of gland cells (Fig. 3.10).[26,27] This alteration is also often associated with the Arias-Stella reaction but can occur independently. Optically clear nuclei usually are focal. They have a clear to glassy appearance that is due to accumulation of a filamentous material in the nuclei. Recent study indicates that optically clear change is related to the intranuclear accumulation of biotin.[26] Clear nuclei can mimic the changes seen in herpesvirus infection, although with the pregnancy-associated optically clear nuclei, the cells lack the Cowdry type A eosinophilic nuclear inclusions, nuclear molding, and associated necrosis seen in the virus infection. This alteration is infrequent, occurring in less than 10% of first-trimester abortion specimens. These changes may persist until term, however.

As with the Arias-Stella reaction, optically clear nuclei simply reflect the presence of chorionic tissue.

In early pregnancy, endometrial glands become strongly immunoreactive for S-100 protein.[28,29] This immunoreactivity rapidly disappears after the 12th week of gestation. Normal proliferative and secretory endometrium as well as glands in hyperplasia and neoplasia do not stain for S-100 protein. There are no other markers of the glands that are generally practical for identifying pregnancy-related changes.

Trophoblast and Villi

In early pregnancy the trophoblastic proliferation begins with the development of the blastocyst, the outer layer of which is termed the trophoblastic shell. Villous formation does not

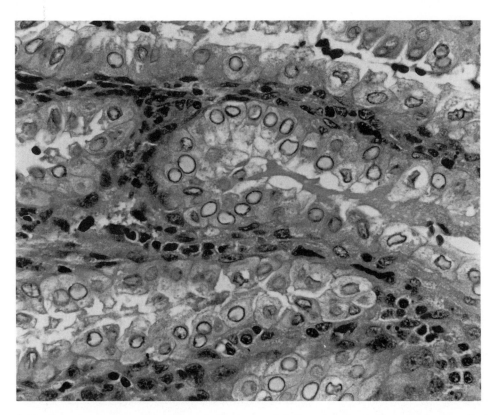

FIGURE 3.10. Gestational endomtrium with optically clear nuclei. Crowded glands show prominent optically clear nuclei. This gland cell change is infrequent and usually is focal. It may be seen throughout pregnancy, however.

begin until about 7 days after implantation of the blastocyst (13 days following conception).[4] For morphologic identification, the products of conception are divided into three components: 1) the villi and their trophoblast ("villous" trophoblast), 2) the implantation site ("extravillous" trophoblast), and 3) fetal tissues. Usually these tissues are easy to recognize.

Identifying trophoblast and villi is essential for confirming the diagnosis of an abortion. Also, the presence of placental and fetal tissue in curettings, for all practical purposes, rules out an ectopic pregnancy. These abortion specimens can be highly varied in their morphologic features. Occasionally the diagnostic features of the products of conception are difficult to identify, especially in early pregnancy when the placental component is very small and often missed in small biopsies, or if most of the products of conception were expelled

prior to the curettage. When villi and fetal parts are not present in curettings, trophoblastic cells should be searched for to confirm the diagnosis of intrauterine pregnancy. Learning to recognize the full morphologic spectrum of normal trophoblastic cells is important not only for establishing the presence of an intrauterine pregnancy but also for distinguishing exaggerated but physiologic changes from gestational trophoblastic disease.

Trophoblastic Cells

The trophoblast is extraembryonic but fetal in origin, growing in intimate association with host maternal tissues. Very early in pregnancy trophoblastic cells differentiate and invade decidua even before villi form.[4] At this stage of early gestation, implanting trophoblast is the predominant component of placental tissue. The trophoblast con-

TABLE 3.3. Morphologic features of normal trophoblastic cells.[a]

Feature	CT cells	IT cells	ST cells
Nucleus	Single	One to several	Multiple
Mitotic activity	Moderate	Low	Absent
Shape	Round	Variable; polyhedral to spindle	Irregular; highly variable
Cytoplasm	Scant; clear to granular; prominent cell borders	Abundant; amphophilic; occasional vacuoles	Abundant; dense; multiple vacuoles; lacunae; red cell lakes
Growth pattern	Often associated with villi; usually dimorphic, mixed with ST cells	Extravillous infiltration of decidua and vessel walls; extracellular fibrinoid	Often associated with villi; usually dimorphic, mixed with CT cells
Immunostaining[b]			
hCG	−	+	+ + + +
hPL	−	+ + + +	+ +
Keratin	+ + + +	+ + + +	+ + + +

[a] Abbreviations: hCG, human chorionic gonadotropin; hPL, human placental lactogen; ST, syncytiotrophoblastic; CT, cytotrophoblastic; IT, intermediate trophoblastic.
[b] $- \rightarrow + + + +$ denotes semiquantitative scoring of proportion of cells showing a positive reaction.

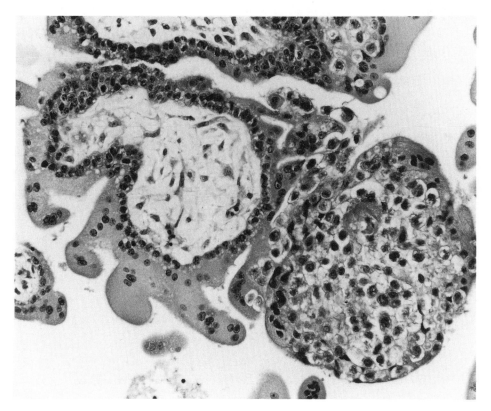

FIGURE 3.11. Immature chorionic villi with tropho-blast. Syncytiotrophoblast and cytotrophoblast grow from the surface of immature first-trimester villi. The villi are lined by an inner layer of mononucleated CT cells capped by ST cells. To the right of the villus a dimorphic mixture of ST and IT cells proliferates toward the implanting margin of the placental tissue.

tinues to grow along this interface of maternal and placental tissue throughout pregnancy. The decidua basalis where trophoblast interfaces with the endometrium and myometrium becomes the placental implantation site. The trophoblastic cells are the epithelial component of the placenta and are divided into three cytologically and functionally distinct populations: cytotrophoblastic (CT) cells, syncytiotrophoblastic (ST) cells, and intermediate trophoblastic (IT) cells (Table 3.3).[30-34] Trophoblast can also be classified according to its anatomic location into "villous" and "extravillous" trophoblast.[35]

CT cells are the germinative cells from which other trophoblastic cells differentiate. Accordingly, they are mitotically active. They are uniform cells about the size of a decidualized stromal cell, with a single nucleus, one or two nucleoli,

pale to faintly granular cytoplasm, and prominent cell borders (Fig. 3.11). ST cells, in contrast, are larger and multinucleate with dense amphophilic to basophilic cytoplasm. The nuclei of ST cells are dark and often appear pyknotic; they do not contain mitoses. The cytoplasm also typically contains small vacuoles and larger lacunae in which maternal erythrocytes can be identified. A microvillous brush border sometimes lines the lacunae of the ST cells. CT and ST cells typically display a dimorphic growth pattern with the two cell types growing in close proximity. In early abortions the CT and ST cells are quite prominent compared with the amount of villi present. In very early, unanticipated abortions, the entire products of conception consist of previllous trophoblast that can be easily confused with choriocarcinoma (Fig. 3.12) (Chapter 4). In

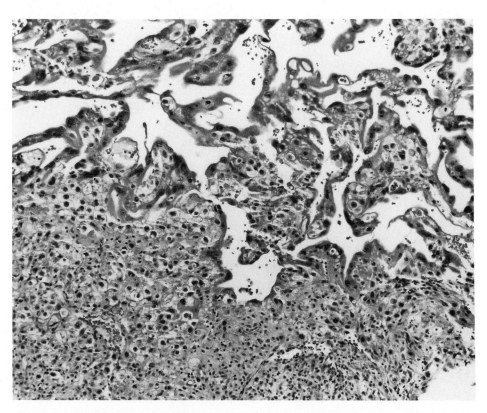

FIGURE 3.12. Trophoblast of early pregnancy. A prominent network of ST and CT cells encountered in inadvertent endometrial biopsy during early pregnancy. The cells with pleomorphic, hyperchromatic nuclei in the lower left part of the field are IT cells that are infiltrating the decidua. No villi are present.

Despite the biopsy, the pregnancy continued to term and uneventful delivery. In the absence of villi, this pattern resembles choriocarcinoma, and clinical history may be required to determine the significance of the finding.

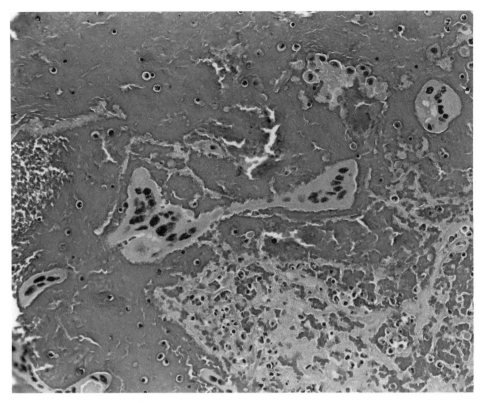

FIGURE 3.13. Isolated ST cells in abortion specimen. A few ST cells mixed with fibrin and blood are the only evidence of intrauterine pregnancy in this curettage specimen from a patient with a spontaneous abortion. Isolated ST cells such as this are often found in areas of hemorrhage.

curettings for suspected abortions, sometimes the only evidence of an intrauterine pregnancy is a few isolated trophoblastic cells mixed with blood, and these may be necrotic (Fig. 3.13). Careful scrutiny may be necessary to identify these diagnostic cells.

The intermediate trophoblast develops from cytotrophoblast on the villous surface and is manifested as sprouts and columns that extend to and extensively infiltrate the underlying decidua at the implantation site (see below). In fact, the predominant location of the intermediate trophoblast is at the implantation site, explaining why it is often called "extravillous cytotrophoblast."[35] The latter term is less precise, however, since these cells also occur in association with villi (Fig. 3.11), and they are immunohistochemically and physiologically different from cytotrophoblast. Another term used for IT cells is "X cells."[4]

Placental Implantation Site

The placental implantation site is largely composed of IT cells that infiltrate the decidua basalis, mixing with decidualized stromal cells, glands, and vessels.[4,30,32,35–38] This site begins as a microscopic focus where the blastocyst implants into secretory endometrium, and it expands with the growing placenta to cover the entire area of decidua and superficial myometrium to which the placenta is attached. It can be diffuse or focal in endometrial biopsies. Previous terminology for the trophoblastic infiltrate in decidual and myometrial tissue included "syncytial endometritis," "syncytial endomyometritis," and "placental giant cell reaction." None of these terms is correct, however, because the process is physiologic, not inflammatory, the majority of the cells are not giant cells, and the change is not con-

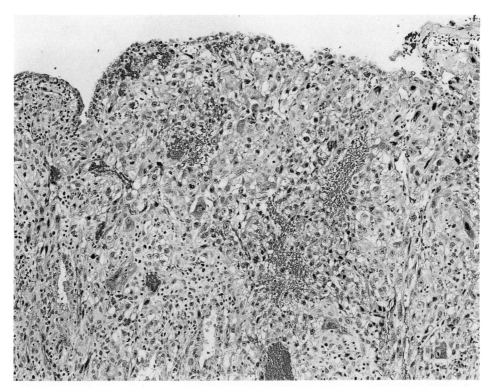

FIGURE 3.14. Placental implantation site. Large numbers of IT cells with irregular, hyperchromatic nuclei and cytoplasmic vacuoles are interspersed among decidual cells. Chorionic villi are not seen, but the presence of intermediate trophoblast in decidua establishes the diagnosis of intrauterine pregnancy.

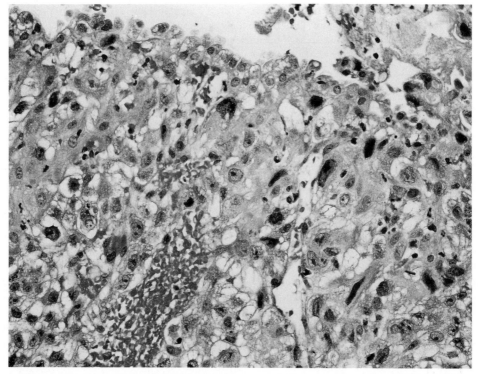

FIGURE 3.15. IT cells and decidua. Placental implantation site in an abortion specimen contains numerous IT cells that infiltrate the decidua. IT cells have characteristic large, irregular, hyperchromatic nuclei. Some of the IT cells have prominent nucleoli.

fined to the endometrium but also involves the myometrium.

At the placental site intermediate trophoblast characteristically shows diffuse permeation of the decidua (Figs. 3.14 and 3.15). In decidua IT cells often are difficult to recognize. In fact, IT cells have been misinterpreted as degenerating decidual cells because of their intimate association with the latter (Figs. 3.16 and 3.17). The IT cells have variable size and shape, with a moderate amount of eosinophilic to amphophilic cytoplasm.[37] They are larger than decidualized stromal cells, with which they are intimately admixed. They may have sharply outlined cytoplasmic vacuoles. The nuclear morphology of IT cells, however, is the most important feature that distinguishes these cells from decidua. The nuclei of IT cells are enlarged, lobated, and hyperchromatic with irregular nuclear membranes. Sometimes they have deep clefts, and some nuclei appear smudged.[39] Most IT cells contain a single nucleus, but bi- or multinucleate cells with similar nuclear and cytoplasmic features occur, too. The dark and irregular IT cell nuclei, which often contain a prominent nucleolus, contrast with the nuclei of decidualized stromal cells, which are uniform and round to oval with an even, delicate chromatin distribution. Immunohistochemical stains for keratin and human placental lactogen (hPL) help identify intermediate trophoblast (see below).[31,40]

At the implantation site intermediate trophoblast also extends into myometrium (Fig. 3.18). IT cells are often more conspicuous here, where they are multinucleated and contrast sharply with myometrial smooth muscle cells. They infiltrate between muscle bundles and fibers, often with no evidence of a tissue reaction. It is very com-

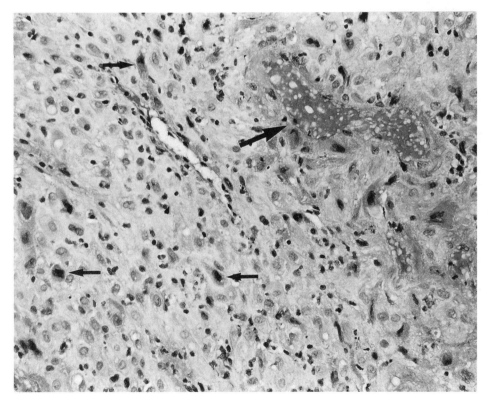

FIGURE 3.16. IT cells and decidua. Scattered IT cells (*small arrows*) with enlarged, hyperchromatic nuclei infiltrate decidua in an abortion specimen. In contrast to IT cells, decidual cells have pale, rounded, uniform nuclei with delicate chromatin. Decidual cells have more abundant cytoplasm and better-defined cell membranes than IT cells. A spiral artery (*large arrow*) in the right upper portion of the micrograph is partially infiltrated by IT cells.

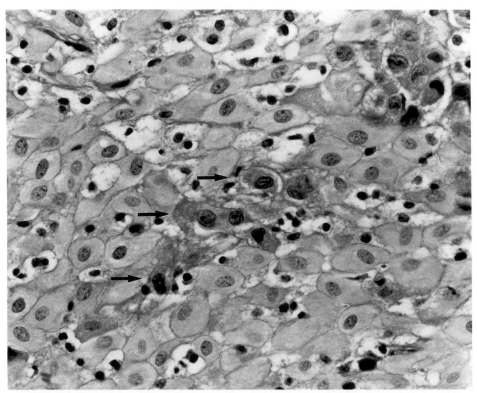

FIGURE 3.17. IT cells and decidua. The IT cells (*arrows*) have irregular, hyperchromatic nuclei that contrast with the round to oval, uniform nuclei of the surrounding decidualized stromal cells.

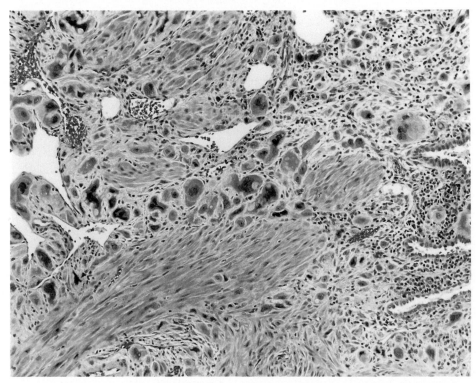

FIGURE 3.18. IT cells in myometrium. Curetted placental site from an abortion includes a fragment of myometrial smooth muscle infiltrated by large IT cells. These cells often become multinucleated when they invade the myometrium.

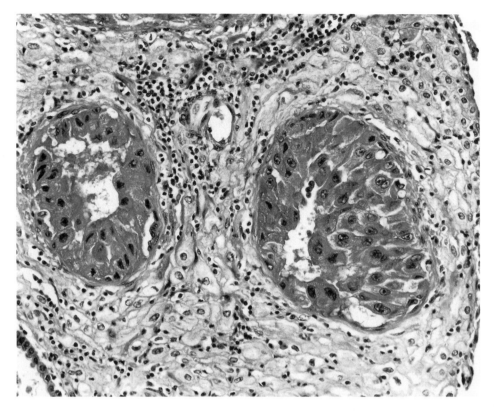

FIGURE 3.19. IT cells. Prominent infiltration of blood vessels in the decidua by IT cells in an abortion specimen. The cells infiltrate and replace the wall but preserve the lumen.

mon to see fragments of myometrium infiltrated by intermediate trophoblast in curettings from abortion specimens.

In addition to permeating decidua and myometrium, the IT cells invade blood vessels, extensively replacing the wall and endothelium while maintaining the integrity of the lumen (Fig. 3.19). When vascular infiltration is extensive, the IT may partially fill the lumen of the vessel. This infiltration of vessels contributes to the enlargement of the spiral arteries.

Besides their characteristic growth pattern and cytologic features, IT cells can be recognized because they typically are associated with patches of extracellular eosinophilic fibrinoid material (Fig. 3.20). This fibrinoid matrix in the placental bed eventually becomes the so-called Nitabuch's layer. When this fibrinoid material becomes disrupted in abortions, it forms hyaline, eosinophilic strands termed Rohr's stria. The origin of this fibrinoid, hyaline material is not fully under-

stood, although it appears to be partly composed of fibronectin and type IV collagen. In any event, fibrinoid is a distinctive part of the implantation site.

Placental site fibrinoid can resemble fibrin thrombi that occur as a result of chronic bleeding from a variety of causes. Also, endometrial stroma can become hyalinized and fibrotic in areas of continued breakdown such as the surface of polyps, and this change, too, can mimic the fibrinoid deposition of the implantation site. Fibrin thrombi and hyalinized endometrial stroma are distinguished from fibrinoid by the absence of interspersed intermediate trophobleast and the lack of the linear deposits of eosinophilic implantation site fibrinoid.

Changes in the spiral arteries of the placental site are significant. The presence of enlarged, hyalinized spiral arteries from the decidua basalis is a valuable adjunct in diagnosing intrauterine gestation.[40] These vessels have thickened hyalin-

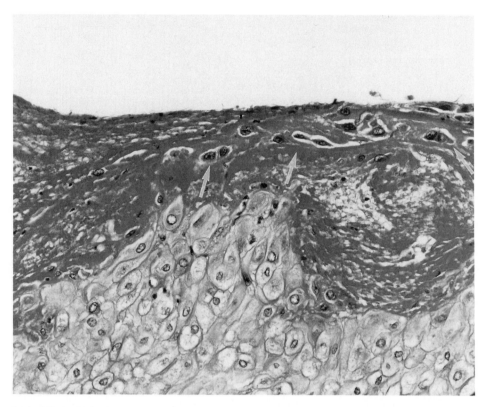

FIGURE 3.20. Fibrinoid (Rohr's stria). A strand of densely eosinophilic fibrinoid material of the placental implantation site overlies the decidua in curettings from an abortion specimen. A few IT cells are enmeshed in the fibrinoid (*arrows*).

ized walls that are partially infiltrated by IT cells and show an increased luminal diameter (Figs. 3.16 and 3.19). Often several implantation site vessels are seen in cross section, forming a prominent cluster. These vascular changes, like the presence of IT cells in the decidua, are characteristic of the implantation site and are not found in endometrium associated with ectopic pregnancy.

Histologic recognition of the placental implantation site usually is straightforward. Sometimes IT cells are indistinct, however, and ancillary immunohistochemical techniques are useful for their detection. Since intermediate trophoblast is epithelial, it reacts with broad-spectrum keratin antibodies.[31,40-42] Endometrial glands also stain with keratin, so all keratin-positive cells do not represent IT cells. It is the growth pattern along with immunoreactivity for keratin that identifies IT cells. With the keratin immuno-

stain, IT cells appear as intensely staining single cells or irregular clusters of cells with intervening decidua or smooth muscle that is nonreactive for keratin (Fig. 3.21). The IT cells produce hPL and, to a lesser degree, human chorionic gonadotropin (hCG). Immunostains for these proteins, especially hPL, also are useful for detecting IT cells.[31,40-42]

Exaggerated Placental (Implantation) Site

An exaggerated placental site represents one end of the spectrum of the morphologic features of the normal implantation site.[36,37] It is not a tumor. Instead it is an unusually prominent but physiologic placental site that may be difficult to distinguish from a placental site trophoblastic tumor (PSTT) (see Chapter 4). In molar pregnancy the placental site is exaggerated, but exaggerated pla-

FIGURE 3.21. Keratin immunore-activity of intermediate tropho-blast. Scattered IT cells in decidua show cytoplasmic staining for kera-tin (*arrows*).

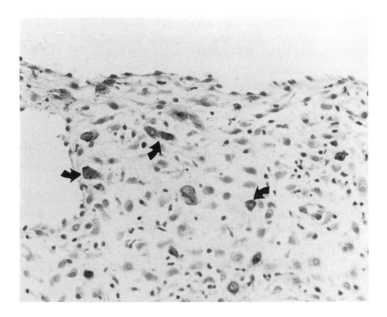

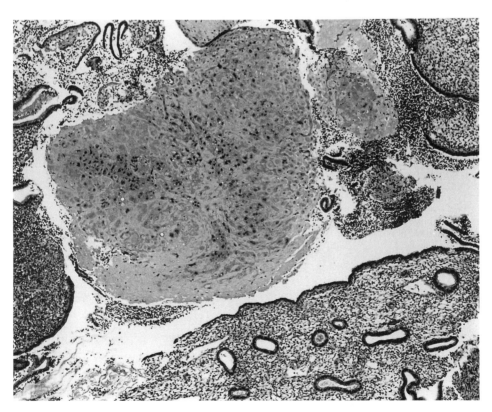

FIGURE 3.22. Placental site nodule. Well-circumscribed fragment of placental site nodule is present in endometrial curettings. This microscopic focus is composed of hyaline material with entrapped, degenerate IT cells.

cental site can occur in association with a normal gestation as well. The exaggerated placental site is characterized by an increase in the number and size of individual IT cells. In addition, widely dispersed multinucleated ST cells are a component of the trophoblastic infiltrate. Often several fragments of tissue in curettings contain portions of the lesion, and this process can extensively infiltrate fragments of myometrium. A few chorionic villi may be present. In the exaggerated placental site, IT cells appear larger and more hyperchromatic than normal. Despite their apparent prominence, these IT cells show virtually no mitotic activity. Necrosis is not a feature of the exaggerated placental site, although the surrounding decidua often shows degeneration and necrosis typical of spontaneous abortions. PSTT is an important consideration in the differential diagnosis of this lesion. The distinction is largely a matter of degree, as discussed in Chapter 4.

Placental Site Nodules

Placental site nodules are small, circumscribed foci of hyalinized implantation site with IT cells that occasionally present in an endometrial biopsy or curettage.[36,37,43] These benign lesions occur in women of reproductive age, although often the pregnancy history is remote.[43,44] The nodules may be present in biopsies taken several years after tubal ligation, suggesting that they are retained in the endometrium for extended periods of time.[43,44] Generally these lesions are microscopic, although hysterectomies may yield gross lesions as much as 1 or 2 cm in diameter. Some cases are incidental findings, but they frequently cause abnormal bleeding. They show a propensity for lower uterine segment and cervical involvement. The surrounding endometrium often is proliferative or secretory, and it usually is not decidualized.

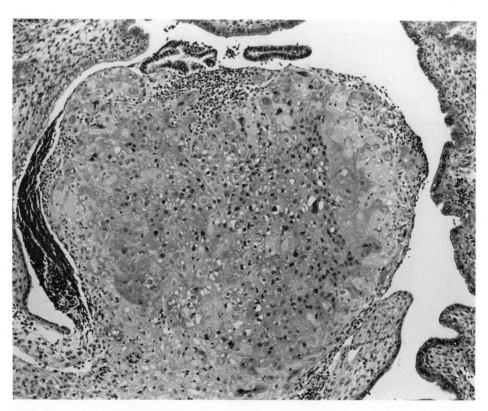

FIGURE 3.23. Placental site nodule. Placental site nodule shows degenerate, vacuolated IT cells with smudged nuclear chromatin surrounded by dense, hyaline stroma. A chronic inflammatory infiltrate is present at the periphery of the lesion.

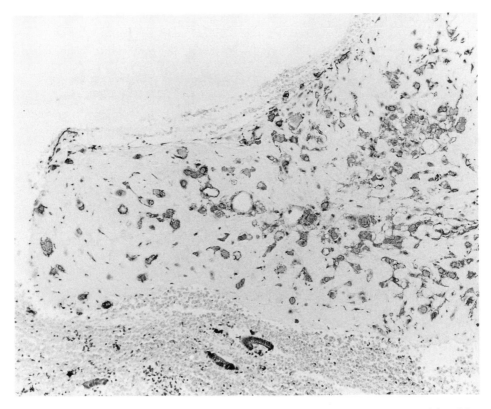

FIGURE 3.24. Placental site nodule. Immunohistochemical stain for keratin shows strong reactivity of the trophoblast.

The lesion itself is circumscribed, nodular, or plaque-like with densely eosinophilic, hyalinized stroma containing aggregates of IT cells (Fig. 3.22). Often focal chronic inflammation including plasma cells surrounds the nodule, while the rest of the endometrium shows no inflammation. The trophoblastic cell nuclei are dark, irregular, and hyperchromatic, and they appear degenerated (Fig. 3.23). Mitoses are rare or absent. In the past these nodules and plaques were considered hyalinized decidua, but strong reactivity for keratin and epithelial membrane antigen, along with focal reactivity for hPL in the cells that constitute the nodule, indicates that they are IT cells (Fig. 3.24).[43–45] Not all cases are immunoreactive for hPL, however, and hCG reactivity usually is absent. The trophoblast in these nodules also frequently shows reactivity for pregnancy-specific beta-1-glycoprotein (SP-1), placental alkaline phosphatase (PLAP), and vimentin.[45] The small size, circumscription, and extensive hyalinization are consistent features of the lesions that help to separate them from the placental site trophoblastic tumor discussed in Chapter 4.

Chorionic Villi and Villous Trophoblast in the First Trimester

Villus formation in very early pregnancy depends on the existence of the embryonic disc. Villi begin to develop on the 12th to 13th day postfertilization, and by days 12 to 15 the placenta can develop for a while independently, without the presence of an embryo.[4,46] In fact, in spontaneous abortions the placenta can persist for several weeks after the death of the embryo. In the early stages of pregnancy, villi have a loose, edematous stroma with few well-developed capillaries (Figs. 3.11 and 3.25). Once the yolk sac and embryo develop, vascular circulation is established in the villous stroma and these vessels contain nucleated red blood cells. During this early pe-

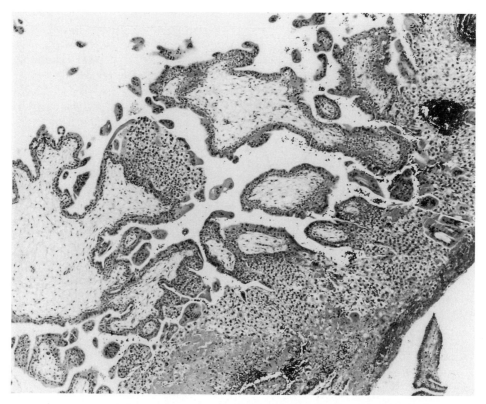

FIGURE 3.25. Immature chorionic villi. Immature villi from an abortion specimen show loose, edematous stroma containing a few capillaries with nucleated erythrocytes. Trophoblast emanates from one pole of several villi, which is the implanting portion of the anchoring villi.

riod of placental development, the trophoblastic covering of the villi consists of an inner layer of CT cells and an outer layer of ST cells. The CT and IT cells also proliferate at the implanting end of the anchoring villi that grow along the basal plate of the developing placenta.

A few histologic changes in the placenta help to determine the age of the developing conceptus (Table 3.4), although the length of gestation is an infrequent clinical question. These developmental intervals are stated in relation to the time of fertilization, also known as the postcoital or postconception date. Menstrual age from the last known menstrual period adds 2 weeks to these figures. The conceptus is traditionally called an embryo in the first 2 months of development; thereafter it is called a fetus.

As placental development proceeds, the presence of nucleated erythrocytes produced in the yolk sac helps determine the approximate gesta-

tional age.[46] The nucleated erythrocytes from the yolk sac appear in the villous circulation at 4.5 weeks. By 5 to 6 weeks, non-nucleated erythrocytes from the embryonic liver also begin to appear in the villi, and from this point on there is a shift in the proportion of nucleated to non-nucleated erythrocytes. By 9 weeks postfertilization the percentage of nucleated erythrocytes in the villi decreases from 100% to only 10%. Consequently, if the embryo dies before 4.5 weeks postfertilization, the villi contain no red blood cells. Death of the embryo between 4.5 and 10 weeks leaves a mixture of nucleated and non-nucleated erythrocytes in villous capillaries, and later death of the embryo usually leaves non-nucleated red cells in the stroma.

Other features also help to determine the relative length of gestation. For example, normally developing immature villi are relatively larger than those of later pregnancy. They have a

TABLE 3.4. Events in first-trimester placental development.[a]

Development of placenta	Time after fertilization
Blastocyst implantation	6–7 days
Villus formation begins[b]	12 days
Nucleated RBCs from yolk sac appear in villi	4.5 weeks
Non-nucleated RBCs from liver appear in villi	5–6 weeks
Proportion of nucleated RBCs decreases from 100% to 10% in villi	4.5–9 weeks
Decrease in prominence of inner cytotrophoblast layer	16–18 weeks

Abbreviation: RBCs, red blood cells.
[a] From time of ovulation. For menstrual age add 2 weeks.
[b] After 12–15 days, placental development proceeds even if embryo dies.

loose, myxoid stroma with widely spaced capillaries. As pregnancy progresses, the villi become smaller but more vascular and their stroma loses its edematous appearance. The morphologic features of the trophoblast covering the villi change along with growth of the placenta. The bilayered CT and ST covering of the villi persists to some extent throughout gestation, but a visible inner layer of CT cells starts to disppear at about 14 weeks of gestation. Between weeks 14 and 18, the percentage of villi showing an inner layer of CT cells decreases from 80% to 60%.[4] From then on there is a continuing gradual decrease in the CT layer. The large decrease in identifiable CT cells by week 18 is especially useful for determining the relative duration of early pregnancy.

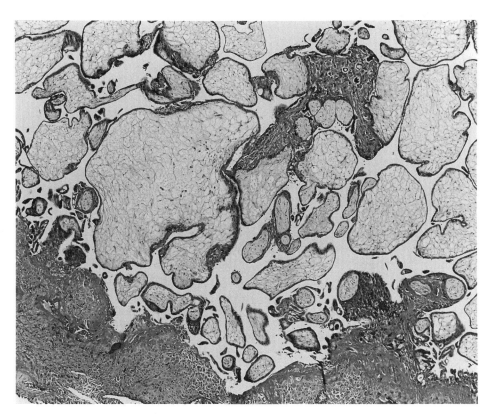

FIGURE 3.26. Immature chorionic villi with hydropic change. Abortion specimen shows avascular, edematous chorionic villi. This change is associated with the so-called blighted ovum and usually indicates very early demise of the embryo. Although the villi are edematous, the change is microscopic and not associated with hyperplasia of trophoblast. Furthermore, there is a polar distribution of the trophoblast toward the placental implantation site at the bottom of the field. These features distinguish this hydropic abortus from a partial mole.

Hydropic Change and Other Pathologic Changes in Abortions

The microscopic features of the decidua and the products of conception in curettings vary depending on the type of abortion.[4,47,48] Villi are usually normal in therapeutic abortions, whereas they tend to reflect early death of the embryo in spontaneous or missed abortions. Therapeutic abortion specimens may show pathologic changes in the villi, however.[49] In spontaneous or missed abortions, placental morphology is influenced by gestational age, karyotype, and regressive changes.[4,47,48,50-52] With the death of the embryo, the villi often show hydropic change because of loss of the villous vascular supply, especially with embryonic death occurring very early, often before 4.5 weeks postfertilization age.[46] The avascular villi are mildly distended with fluid and the curettings do not contain fetal parts, giving the changes of the so-called blighted ovum (Fig. 3.26). This pattern of mild villous edema and no evidence of fetal development indicates that the embryo either never developed or ceased development at a very early stage of gestation. Microscopically, villous edema in a hydropic abortion can appear especially prominent at first glance. Hydropic change affects most villi but is minimal and microscopic; cistern formation in the villi is rare but does occur (Fig. 3.27). There is no associated trophoblastic hyperplasia except the normal growth at one pole of the anchoring villi. Usually these microscopic abnormalities are less impressive when the gross, quantitative aspects are considered, too. Hydropic abortions usually consist of one or two cassettes of tissue with villi, whereas moles yield multiple cassettes. The changes of the blighted ovum are important to recognize in order to separate an abortion with hydropic changes from a hydatidiform mole

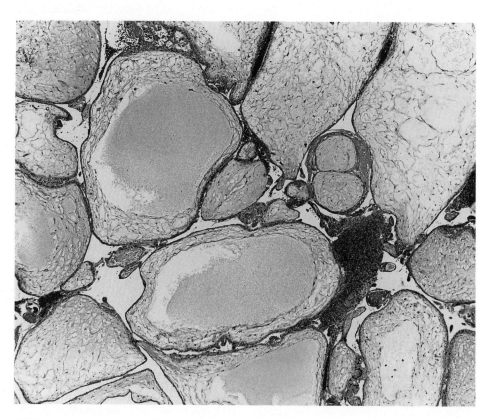

FIGURE 3.27. Immature chorionic villi with hydropic change. This hydropic abortus shows scattered cisterns. Despite the edema, this is a microscopic finding. There is no associated hyperplasia of the trophoblast, and this does not represent a hydatidiform mole.

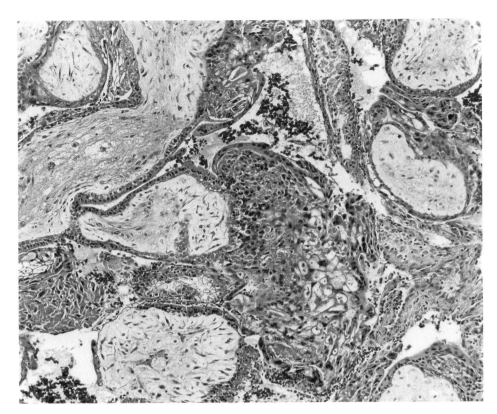

FIGURE 3.28. Immature chorionic villi with villous fibrosis. Abortion specimen showing immature villi with absence of vessels and stromal fibrosis. Hyperplastic trophoblast remains confined to one pole of the villi.

(Chapter 4). Hydropic change also may be focally present in therapeutic abortions,[49,53] especially if the blocks of sample villi of the chorion leave, where the villi normally degenerate, and mild hydropic change often is difficult to distinguish from the loose, myxoid stroma of the normal early placenta.

Other morphologic changes in chorionic villi from first-trimester abortion specimens may be found.[4] Irregular outlines of villi yielding a scalloped appearance and trophoblastic invagination into the villous stroma forming pseudoinclusions often are associated with abnormal karyotypes of the conceptus, particularly triploidy, but the findings are not sufficiently specific by themselves to be diagnostic of a chromosomal abnormality. Karyotyping is necessary to determine whether a chromosomal abnormality is present.[50,51,54,54a]

With incomplete abortions, the amount of villous tissue may be greatly reduced or even absent if portions of the placenta spontaneously pass before curettage. The implantation site, however, with its characteristic features, usually is present. In missed abortions the villi often are necrotic or hyalinized and the decidua is necrotic. Another change in villi associated with death of the embryo is loss of villous vascularity and fibrosis of the villous stroma (Fig. 3.28).[52,55,56] This change occurs more frequently in missed abortions. Some or many villi may be necrotic. These villous changes have little if any clinical significance.

Chorionic Villi and Villous Trophoblast After the First Trimester

After the first trimester or early second trimester, the placenta is sufficiently large that it is delivered spontaneously or by induction, and curettage specimens are rare. The villi are more numerous and become more complex. By this time there is a mixture of larger stem villi with prominent vessels

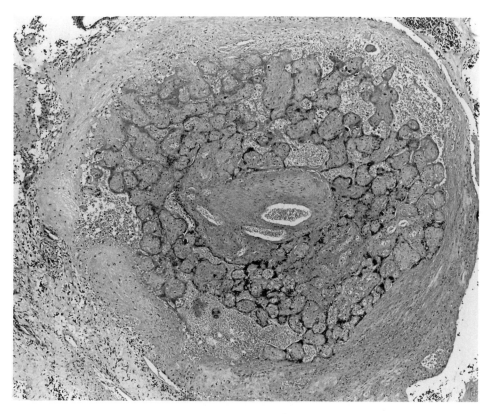

FIGURE 3.29. Placental polyp. Polypoid fragment of retained placental tissue removed by curettage several weeks after term delivery. The mature villi are degenerate and hyalinized.

and central stromal fibrosis, and many smaller tertiary villi containing numerous capillaries.[4] By late in the second trimester, the inner CT cells are indistinct over most villi and the trophoblastic proliferation along the anchoring villi has largely ceased. Some abortion specimens present early in the second trimester following intrauterine fetal death. In these cases the villous stroma often is fibrotic and hypovascular, with either no residual erythrocytes or a few residual degenerating red blood cells present.

Following delivery of the term or near-term placenta, abnormal bleeding may require curettage. The histologic findings in the postpartum endometrium vary. Failure of the implantation site to resolve quickly is called subinvolution. With subinvolution the uterus contains remnants of necrotic decidua and the placental site with eosinophilic fibrinoid, trophoblastic cells and enlarged vessels that often are infiltrated by the intermediate trophoblast. Retained placental site also serves as a nidus for inflammation, yielding inflamed and necrotic endometrium and implantation site. Immunohistochemical stains for keratin help to demonstrate the residual intermediate trophoblastic cells.

Placental Polyps

Placental polyps are a form of retained product of conception that represent polypoid portions of chorionic villi from an incomplete abortion or a term gestation retained in the uterine cavity.[4,57,57a] The villi may be necrotic, hyalinized, or partially calcified (Fig. 3.29). These polyps are not tumors, but they do form a nidus for inflammation and bleeding. Often these pedunculated masses of villi are found within days to weeks following abortion or delivery of a term placenta. Rarely, they persist for months or years after pregnancy.

Placenta Accreta

Placenta accreta is a form of abnormal implantation in which the placenta implants directly onto the myometrium with no intervening decidua; it may grow into or through the myometrium (placenta increta and percreta, respectively).[4,52] Usually placenta accreta presents immediately following delivery of a term pregnancy when the placenta or portions of the placenta cannot be delivered. The placental tissue fails to detach from the implantation site in the myometrium and cannot be manually removed. The usual management of placenta accreta is hysterectomy, but on occasion focal placenta accreta is encountered in curettings for postpartum hemorrhage. The diagnostic feature is villi in direct apposition to myometrium without intervening decidua. Hyaline fibrinoid material with scattered IT cells are interposed between the villi and myometrium, but decidual cells are absent. Some placental polyps may represent focal placenta accreta, although the latter are diagnosed only when villi are contiguous with myometrium. Scattered IT cells without villi in the myometrium are a physiologic phenomenon and not placenta accreta.

Endometrium Associated with Ectopic Pregnancy

In most circumstances, the endometrium associated with an ectopic pregnancy shows the typical features of early gestation, yet trophoblastic tissue is not present. A decidualized stroma, hypersecretory to atrophic glands, and thick-walled spiral arterioles usually are present.[18–20,24,57,58] Often the Arias-Stella reaction is present, at least focally. The endometrium associated with ectopic gestation can be highly variable, however, depending on the status of the trophoblastic tissue. If ectopic trophoblast is actively proliferating, the endometrium continues to show the changes of pregnancy. If the trophoblast begins to regress, the endometrium can display a variety of patterns ranging from proliferative to secretory changes. The endometrium can show features seen in dysfunctional bleeding, including anovulatory bleeding patterns, abnormal secretory patterns, or progestin effects. Subtle clues, such as a focal Arias-Stella reaction or a small aggregate of gland cells with clear cytoplasm, can suggest an ectopic pregnancy.

Establishing the presence of an intrauterine pregnancy effectively rules out an ectopic pregnancy. Evidence of an intrauterine pregnancy includes chorionic villi, trophoblastic cells, or the placental implantation site. Occasionally individual ST giant cells may be detected enmeshed in blood or fibrin. In cases where there are no villi or ST cells, an attempt should be made to identify IT cells scattered in partially necrotic decidua, often around spiral arterioles. Identification of IT cells of the placental site is crucial, and in such cases immunostaining for keratin can help show scattered trophoblast, usually intermediate trophoblast, in the decidua.[40,41,42,59,60] Immunostains for hPL and hCG specifically identify trophoblast, but the reactivity is less sensitive than that seen with keratin antibodies. Accordingly a panel of keratin, hPL, and hCG antibodies is most helpful for identifying trophoblastic cells.

Clearly, adequate sampling of endometrial tissue is important to ensure recognition of chorionic tissue. We have empirically found that three cassettes from abortion specimens are usually sufficient to establish the presence of chorionic tissue. If no trophoblast or villi are present in the first three tissue blocks, all of the residual tissue should be processed.

Clinical Queries and Reporting

For most endometrial biopsies or curettings related to pregnancy, there are three clinical questions to be answered by pathologic examination: 1) Does the endometrium show features of pregnancy? 2) If the changes indicate pregnancy, are chorionic villi and/or trophoblast present? 3) If villi and/or trophoblast are present, do they appear normal? For example, endometrial changes of pregnancy without the presence of chorionic villi or trophoblast suggest the possibility of an ectopic pregnancy. In spontaneous abortion the villi may reflect pathologic development of the embryo, a feature that helps explain the occurrence of the abortion. In other cases, edematous villi or proliferative trophoblast can raise the question of a hydatidiform mole, choriocarcinoma, or placental site trophoblastic tumor (Chapter 4).

The pathology report should consider the clinical questions asked regarding pregnancy as well as the pathologic findings. Most cases only require documentation of the presence of placental or fetal tissue. The most urgent question is that of an ectopic pregnancy. If pregnancy is suspected, or if the morphology shows pregnancy-induced endometrial patterns but there is no evidence of chorionic villi, placental site trophoblast, or fetal tissue, then an ectopic pregnancy must be considered. Occasionally the entire placenta with implantation site is expelled before the curettage, so lack of identifiable products of conception does not unequivocally indicate ectopic pregnancy. Nonetheless, an ectopic pregnancy can result in sudden, life-threatening intraabdominal hemorrhage, so immediate notification of the clinician managing the patient is imperative. Also, all the residual tissue should be processed. The clinician should be informed if immunohistochemical stains to identify trophoblast are pending or if residual tissue is being processed. Another call should follow as soon as the results are available.

Occasional spontaneous abortion specimens show only a small amount of early placental site with intermediate trophoblast and no chorionic villi. This finding is sufficient to establish the diagnosis of an intrauterine pregnancy. The specimen represents products of conception, and a descriptive diagnosis such as "implantation site and decidua" or "intermediate trophoblast" serves to verify the presence of an intrauterine gestation.

When villi are present in first-trimester specimens, some morphologic findings may be clinically relevant. In spontaneous abortions, for example, mild villous edema (hydropic change) and absence of fetal tissues including erythrocytes in villous vessels indicates that the gestation was abnormal and may help the clinician in the counseling of a patient. Although the microscopic findings can help indicate early death of the embryo, cytogenetic analysis of tissue has more value for assessing significant abnormalities that may lead to recurrent abortion. Sometimes the term "hy-

dropic villi" raises the specter of hydatidiform mole, so this term should be used cautiously unless the clinician fully understands the significance. If hydropic change is diagnosed, it may be useful to add a comment to indicate that this does not represent a mole.

Since pregnancy can be complicated by gestational trophoblastic disease, the status of the trophoblast, especially any abnormal proliferative activity, deserves comment. A specimen containing more than a small amount of trophoblast without villi, an exaggerated placental site without villi or unusually hydropic villi that are not clearly molar (Chapter 4) should be reported. In such cases, a comment regarding the uncertainty of the finding and recommendation for follow-up with serum hCG titers helps in the management of the patient.

The placental site nodule can be a confusing diagnosis to the gynecologist. The terminology for this lesion is relatively new. Although these lesions are almost always microscopic and incidental, confusion with PSTT may arise. It is therefore important to indicate clearly the small and benign appearance of the usual lesion. Some also use the term "hyalinized implantation site" to describe this change.

References

1. Mishell DR, Jr: Abortion. In: Comprehensive Gynecology. Herbst AL, Mishell DR, Jr., Stenchever MA, Droegemueller W, eds. St. Louis: Mosby, 1992;425–455.
2. Kalousek DK: Pathology of abortion: Chromosomal and genetic correlations. In: Pathology of Reproductive Failure. Kraus FT, Damjanov I, Kaufman N, eds. Baltimore: Williams & Wilkins, 1991; 228–256.
3. Miller JF, Williamson E, Glue J, Gordon YB, Grudzinskas JG, et al: Fetal loss after implantation. A prospective study. Lancet 1980;2:554–556.
4. Benirschke K, Kaufmann P: Pathology of the Human Placenta. 2nd ed. New York: Springer-Verlag, 1990.
5. Wilcox AJ, Weinberg CR, O'Conner JF, Baird DD, Schlatterer JP, et al: Incidence of early loss of pregnancy. N Engl J Med 1988;319:189–194.
6. Simpson JL: Incidence and timing of pregnancy losses. Am J Med Genet 1990;35:165–173.

7. Mazur MT, Duncan DA, Younger JB: Endometrial biopsy in the cycle of conception: Histologic and lectin histochemical evaluation. Fertil Steril 1989;51:764–767.

8. Foss BA, Horne HW, Hertig AT: The endometrium and sterility. Fertil Steril 1958;9:193–206.

9. Karow WG, Gentry WC, Skeels RF, Payne SA: Endometrial biopsy in the luteal phase of the cycle of conception. Fertil Steril 1971;22:482–495.

10. Hertig AT: Gestational hyperplasia of endometrium. A morphologic correlation of ova, endometrium, and corpora lutea during early pregnancy. Lab Invest 1964;13:1153–1191.

11. Wentz AC, Herbert CM III, Maxson WS, Hill GA, Pittaway DE: Cycle of conception endometrial biopsy. Fertil Steril 1986;46:196–199.

12. Andoh K, Yamada K, Mizunuma H, Michishita M, Nakazato Y, et al: Endometrial dating in the conception cycle. Fertil Steril 1992;58:1127–1130.

13. Arronet GH, Bergquist CA, Parekh MC, Latour JPA, Marshall KG: Evaluation of endometrial biopsy in the cycle of conception. Int J Fertil 1973;18:220–225.

14. Sulewski JM, Ward SP, McGaffic W: Endometrial biopsy during a cycle of conception. Fertil Steril 1980;34:548–551.

15. Lichtig C, Korat A, Deutch M, Brandes JM: Decidual vascular changes in early pregnancy as a marker for intrauterine pregnancy. Am J Clin Pathol 1988;90:284–288.

16. Clement PB, Young RH, Scully RE: Nontrophoblastic pathology of the female genital tract and peritoneum associated with pregnancy. Semin Diagn Pathol 1989;6:372–406.

17. Holmes EJ, Lyle WH: How early in pregnancy does the Arias-Stella reaction occur? Arch Pathol 1973;95:302–303.

18. Arias-Stella J: Atypical endometrial changes produced by chorionic tissue. Hum Pathol 1972;3:450–453.

19. Arias-Stella J: Atypical endometrial changes associated with the presence of chorionic tissue. AMA Arch Pathol 1954;58:112–128.

20. Arias-Stella J: Gestational endometrium. In: The Uterus. Norris HJ, Hertig AT, Abell MR, eds. Baltimore: Williams & Wilkins, 1973;185–212.

21. Dardi LE, Ariano L, Ariano MC, Gould VE: Arias-Stella reaction with prominent nuclear pseudoinclusions simulating herpetic endometritis. Diagn Gynecol Obstet 1982;4:127–132.

22. Beswick IP, Gregory MM: The Arias-Stella phenomenon and the diagnosis of pregnancy. J Obstet Gynaecol 1971;78:143–148.

23. Bernhardt RN, Bruns PD, Drose VE: Atypical endometrium associated with ectopic pregnancy. The Arias-Stella phenomenon. Obstet Gynecol 1966;23:849–853.

24. LaIuppa MA, Cavanagh D: The endometrium in ectopic pregnancy. A study based on 35 patients treated by hysterectomy. Obstet Gynecol 1963; 21:155–164.

25. Roach WR, Guderian AM, Brewer JI: Endometrial gland cell atypism in the presence of trophoblast. Am J Obstet Gynecol 1960;79:680–691.

26. Yokoyama S, Kashima K, Inoue S, Daa T, Nakayama I, et al: Biotin-containing intranuclear inclusions in endometrial glands during gestation and puerperium. Am J Clin Pathol 1993; 99:13-17.

27. Mazur MT, Hendrickson MR, Kempson RL: Optically clear nuclei. An alteration of endometrial epithelium in the presence of trophoblast. Am J Surg Pathol 1983;7:415–423.

28. Nakamura Y, Moritsuka Y, Ohta Y, Itoh S, Haratake A, et al: S-100 protein in glands within decidua and cervical glands during early pregnancy. Hum Pathol 1989;20:1204–1209.

29. Agarwal S, Singh UR: Immunoreactivity with S100 protein as an indicator of pregnancy. Indian J Med Res 1992;96:24–26.

30. Mazur MT, Kurman RJ: Gestational trophoblastic disease and related lesions. In: Blaustein's Pathology of the Female Genital Tract. 4th ed. Kurman RJ, ed. New York: Springer-Verlag, 1994:1049–1093.

31. Kurman RJ, Main CS, Chen HC: Intermediate trophoblast: A distinctive form of trophoblast with specific morphological, biochemical and functional features. Placenta 1984;5:349–370.

32. Kurman RJ, Young RH, Norris HJ, Main CS, Lawrence WD, et al: Immunocytochemical localization of placental lactogen and chorionic gonadotropin in the normal placenta and trophoblastic tumors, with emphasis on intermediate trophoblast and the placental site trophoblastic tumor. Int J Gynecol Pathol 1984;3:101–121.

33. Yeh IT, O'Connor DM, Kurman RJ: Intermediate trophoblast: Further immunocytochemical characterization. Mod Pathol 1990;3:282–287.

34. Yeh IT, Kurman RJ: Functional and morphologic expressions of trophoblast. Lab Invest 1989;61:1–4.

35. Wells M, Bulmer JN: The human placental bed: Histology, immunohistochemistry and pathology. Histopathology 1988;13:483–498.

36. Silverberg SG, Kurman RJ: Tumors of the uterine corpus and gestational trophoblastic disease. Atlas of Tumor Pathology, 3rd series, Fascicle 3. Wash-

ington, D.C.: Armed Forces Institute of Pathology, 1992.

37. Kurman RJ: The morphology, biology, and pathology of intermediate trophoblast—A look back to the present. Hum Pathol 1991:22:847–855.

38. Young RE, Kurman RJ, Scully RE: Proliferations and tumors of intermediate trophoblast of the placental site. Semin Diagn Pathol 1988;5: 223–237.

39. Wan SK, Lam PWY, Pau MY, Chan JKC: Multiclefted nuclei. A helpful feature for indentification of intermediate trophoblastic cells in uterine curetting specimens. Am J Surg Pathol 1992; 16:1226–1232.

40. O'Connor DM, Kurman RJ: Intermediate trophoblast in uterine curettings in the diagnosis of ectopic pregnancy. Obstet Gynecol 1988;72: 665–670.

41. Daya D, Sabet L: The use of cytokeratin as a sensitive and reliable marker for trophoblastic tissue. Am J Clin Pathol 1991;95:137–141.

42. Angel E, Davis JR, Nagle RB: Immunohistochemical demonstration of placental hormones in the diagnosis of uterine versus ectopic pregnancy. Am J Clin Pathol 1985;84:705–709.

43. Young RH, Kurman RJ, Scully RE: Placental site nodules and plaques. A clinicopathologic analysis of 20 cases. Am J Surg Pathol 1990;14:1001–1009.

44. Huettner PC, Gersell DJ: Placental site nodule: A clinicopathologic study of 38 cases. Int J Gynecol Pathol 1994;13:191–198.

45. Shitabata PK, Rutgers JL: The placental site nodule. An immunohistochemical study. Mod Pathol 1993;6:78A. (Abstract)

46. Szulman AE: Examination of the early conceptus. Arch Pathol Lab Med 1991;115:696–700.

47. Rushton DI: Examination of products of conception from previable human pregnancies. J Clin Pathol 1981;34:819–835.

48. Rushton DI: Pathology of abortion. In: Haines and Taylor: Obstetrical and Gynecologic Pathology. Fox H, ed. Edinburgh: Churchill Livingstone, 1987;1131–1136.

49. Jurkovic I, Muzelak R: Frequency of pathologic changes in the young human chorion in therapeutic abortions of normal pregnancies: A report of 500 cases studied histologically. Am J Obstet Gynecol 1970;108:382–386.

50. Vanlijnschoten G, Arends JW, Delafuente AA, Schouten HJA, Geraedts JPM: Intra-observer and inter-observer variation in the interpretation of histological features suggesting chromosomal abnormality in early abortion specimens. Histopathology 1993;22:25–29.

51. Novak R, Agamanolis D, Dasu S, Igel H, Platt M, et al: Histologic analysis of placental tissue in first trimester abortions. Pediatr Pathol 1988; 8:477–482.

52. Gersell DJ, Kraus FT: Diseases of the placenta. In: Blaustein's Pathology of the Female Genital Tract. 4th ed. Kurman RJ, ed. New York: Springer-Verlag, 1994;975–1048.

53. Ladefoged C: Hydrop degeneration: A histopathological investigation of 260 early abortions. Acta Obstet Gynecol Scand 1980;59:509–512.

54. Rehder H, Coerdt W, Eggers R, Klink F, Schwinger E: Is there a correlation between morphological and cytogenetic findings in placental tissue from early missed abortions? Hum Genet 1989;82:377–385.

54a. Fukunaga, M, Ushigome S: Spontaneous abortions and DNA ploidy. An application of flow cytometric DNA analysis in detection of non-diploidy in early abortions. Mod Pathol 1993; 6:619–624.

55. Fox H: Morphological changes in the human placenta following fetal death. J Obstet Gynaecol Br Commonw 1968;75:839–843.

56. Hustin J, Gaspard U: Comparison of histological changes seen in placental tissue cultures and in placentae obtained after fetal death. Br J Obstet Gynaecol 1977;84:210–215.

57. Buckley CH, Fox H: Biopsy Pathology of the Endometrium. New York: Raven Press, 1989; 234–247.

57a. Lawrence, WD, Quresh: F, Bonakdar MI: "Placental polyp": Light microscopic and immunohistochemical observations. Hum Pathol 1988;19:1467–1470.

58. Romney SL, Hertig AT, Reid DE: The endometria associated with ectopic pregnancy. A study of 115 cases. Surg Gynecol Obstet 1950;91:605–611.

59. Kaspar HG, To T, Dinh TV: Clinical use of immunoperoxidase markers in excluding ectopic gestation. Obstet Gynecol 1991;78:433–437.

60. Sorensen FB, Marcussen N, Daugaard HO, Kristiansen JD, Moller J, Ingerslev HJ: Immunohistochemical demonstration of intermediate trophoblast in the diagnosis of uterine versus ectopic pregnancy—A retrospective survey and results of a prospective trial. Br J Obstet Gynaecol 1991; 98:463–469.

4
Gestational Trophoblastic Disease

Gestational trophoblastic disease (GTD) includes disorders of placental development (hydatidiform mole) and neoplasms of the trophoblast [choriocarcinoma and placental site trophoblastic tumor (PSTT)].[1,2] The recent classification of these lesions by the World Health Organization (WHO) clearly defines the different histologic forms of GTD (Table 4.1).[3] A common feature of all of these trophoblastic lesions is that they produce human chorionic gonadotropin (hCG), which serves as a marker for the presence of persistent or progressive trophoblastic tissue. Because these

lesions are often treated in the absence of a histologic diagnosis, they are clinically classified as GTD without designation of the morphologic subtype. Nonetheless, identification and separation of the different pathologic forms of the disease are important, since they have different clinical presentations and behavior.

Hydatidiform mole, either partial or complete, is the most common form of GTD, and this is also the trophoblastic lesion most commonly encountered in endometrial curettings.[2] Choriocarcinoma and PSTT are infrequent. Recognition of any of these lesions can be difficult, however, because the morphologic features of all forms of GTD overlap with the features of placental and trophoblastic growth encountered in early pregnancy, abortion, and persistent placental implantation sites.

TABLE 4.1. Modified WHO classification of gestational trophoblastic disease.

Hydatidiform mole
  Complete
  Partial
Invasive mole
Choriocarcinoma
Epithelioid trophoblastic tumor
Placental site trophoblastic tumor (PSTT)
Trophoblastic lesions, miscellaneous
  Exaggerated placental site[a]
  Placental site nodule or plaque[a]
Unclassified trophoblastic lesion

[a]See Chapter 3 for a description of these lesions.

Hydatidiform Mole

General Features

Hydatidiform mole, either partial or complete, is infrequent in the United States and Europe, occurring in about one in 2,000 pregnancies.[4-7] In other parts of the world, including Asia and Latin America, these disorders are more common, although problems in methodology often complicate studies of their frequency when uncomplicated deliveries take place at home.[2,8,9]

The separation of hydatidiform mole into two subtypes, complete and partial, represents a significant advance in our understanding of molar pregnancy. These two forms of hydatidiform mole have different cytogenetic patterns that are accompanied by different clinicopathologic profiles and different degrees of risk for the development of persistent GTD (Table 4.2).[1,2,7,10-13] Both forms of mole typically present in the first trimester, often as an abortion.

Complete mole, also known as "classical" hydatidiform mole, has been recognized and studied for many years.[4] The typical complete mole used to present around the 16th week of pregnancy, but with the widespread use of ultrasound in prenatal assessment, many moles are now detected earlier in gestation. Complete moles commonly present with uterine enlargement greater than that expected for the gestational age, and the patient often has signs or symptoms of toxemia of pregnancy. Abortion with abnormal bleeding and passage of molar tissue is a frequent presentation. Because of the symptomatology, many complete moles are diagnosed before curettage. The serum beta-hCG titers typically are markedly elevated, and a beta-hCG titer above 82,350 mIU/ml, coupled with absence of fetal heart movement, is correlated with the presence of hydatidiform mole.[14]

Partial moles tend to present a little later in gestation, often at 18-19 weeks and sometimes after 20 weeks as a spontaneous or missed abortion (Table 4.2).[10,11] As with complete mole, however, with improved prenatal care and ultrasound assessment, many partial moles are detected much earlier in pregnancy. In these patients the uterus often is small for gestational age. The diagnosis of a partial hydatidiform mole often is unsuspected before curettage. Serum beta-hCG titers are in the low or normal range for that time in pregnancy, and toxemia is less frequent in comparison to complete moles.

Persistent GTD following a complete or partial mole is detected by serum hCG titers that fail to return to normal. The risk of persistent GTD is greater with complete mole. Up to 20% or more of patients with complete mole require further therapy, usually chemotherapy, for a plateau or increase in the serum hCG titer after evacuation.[2,15-17] About 2% to 3% of patients with com-

TABLE 4.2. Clinical and laboratory features of complete mole, partial mole, and hydropic abortus.[a]

	Complete mole	Partial mole	Hydropic abortus
Preoperative diagnosis			
Mole	+ + +	+ / −	−
Spontaneous abortion	+ +	+ +	+ +
Missed abortion	+ / −	+ + +	+ +
Heavy bleeding	+ + +	+	+ / −
Toxemia	+ +	+ / −	−
Uterus large for dates	+ +	+ / −	−
Uterus small for dates	+ / −	+ +	+ +
Serum hCG level	+ + +	+ / + +	+
Cytogenetics (karyotype)	46XX	69XXY or XXX	Variable, often
	(all paternal)	(2:1, paternal:maternal)	abnormal

Abbreviation: hCG, human chorionic gonadotropin.

[a] − → + + + = comparative frequency of clinical features or semiquantitative serum hCG titer between moles and hydropic abortus.

plete mole will develop choriocarcinoma. Among patients with partial mole, most studies indicate that about 5% develop persistent GTD.[2,10,11,18-20] Most of these cases represent persistent mole in the uterine cavity or invasive mole in the myometrium. Less often a patient has invasive mole with villi and trophoblast deported to the lungs, vulva, or vagina. Development of choriocarcinoma following a partial mole is a very rare sequela.[21]

Cytogenetics

Cytogenetic studies show that complete mole is diploid, usually 46XX. The entire chromosomal complement comes from the father by duplication of a haploid paternal genome (23X); the complete mole lacks maternal DNA.[22] Over 90% of complete moles contain this composition of paternal chromosomes.[12,23-25] The remaining complete moles also are androgenetic but are 46XY and formed by dispermy, i.e., fertilization of an ovum lacking functional maternal chromosomes by two spermatozoa.[24,26,27]

Cytogenetically, partial mole usually is triploid with two sets of chromosomes of paternal origin (diandric) and a haploid maternal set.[12,27,28] Usually the triploid chromosomal composition is 69XXY (58%); less often it is XXX (40%) or XYY (2%).[27] Cytogenetic distinctions between complete and partial moles are not absolute, however. A few partial moles may be diploid,[29-31] and occasional complete moles are triploid.[29,32] Furthermore, both complete and partial moles can even show marked heterogeneity in ploidy patterns. Haploid, aneuploid, and tetraploid

moles, both partial and complete, rarely occur.[32,33] To date, most studies find no consistent association between DNA ploidy and the subsequent clinical course of either partial or complete mole.[32] One report, however, suggests that aneuploidy predicts persistence in complete moles.[34] DNA ploidy analysis can be helpful in classifying cases that lack clear-cut morphologic features that identify the mole as either complete or partial.[30,32,33,35,36]

Pathologic Features

Most cases of hydatidiform mole have characteristic morphologic features and are readily identified. Hydatidiform mole is one of the few curettage specimens that has distinctive gross features, namely large, translucent villi.[2] Tissue recovered from molar pregnancies often is voluminous, especially in complete mole. The grapelike villi typically range from several millimeters to 2.0 cm or more in the greatest dimension (Table 4.3). Occasionally, however, villi are not grossly visible. This is due to villi being passed spontaneously before curettage or villi collapsing during the suction curettage. Besides the presence of grossly edematous villi, specimens from partial moles may have remnants of a fetus.

Microscopically, the villi in both complete mole and partial mole show circumferential hyperplasia of trophoblast and cistern formation.[1,2] In partial mole, the villous abnormalities affect only a portion of the placenta, resulting in two populations of villi.[1,2,10,13] In complete mole, edema affects all villi, although the degree of enlargement

TABLE 4.3. Comparison of pathologic features of complete mole, partial mole, and hydropic abortus.

	Complete mole	Partial mole	Hydropic abortus
Gross appearance of villi	Usually diffuse, marked enlargement	Focal enlargement, generally smaller than complete	Generally not visible
Fetal tissue	Usually none	Often present	Usually none
Villous swelling	Generalized, involving most villi	Partial: two populations of villi, one hydropic and one not	Microscopic and focal
Trophoblast polarity	Circumferential over villi	Circumferential over villi	Polar, only on anchoring villi
Trophoblast proliferation	Variable amount	Focal, minimal	Limited to anchoring villi
Atypia	Often present	Rare	None

caused by the edema is variable. Sometimes one of the two features, circumferential hyperplasia or edema, predominates, but both features should be present to establish the diagnosis. As a general rule, molar villi should be sufficiently large to at least fill a microscopic field under a 10 × objective.

Complete Mole

In complete mole, the circumferential trophoblastic hyperplasia is characterized by masses of trophoblast, often confluent, that project randomly along the surface of edematous villi (Figs. 4.1 and 4.2).[1,2,4,37,38] The trophoblastic hyperplasia can involve smaller villi as well as the large villi with cisterns. This haphazard trophoblastic proliferation contrasts with the proliferating trophoblast in an immature placenta that maintains polar orientation at the anchoring villi and is not present over the other villi. The degree of tropho-

blastic hyperplasia in a complete mole is highly variable. Often the hyperplasia is moderate to marked with large masses of trophoblast that may be confluent extending from the surface of the villi. Occasional cases, however, have only minimal trophoblastic hyperplasia. The trophoblast that accompanies complete moles also often shows atypia (anaplasia) with enlarged, pleomorphic, and hyperchromatic nuclei. Mitotic activity may be brisk. The amount of trophoblast and the degree of atypia present have no apparent bearing on the subsequent clinical course, so grading the trophoblast is not helpful.[38]

The second change that is associated with a complete mole is marked edema with cistern formation (Figs. 4.1 and 4.3). A cistern is a completely acellular central cavity within a villus that is filled with edema fluid and surrounded by a sharply demarcated stromal border. In complete mole, many but not all of the villi show cistern

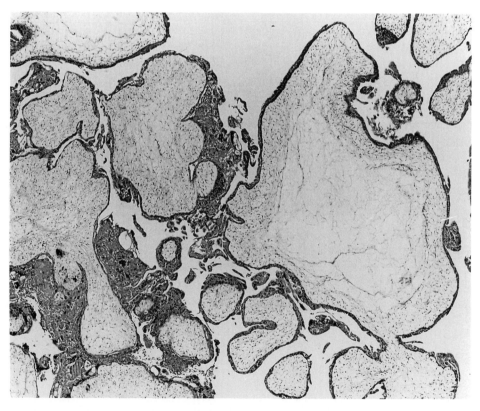

FIGURE 4.1. Complete hydatidiform mole. Low magnification shows generalized villous edema and marked enlargement of many villi. The massively distended villus to the right of center has a central cistern. Irregular, haphazard hyperplasia of trophoblast is present along the surface of several villi.

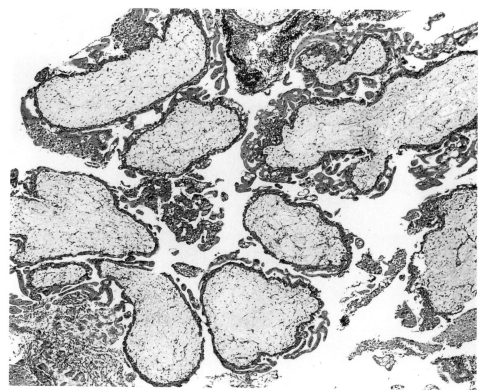

FIGURE 4.2. Complete hydatidiform mole. Circumferential hyperplasia of trophoblast is seen along the surface of most of the edematous villi in this field. Cisterns are ill-defined but all the villi are edematous.

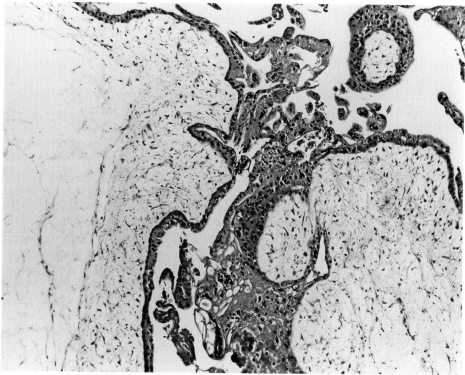

FIGURE 4.3. Complete hydatidiform mole. Portions of edematous, avascular villi in a complete mole show hyperplasia of the trophoblastic covering. A portion of a cistern is present in the villus to the left of center. Note the smaller villus with edema in the right upper corner. Occasional smaller villi such as these are commonly found in complete mole specimens.

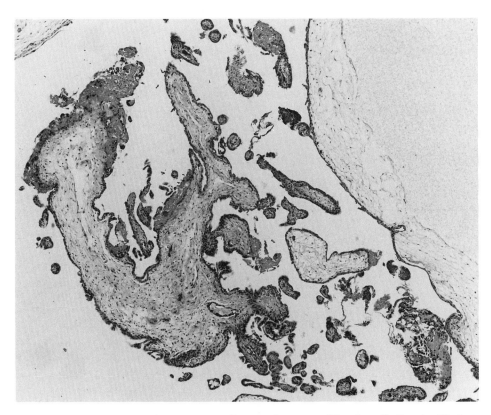

FIGURE 4.4. Partial hydatidiform mole. A mixture of large, edematous villi and small, fibrotic villi characterizes partial mole. A portion of a markedly enlarged villus to the right contains a central cistern. Irregular, patchy hyperplasia of trophoblast is present along the surface of the large villus to the left of center.

formation, although *all* the villi are edematous (Table 4.3). In fact, with the complete mole, scattered small villi without cisterns often are admixed (Fig. 4.1). Even these small villi show edema, however, with sparsely cellular stroma showing widely separated fibroblasts. In addition to these changes, some villi may be necrotic and occasional villi can show partial calcification. Since fetal development does not take place, the villi usually do not have blood vessels. Occasional vessels in the villous stroma can be found, however; these may contain cellular debris.

Partial Mole

Partial mole, as the name implies, shows only partial involvement of villi by edema and trophoblastic hyperplasia (Table 4.3).[1,2,10,13] The result is two populations of villi, one composed of small, nonmolar villi that do not show edema and one

that is enlarged and hydropic (Fig. 4.4). Frequently the nonedematous villi are fibrotic. Typically the enlarged villi have irregular, scalloped borders with deep infoldings (Fig. 4.5). Transverse sectioning of the invaginations yields trophoblastic "inclusions" in the villous stroma. Trophoblastic hyperplasia usually is limited, with only small foci of syncytiotrophoblast projecting randomly from the surface of the affected villi (Fig. 4.6). Another frequent finding in partial moles is microscopic evidence of fetal development, such as fetal parts, erythrocytes in villous capillaries, or fetal membranes. Fetal tissue is not invariably present in partial mole, however, and in some studies has been found in less than one-half of cases.[39]

With hydatidiform mole, especially complete mole, the trophoblastic infiltration of the placental implantation site typically is exaggerated (Chapter 3).[40] Curettage, especially sharp curet-

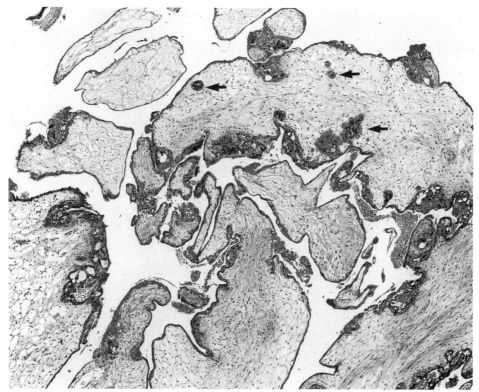

FIGURE 4.5. Partial hydatidiform mole. Many of the enlarged villi show irregular outlines. Note trophoblastic inclusions at the top of the field formed by invaginations of the surface of the villi into the stroma (*arrows*).

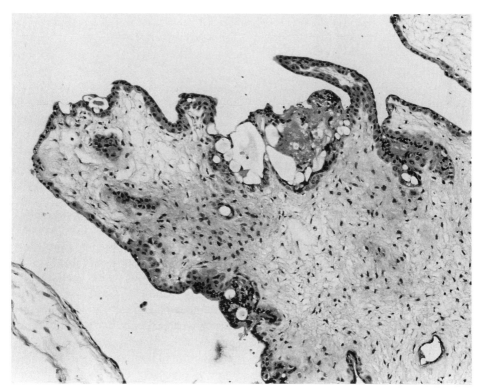

FIGURE 4.6. Partial hydatidiform mole. Portion of an edematous villus shows haphazard foci of trophoblastic hyperplasia along the surface and infoldings that form inclusions in the stroma.

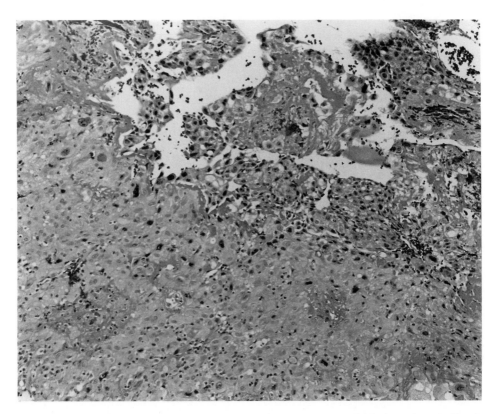

FIGURE 4.7. Exaggerated placental implantation site of complete mole. Abundant, atypical trophoblastic cells are present at the implantation site of a complete mole. The trophoblastic cells in this field are not associated with villi, but other fields showed markedly edematous villi of a complete mole. This exaggerated placental site has no significance by itself.

tage after suction extraction, can yield abundant, atypical trophoblast including many intermediate trophoblastic (IT) cells from the implantation site (Fig. 4.7). This trophoblastic proliferation is a standard feature of hydatidiform moles, and, as with the trophoblastic proliferation that covers the villi, the amount of trophoblast and the atypia do not influence the diagnosis or prognosis of the lesions as long as molar villi are present in the specimen.

Differential Diagnosis

Complete Versus Partial Mole

The distinction between complete and partial mole is straightforward when the characteristic features of either entity are pronounced. Multiple edematous villi with diffuse trophoblastic hyperplasia of complete moles contrast with the more limited villous edema and focal trophoblastic hyperplasia of partial moles. Another feature that separates complete from partial mole is the generalized edema of the villi in the complete mole, in contrast to the mixture of two populations of villi with fibrosis of some of the villi in partial mole.

There are some cases that have obvious features of a mole, yet distinction between a complete mole and a partial mole is not clear-cut. In these cases the morphologic features that allow separation of complete and partial mole may remain ambiguous, even after extensive histologic sampling. Diagnosis of a mole early in pregnancy can be particularly difficult, and more moles are now detected as early as the 7th or the 8th week of pregnancy. In such cases the subclassification of mole is especially difficult, because the cistern formation and trophoblastic hyperplasia are less pronounced than those found several weeks later in gestation.

Rarely a complete mole may occur as a twin gestation in conjunction with a normal placenta.[32,41] In these cases the curettings contain a mixture of normal-sized and molar villi that mimics a partial mole. Thus it may not always be possible to classify a specimen accurately as a complete or a partial mole by morphology alone. Management of either type of mole is similar, with monitoring of serum hCG titers after evacuation, and, therefore, the differential is not critical. Nonetheless, it is important to characterize the type of mole whenever possible, since partial mole more frequently resolves spontaneously and is only very rarely complicated by choriocarcinoma. Because of the relatively low rate of persistent GTD associated with partial mole, future management of this lesion may require shorter-term beta-hCG follow-up than for complete mole.

Usually at least eight cassettes of tissue should be submitted for a molar pregnancy to evaluate the degree of molar change, trophoblastic hyperplasia, and presence or absence of fetal tissues. Flow cytometric analysis of paraffin blocks for ploidy is rarely used in classification because of the cost and the occasional overlap in karyotypes between the two types of mole. Nonetheless, several studies suggest that ploidy may be useful in occasional cases,[36,37,42] especially if the morphologic features are ambiguous and there is a pressing clinical need to determine whether the mole is complete or partial.

Hydatidiform Mole Versus Hydropic Abortus

Another frequent consideration in the differential diagnosis of hydatidiform mole is the nonmolar hydropic abortion with villous edema (Chapter 3).[7,37,43,44] Microscopically, the edema of the hydropic abortus can appear striking. Hydropic abortions generally are smaller gross specimens, however, and villous enlargement cannot be seen by either the clinician or the pathologist (Table 4.3). It is important to keep microscopic observations in context with the gross findings. Most hydropic abortions yield only one or a few cassettes of tissue, whereas moles tend to be voluminous.

These generalizations usually hold, but in some cases of hydatidiform mole the villi are also not grossly visible. This is especially true if part of the molar tissue has been spontaneously aborted prior to curettage, if the mole is evacuated very early in gestation, if there is collapse of villi secondary to suction curettage, or if the specimen is a partial mole with limited tissue.

There are several microscopic features that distinguish a hydropic abortus from a mole.[1,2] In hydropic abortion the villi are edematous and avascular. Some also may shown trophoblastic inclusions.[45] Occasional small cisterns do occur in hydropic abortuses, but they are infrequent and do not cause gross villous enlargement. The most useful feature for separating a mole from a hydropic abortus is the distribution of the villous trophoblast. In a mole at least occasional villi show circumferential hyperplasia of trophoblast along their surface, whereas in the hydropic abortus the proliferating trophoblast has a polar distribution, projecting only from one surface of the anchoring villi. Since trophoblastic hyperplasia may be limited and focal, especially in a partial hydatidiform mole, thorough sampling may be needed to establish the diagnosis. In questionable cases it often is best to process multiple blocks to assess the overall edema and trophoblastic growth pattern. Since nonmolar hydropic abortus specimens may be diploid, triploid, or aneuploid,[32,45] DNA ploidy analysis in not practical for the separation of mole from hydropic abortus in most cases.

Hydatidiform Mole Versus Choriocarcinoma

The marked trophoblastic hyperplasia and cytologic atypia found in some cases of complete moles resembles the patterns found in choriocarcinoma. These cases can show large sheets of trophoblast with an alternating arrangement of cytotrophoblast and syncytiotrophoblast mixed with hemorrhage. Trophoblast may be prominent in the original curettings (Fig. 4.8) or in subsequent curettings done for abnormal elevation of hCG titers (Fig. 4.9). As long as edematous chorionic villi are present, no matter how much trophoblastic proliferation is present, the lesion is a hydatidiform mole.

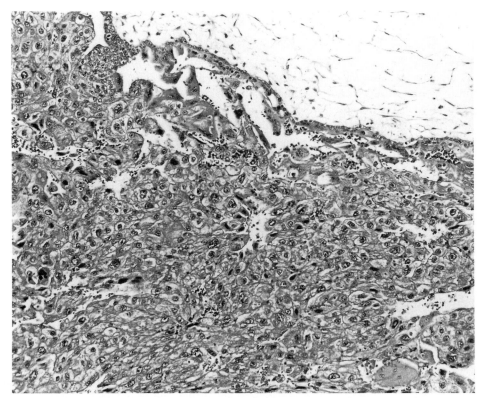

FIGURE 4.8. Hydatidiform mole. Prominent hyperplasia of the trophoblast from the surface of a villus of a complete mole.

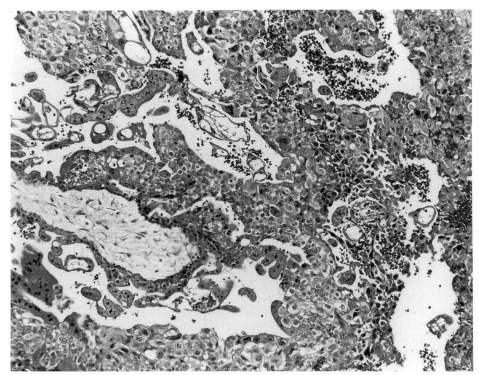

FIGURE 4.9. Persistent complete mole. Persistent mole obtained by curettage several weeks after initial evacuation of a complete hydatidiform mole. The trophoblastic proliferation is striking, but the presence of a villus to the left of center indicates that the diagnosis is persistent mole, not choriocarcinoma.

Persistent Postmolar Gestational Trophoblastic Disease and Invasive Hydatidiform Mole

After a hydatidiform mole has been evacuated, a subsequent curettage may be done for persistence or elevation of follow-up hCG titers or for significant uterine bleeding.[46–48] The repeat curettage may show persistent hydatidiform mole, choriocarcinoma, retained implantation site, no evidence of trophoblastic tissue, or, rarely, a new pregnancy.[46] If the specimen contains persistent hydatidiform mole, it will show residual molar villi mixed with trophoblast (Fig. 4.9). Usually the amount of tissue and villi is greatly reduced compared to the original curettage specimen, but as long as villi are present, the diagnosis remains that of persistent intracavitary mole. Choriocarcinoma is diagnosed when there is abundant trophoblast without villi that shows a dimorphic arrangement of syncytiotrophoblast and cytotrophoblast. In addition it is necessary to see invasion of tissue by trophoblast to make the diagnosis of choriocarcinoma (see below). Scant trophoblastic tissue without villi is not choriocarcinoma but persistent trophoblast (Fig. 4.10).[49]

With invasive hydatidiform mole, hydropic molar villi and hyperplastic trophoblast either invade myometrium or are present at other sites, usually the vulva, vagina, or lungs.[1,2,50] To establish the diagnosis, it is necessary to clearly identify molar villi beyond the endometrium. In curettings this requires finding the villi within myometrial smooth muscle, an extremely rare event. Consequently, invasive mole is almost never diagnosed by endometrial biopsy or curettage. It is important to remember that the presence of residual mole in recurettage specimen does not represent invasive mole in the absence of demonstrable myometrial invasion.

In occasional cases, curettage for bleeding or

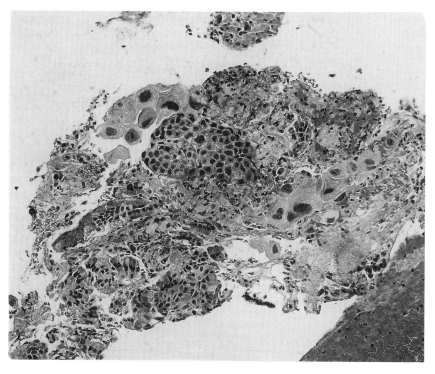

FIGURE 4.10. Persistent trophoblast following hydatidiform mole. A cluster of trophoblastic cells found in curettings after evacuation of a mole. Although no villi are present, the amount of trophoblast is scant and shows no evidence of invasion. The quantity of tissue is not sufficient for a conclusive diagnosis, and this tissue should be diagnosed as "persistent trophoblast."

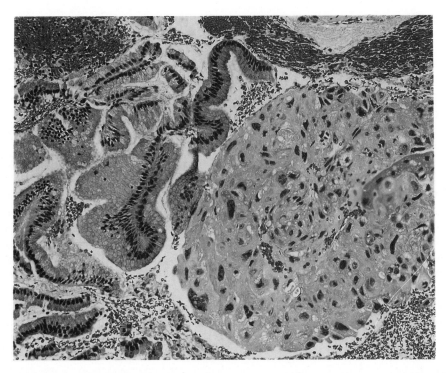

FIGURE 4.11. Nodule of intermediate trophoblast following hydatidiform mole. An aggregate of IT cells in curettings after evacuation of a mole is similar to the placental site nodule. Multiple nodules such as this rarely may be found in curettings, and they generally behave in a benign fashion.

persistent hCG titers after diagnosis of a mole has shown multiple nodules of intermediate trophoblast that are morphologically similar to the placental site nodule (Chapter 3) except for their multiplicity (Fig. 4.11).[51] Up to 65 separate nodules have been found in a curettage specimen. These nodules appear to be a mild form of persistent trophoblastic disease related to lack of complete regression of the exaggerated placental site of a mole. One study describing these lesions showed that they generally behaved in a benign fashion, although in two cases the nodules were associated with the development of choriocarcinoma.[51]

Clinical Queries and Reporting of Hydatidiform Mole

One of the most important clinical questions in the evaluation of an abortion specimen is whether gestational trophoblastic disease is present, since hydatidiform mole, choriocarcinoma, or PSTT can present as a spontaneous or missed abortion. Even a therapeutic abortion for an apparently normal gestation may reveal an unsuspected hydatidiform mole.

Often the clinician suspects a hydatidiform mole from the clinical history and from findings such as rapid uterine enlargement, abnormally high hCG titers, or toxemia in the first trimester. Ultrasound findings may support the clinical impression of a mole. At other times hydatidiform mole is clinically suspected when visibly enlarged, edematous villi are encountered at curettage. In such cases the logical questions are whether a mole is present, and, if so, whether it is a complete or partial mole. This distinction is usually based on the morphologic features; ancillary studies such as ploidy analysis are not sufficiently specific and have limited utility for distinguishing complete mole from partial mole. With either type of mole, the grading of the trophoblast has little clinical significance in terms of the overall risk for persistent GTD.[38] If there is any doubt about whether a specimen should be classified as an abortus with hydropic villi or as a hydatidiform mole, more tissue should be submitted if available. If a case remains equivocal, the gynecologist should be cautioned to follow the patient to be certain that hCG titers return to normal before pregnancy is attempted again.

Patients with known hydatidiform mole who are being followed may undergo repeat curettage for continued bleeding or for abnormally persistent or elevated hCG titers. If the biopsy shows trophoblastic tissue, then the presence or absence of chorionic villi is important and should be clearly reported. Molar villi generally indicate persistent intrauterine mole rather than invasive mole or development of choriocarcinoma.[49] Immature but normal villi indicate a new pregnancy unrelated to GTD.

Trophoblastic Neoplasms

Choriocarcinoma

General Features

Gestational choriocarcinoma can occur in the uterine cavity following any type of pregnancy.[1,2,4] As a rule, the risk of choriocarcinoma increases with the abnormality of the antecedent gestation. Complete hydatidiform mole is a major predisposing factor, and about half the cases of choriocarcinoma follow a complete mole. Choriocarcinoma also can arise from the trophoblast of an abortion or a term pregnancy. Consequently, this lesion may be present whenever abnormal vaginal bleeding occurs during the postpartum period in a young woman who has had a pregnancy of any type. Patients with choriocarci-

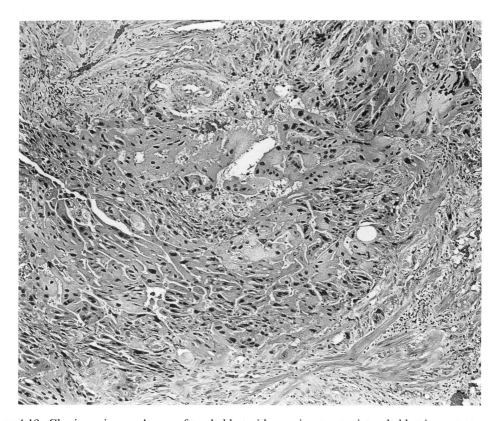

FIGURE 4.12. Choriocarcinoma. A mass of trophoblast with prominent syncytiotrophoblast in a curettage specimen of a young woman with abnormal uterine bleeding. Abundant trophoblastic tissue is present with no associated villi. The trophoblast shows invasion of the myometrium.

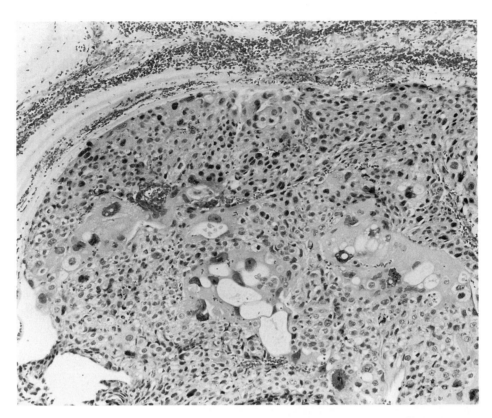

FIGURE 4.13. Choriocarcinoma. Dimorphic population of ST and CT cells in choriocarcinoma. Large ST cells with multiple nuclei and abundant, vacuolated cytoplasm are interspersed among CT cells.

noma also can present with metastatic disease without uterine signs or symptoms. Typically, the patient with choriocarcinoma has markedly elevated serum hCG titers.

Pathologic Features

Characteristically choriocarcinoma is hemorrhagic and necrotic, composed of trophoblastic cells without villi that invade normal tissues (Fig. 4.10). the two main diagnostic features are an absence of chorionic villi and a dimorphic population of trophoblast cells (Figs. 4.12–4.14). The first criterion, absence of villi, is important, since the proliferative trophoblast of hydatidiform moles or of early normal pregnancy can closely simulate the trophoblast of choriocarcinoma. The second criterion of choriocarcinoma, a dimorphic pattern of syncytiotrophoblastic (ST) cells alternating with nests of cytotrophoblastic (CT) or intermediate trophoblastic (IT) cells

should be found, at least focally, to establish a histologic diagnosis of choriocarcinoma. Often, the characteristic pattern of choriocarcinoma is readily apparent, but at times the dimorphic population of trophoblast may be difficult to recognize (Fig. 4.15). The admixture of ST cells with CT or IT cells yields a plexiform pattern. In these cases identification of the ST cells is an important diagnostic feature. These cells contain multiple nuclei, ranging from three to over 20 per cell, that are variable in size. Often the nuclei are pyknotic but they can be vesicular with prominent nucleoli. ST cells have dense eosinophilic to amphophilic cytoplasm with small vacuoles or large lacunae that often contain erythrocytes (Fig. 4.13). In contrast to ST cells, CT cells are small (about the size of a decidualized stromal cell) and uniform. They have a single nucleus with a prominent nucleolus, pale to clear cytoplasm, and distinct cell borders. Usually there is generalized enlargement of the trophoblastic cells with in-

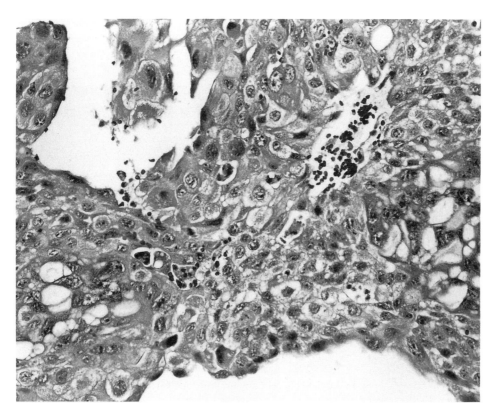

Figure 4.14. Choriocarcinoma. Endometrial curettings following a complete mole show numerous IT cells with interspersed ST cells containing multiple nuclei. Although intermediate trophoblast is prominent, the juxtaposition of syncytiotrophoblast forming a dimorphic population establishes the diagnosis of choriocarcinoma.

creased nuclear atypia in choriocarcinoma compared to normal trophoblastic cell populations in early pregnancy.

The amount of trophoblast in cases of choriocarcinoma is highly variable. There may be abundant neoplastic tissue, but frequently only a small amount of viable tumor associated with extensive hemorrhage is present. Small amounts of tumor may pose problems in diagnosis. While ST cells generally are prominent in uterine gestational choriocarcinoma, in occasional cases these cells are indistinct and CT cells predominate. Immunohistochemical stains for hCG can be very helpful for demonstrating ST cells in such cases. The ST cells stain intensely for hCG, whereas CT cells are nonreactive. The staining pattern will clearly demonstrate the plexiform pattern of ST cells.

Large IT cells with polygonal shapes and one or two large, hyperchromatic nuclei also occur in choriocarcinoma (Fig. 4.14). Their presence does not change the diagnosis of choriocarcinoma as long as the tumor shows the typical pattern of alternating ST and CT cells in other areas along with the complete absence of chorionic villi.

Epithelioid Trophoblastic Tumor

We have tentatively proposed the term "epithelioid trophoblastic tumor" to describe a specific type of trophoblastic tumor that does not appear to have been previously described.[2] This lesion was initially observed in a few patients with persistent lung metastases following intensive chemotherapy for documented choriocarcinoma[52] We have observed similar tumors in the uterus when there was no history of prior chemotherapy for choriocarcinoma, and in at least two cases this tumor merged imperceptibly with typical choriocarcinoma. This lesion also has been found in the

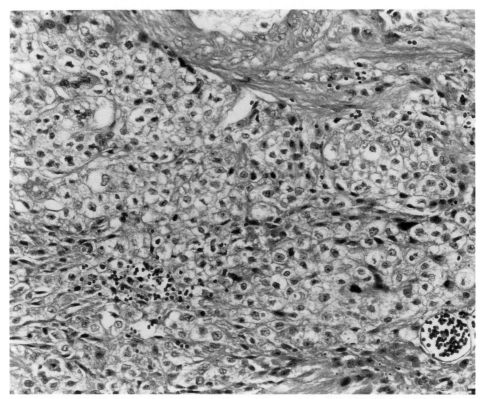

FIGURE 4.15. Choriocarcinoma. In this field ST cells are indistinct and CT cells predominate, yielding a pattern resembling poorly differentiated carcinoma.

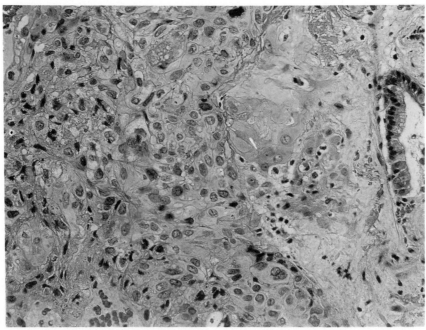

FIGURE 4.16. Epithelioid trophoblastic tumor. The tumor lacks a dimorphic pattern of CT and ST cells but is composed of a popoulation of relatively uniform, polygonal, mononucleate trophoblastic cells with promi- nent cellular membranes. A transition to choriocarcinoma with a typical biphasic pattern was identified in other areas of the tumor.

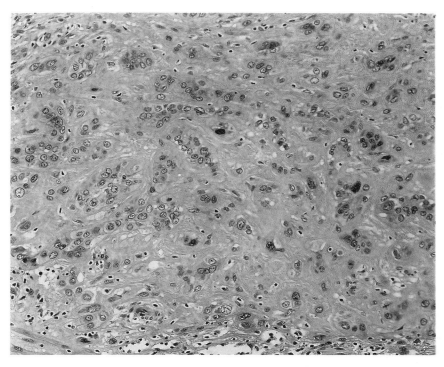

FIGURE 4.17. Epithelioid trophoblastic tumor. In this field the tumor is composed of cords and nests of monotonous cells in a hyaline matrix.

uterus adjacent to placental site nodules following hydatidiform mole.

These tumors lack the dimorphic pattern of classical choriocarcinoma and are composed predominantly of highly atypical mononucleate trophoblastic cells (Fig. 4.16). ST cells are indistinct. The tumor has a striking epithelioid appearance both in its cytologic features and in its pattern of invasion. The predominant cells are relatively uniform in size and are mononucleate. They are larger than et cells but smaller than IT cells. These trophoblastic cells have single, convoluted nuclei with a moderate amount of eosinophilic cytoplasm.

The neoplasm is composed of small nests and cords of cells. The nests often contain dense central hyaline material and necrotic debris, and the cords are encompassed by a hyaline matrix (Fig. 4.17). The hyaline material and necrotic debris simulate keratin, and these tumors may be confused with a poorly differentiated squamous carcinoma, particularly since the ST component is indistinct. Immunohistochemistry for hCG is

therefore particularly helpful in identifying syncytiotrophoblast in these tumors.

Because we have seen only a few cases, it is difficult to draw conclusions concerning the biologic behavior of these neoplasms, although they appear to have a somewhat more favorable prognosis than the usual dimorphic choriocarcinoma. The term "epithelioid trophoblastic tumor" seems appropriate for this lesion, since its distinctive epithelioid appearance sets it apart from choriocarcinoma and PSTT.

Differential Diagnosis

The differential diagnosis of choriocarcinoma includes physiologic trophoblastic proliferations associated with normal pregnancies and the trophoblast associated with hydatidiform moles, as well as PSTT and nontrophoblastic tumors. Trophoblast of normal pregnancy can be highly proliferative, especially at the implantation site of anchoring villi. In contrast to choriocarcinoma, the trophoblast in normal pregnancy usually is associated with small, immature chorionic villi and decidua. Occasionally, only trophoblast without villi is present in an abortion specimen. In such cases the trophoblast should be small in amount and focal, and should lack necrosis, significant hemorrhage, and atypical nuclear features. The finding of a significant amount of secretory endometrium, decidua, or placental implantation site favors the presence of normal trophoblast and not choriocarcinoma. The presence of atypia, including nuclear pleomorphism, macronucleoli, and abnormal mitotic figures, suggests choriocarcinoma.

The marked trophoblastic proliferation that may accompany some hydatidiform moles also resembles choriocarcinoma (Figs. 4.8 and 4.9). This feature can be particularly problematic in persistent hydatidiform mole that is found in a repeat curettage, since villi often are sparse in these specimens. Nonetheless, as long as villi are present, at least focally, the diagnosis is that of hydatidiform mole. Even without villi, a diagnosis of choriocarcinoma should be made only if there is a large amount of atypical, dimorphic trophoblast, hemorrhage, and tumor necrosis, or unequivocal invasion of the myometrium by a dimorphic population of trophoblastic cells. In the absence of these features, a diagnosis of persistent trophoblast is appropriate.

Nontrophoblastic tumors may mimic choriocarcinoma when they show a large component of giant cells. Anaplastic carcinomas and sarcomas with tumor giant cells may simulate choriocarcinoma, at least focally, and may even show choriocarcinomatous dedifferentiation. Usually the clinical history helps resolve this question, since high-grade carcinomas and sarcomas generally occur in older postmenopausal patients, whereas trophoblastic tumors occur during the reproductive years. Furthermore, many patients with choriocarcinoma have a history of a prior hydatidiform mole. In equivocal cases, immunohistochemical stains for beta-hCG are especially useful for demonstrating true syncytiotrophoblast. Since both choriocarcinoma and anaplastic carcinoma are epithelial tumors, immunostains for cytokeratin are less useful in establishing the diagnosis.

Rarely choriocarcinoma may be found in a postmenopausal patient. In such cases the tumor may represent gestational choriocarcinoma with a long latent period or it may represent somatic carcinoma with choriocarcinomatous transformation.[53,54]

Since the epithelioid trophoblastic tumor lacks the dimorphic pattern of typical choriocarcinoma, this lesion by itself could be difficult to distinguish from nontrophoblastic carcinomas. To date, epithelioid trophoblastic tumor has been seen only in cases where there is clear evidence of GTD, such as a recent hydatidiform mole or a pattern of definite choriocarcinoma with a component of syncytiotrophoblast in a premenopausal woman. Until this lesion is better characterized, it should be diagnosed only when it occurs in the presence of forms of well-established GTD.

PSTT is discussed and compared with choriocarcinoma below (Table 4.4).

TABLE 4.4. Comparison of microscopic features, Choriocarcinoma, PSTT, and exaggerated placental site.[a]

	Choriocarcinoma	PSTT	Exaggerated placental site
Amount of lesional tissue	Variable, often abundant	Variable, often abundant	Usually limited
Villi	Absent	Absent[b]	Usually present, focal
Trophoblast growth pattern and cell types	Dimorphic: ST with CT or IT cells	Monomorphic: IT cells	Monomorphic: IT cells
Mitoses	Present, usually high rate	Present, usually low rate	Absent or rare
Nuclear atypia	Variable, may be marked	Moderate to marked	Moderate
Necrosis	Usually present	Usually present	Absent

[a] Abbreviations: PSTT, placental site trophoblastic tumor; ST, syncytiotrophoblastic; CT, cytotrophoblastic; IT, intermediate trophoblastic.
[b] Rarely present and, if so, very focal.

Placental Site Trophoblastic Tumor

General Features

PSTT is a rare form of trophoblastic tumor composed predominantly of intermediate trophoblast.[1,2,40,55–58] Like other forms of GTD, it almost always occurs during the reproductive years. In contrast to choriocarcinoma, this tumor rarely is associated with a recent pregnancy, and a few have occurred after a hydatidiform mole. The hCG titer is generally low and may not be noticeably elevated if a sensitive assay method is not used. These neoplasms usually are benign, despite destructive growth in the myometrium. Because they extensively infiltrate the myometrium, the uterus can be perforated during curettage. About 15% to 20% of reported tumors have shown aggressive malignant behavior with disseminated metastases.

Pathologic Features

PSTT typically produces a mass lesion. These tumors range from focal lesions 1 to 2 cm in diameter to large masses that replace much of the corpus. As a consequence, curettings of PSTT typically yield multiple fragments of neoplastic tissue. Microscopically the PSTT is composed predominantly of IT cells that invade normal tissues (Fig. 4.18). These cells generally are polyhedral and grow in cohesive masses that often show areas of necrosis (Fig. 4.19). The curettings usually include fragments of myometrium infiltrated by IT cells. The IT cell cytoplasm is generally amphophilic with occasional clear vacuoles and distinct cell borders. Some parts of the tumor, especially in areas of myometrial invasion, are composed of spindle-shaped cells. Most cells have a single irregular and hyperchromatic nucleus, but binucleate and multinucleate IT cells are also present. Marked variation in nuclear size

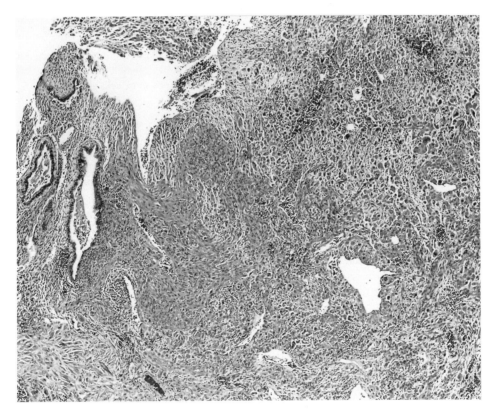

FIGURE 4.18. Placental site trophoblastic tumor. Low magnification shows PSTT invading endometrium and myometrium. Residual endometrium is present on the left side of the micrograph.

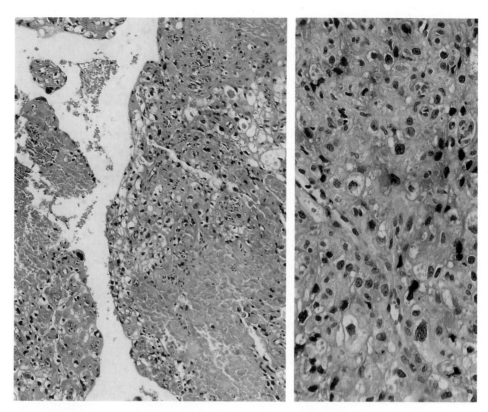

FIGURE 4.19. Placental site trophoblastic tumor. *Left*: Fragments of a PSTT in a curettage specimen show sheets of intermediate trophoblast with associated necrosis. The presence of necrosis is a helpful feature for distinguishing this tumor from an exaggerated placental site. *Right*: Higher magnification of the tumor shows characteristic IT cells.

and shape is often a feature of the tumor (Fig. 4.20). Some nuclei have deep folds or grooves, and others may have pseudoinclusions due to large cytoplasmic invaginations. Scattered ST cells with several nuclei and vacuolated cytoplasm are also present. Mitotic activity is variable but can be brisk with occasional abnormal forms.

Besides the characteristic cytologic features of the individual cells, the growth pattern of intermediate trophoblast in PSTT is also an important diagnostic feature. When myometrium is present in the biopsy, the cells infiltrate and dissect between smooth muscle fibers (Fig. 4.21). Furthermore, in PSTT there is a characteristic pattern of vascular invasion in which the intermediate trophoblast surrounds and replaces the vessel wall while preserving the lumen (Figs. 4.22 and 4.23). One other constant finding in this tumor

is patchy deposition of eosinophilic fibrinoid material (Fig. 4.22). The hyaline, amorphous deposits of fibrinoid occur randomly throughout the tumor, often entrapping individual cells. Fibrinoid also accumulates in the walls of vessels invaded by intermediate trophoblast (Fig. 4.23).

PSTT is immunoreactive for human placental lactogen (hPL), beta-hCG, and cytokeratins. Immunohistochemical stains for these antigens can be helpful in the differential diagnosis. Immunoreactivity for hPL usually is widespread in most of the IT cells. In contrast, hCG immunostaining is limited, with only focal reactivity, usually for cells that resemble syncytiotrophoblast. Keratin immunoreactivity is diffuse and intense.

It is difficult to reliably predict the behavior of PSTT based on the microscopic features, and therefore this neoplasm is not divided into be-

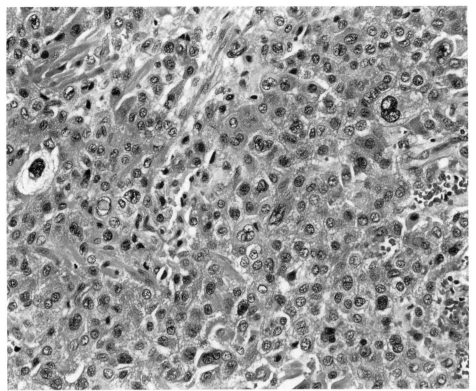

FIGURE 4.20. Placental site trophoblastic tumor. The tumor is composed of a monomorphic population of IT cells with hyperchromatic, irregular nuclei and a moderate amount of eosinophilic cytoplasm. The nuclei vary in size.

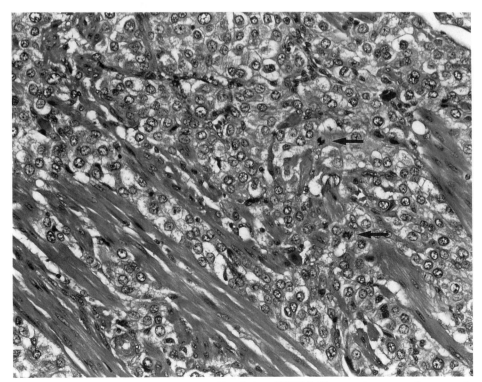

FIGURE 4.21. Placental site trophoblastic tumor. IT cells in a PSTT infiltrate a fragment of myometrium. The neoplastic cells dissect between the smooth muscle fibers. Several mitotic figures are present (*arrows*).

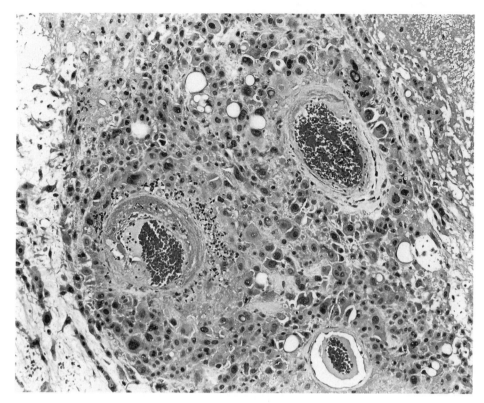

FIGURE 4.22. Placental site trophoblastic tumor. In this field the IT cells invade blood vessel walls in a characteristic fashion, preserving the lumen. In addition, amorphous fibrinoid material is deposited in the walls and in the interstitium. Several of the cells have vacuolated cytoplasm.

nign and malignant categories. The reported malignant cases of PSTT generally show some features that predict aggressive behavior. These clinically malignant tumors are composed of larger sheets and masses of cells with more extensive necrosis than benign tumors.[1,2,40,57,58] In malignant PSTT the cells also tend to have clear instead of amphophilic cytoplasm. Finally, the mitotic rate usually is higher in the malignant tumors, greater than five mitoses per 10 high-power fields (HPFs) in most malignant cases. In contrast, the benign tumors usually show a mitotic rate of about two mitoses per 10 HPFs, with the highest reported rate being five mitoses per 10 HPFs. In several clinically malignant PSTTs, the mitotic rate was only two per 10 HPFs,[59,60] so it appears that some overlap exists in the mitotic rates of malignant and benign PSTT. Abnormal mitotic figures occur in benign as well as malignant PSTT.

Differential Diagnosis

The differential diagnosis of PSTT includes choriocarcinoma, exaggerated implantation site, placental site nodule and plaque, and other, nontrophoblastic tumors. Separation of PSTT from choriocarcinoma is important, since these two tumors behave differently and are treated differently. Choriocarcinoma may have a monomorphic appearance in some areas and may have large numbers of IT cells. In contrast to PSTT, however, a network of syncytiotrophoblast in choriocarcinoma results in a dimorphic population, at least focally (Table 4.4). The syncytiotrophoblast in the PSTT is composed of isolated giant cells that do not show the dimorphic pattern found in choriocarcinoma. Immunohistochemical stains for beta-hCG can be especially helpful in highlighting the network of syncytiotrophoblast in choriocarcinoma. Although both

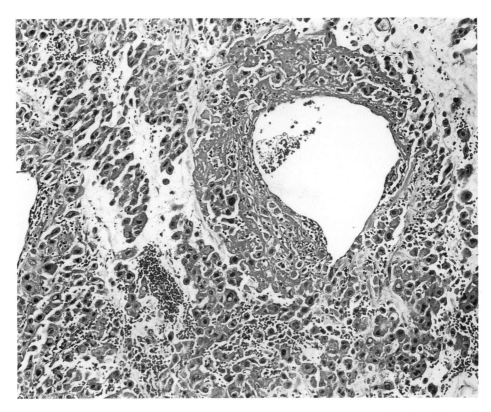

FIGURE 4.23. Placental site trophoblastic tumor. In this field the IT cells are relatively uniform with dense cytoplasm. IT cells embedded in fibrinoid material replace the wall of a large blood vessel.

PSTT and choriocarcinoma show immunostaining for hPL and hCG, the ratio of the number of immunoreactive cells for each marker differs in the two tumors. In PSTT the hPL/hCG ratio is typically 3:1, whereas in choriocarcinoma it is 1:3. Occasionally, however, PSTT, especially one that behaves in a malignant fashion, shows a ratio of hPL and hCG staining that more closely resembles that of choriocarcinoma.

Rarely, a trophoblastic tumor may show features of both choriocarcinoma and PSTT. This is called a mixed PSTT–choriocarcinoma. There is insufficient experience with these tumors to accurately predict their behavior.

An exaggerated placental implantation site can have features that are very similar to those of PSTT (Chapter 3). The distinction is largely one of degree (Table 4.4). The exaggerated placental site usually is focal, maintaining the overall architecture, and in other portions of the tissue there is decidua and/or chorionic villi. PSTT, in con-

trast, produces sheets and masses of cells typically accompanied by necrosis with little normal tissue in the sections. In addition, the exaggerated placental site tends to have more ST giant cells, the nuclei tend to have smudged (degenerative) chromatin, and mitotic activity is extremely rare or absent. Evidence of unequivocal mitotic figures is suspicious for PSTT.

Placental site nodules also are focal abnormalities, usually associated with proliferative or secretory endometrium elsewhere in the sections (Chapter 3). In comparison to PSTT, these lesions tend to be circumscribed and small. The IT cells in placental site nodules are bland and are widely spaced in a hyalinized stroma. This distribution of IT cells contrasts with the sheetlike growth of IT cells in the PSTT. As noted earlier, multiple placental site nodules may be found in the endometrium during follow-up of a hydatidiform mole.

Now that the histologic features of intermediate trophoblast are better recognized, the problem of distinguishing PSTT from other forms of malignancy has decreased. PSTT is a tumor of the reproductive years, whereas many of the malignant tumors that enter into the differential diagnosis tend to occur at a more advanced age. Cytologic features of intermediate trophoblast combined with the typical patterns of vascular invasion and fibrinoid deposition usually allow differentiation of PSTT from other neoplasms. In biopsies PSTT may be confused with keratinizing squamous cell carcinoma when the keratin has an amorphous eosinophilic appearance that superficially resembles the fibrinoid of PSTT. Squamous carcinoma usually arises in the cervix, whereas PSTT occurs in the corpus and clinical features can help to distinguish the neoplasms (Chapter 9). Furthermore, with squamous carcinoma a transition to a more obvious squamous pattern or normal endocervix often is found. Conversely, with PSTT the curettings often show endometrium or myometrial smooth muscle that has been invaded by the tumor.

On occasion PSTT can mimic leiomyosarcoma, especially in areas where intermediate trophoblast invades myometrium and becomes intimately admixed with smooth muscle cells. The trophoblastic cells of the PSTT are strongly immunoreactive for cytokeratin, and this feature can be very helpful in distinguishing PSTT from a smooth muscle tumor. The epithelioid appearance of intermediate trophoblast can also resemble patterns seen in high-grade nontrophoblastic carcinomas. In questionable cases, immunohistochemical stains for hPL and hCG are very helpful in distinguishing PSTT from a nontrophoblastic neoplasm.

Clinical Queries and Reporting of Trophoblastic Neoplasms

In curettings, choriocarcinoma is most commonly found in repeat curettage during follow-up of a hydatidiform mole. Sometimes, however, this neoplasm is an unsuspected finding in a reproductive-age patient with abnormal uterine bleeding. PSTT, because of its rarity, often is not clinically suspected, and the patient presents with amenorrhea or an apparent missed abortion.

Obvious cases of either choriocarcinoma or PSTT do not require more than a concise diagnosis. Because of its rarity, the diagnosis of PSTT should be accompanied by an explanatory comment that describes this as a form of GTD derived from intermediate trophoblast. Furthermore, for PSTT the mitotic count should be stated, since this feature may help to predict aggressive behavior. Because of the rarity and the potential for highly aggressive growth of any trophoblastic tumor, but especially choriocarcinoma, we also recommend oral communication with the gynecologist whenever possible.

At times a specific diagnosis of a trophoblastic tumor may not be possible, yet the lesion is suspicious for neoplasia. WHO does, in fact, have a category of "unclassified" trophoblastic lesion (Table 4.1), a term reserved for those unusual cases that cannot clearly be placed in one of the defined subgroups of the disease. An example of such a case would be a small amount of proliferative trophoblast without villi that can lead to a difficult differential diagnosis of choriocarcinoma versus trophoblast of a normal pregnancy. Also, prominent IT cells within decidua and myometrium may lead to a differential diagnosis of exaggerated placental site versus PSTT. When the diagnosis is not straightforward, a descriptive diagnosis of atypical trophoblast is best. With this type of diagnosis, the clinician is alerted to the possibility of trophoblastic disease. Then the patient can be followed with hCG titers or rebiopsied if symptoms persist.

References

1. Silverberg SG, Kurman RJ: Tumors of the uterine corpus and gestational trophoblastic disease. Atlas of Tumor Pathology, 3rd series, Fascicle 3. Washington, DC: Armed Forces Institute of Pathology, 1992.
2. Mazur MT, Kurman RJ: Gestational trophoblastic disease and related lesions. In: Blaustein's Pathology of the Female Genital Tract. 4th ed. Kurman RJ ed. New York: Springer-Verlag, 1994;1049–1093.
3. Scully RE, Bonfiglio TA, Kurman RJ, Silverberg SG, Wilkinson EJ: International Histological Classification and Typing of Female Genital Tract Tumours. Berlin: Springer-Verlag, 1994.
4. Hertig AT, Mansell H: Tumors of the female sex organs. Part I. Hydatidiform mole and choriocar-

cinoma. Atlas of Tumor Pathology, section 9, Fascicle 33. Washington, DC: Armed Forces Institute of Pathology, 1956.

5. Craighill MC, Cramer DW: Epidemiology of complete molar pregnancy. J Reprod Med 1984;29: 784–787.

6. Womack C, Elston W: Hydatidiform mole in Nottingham: A 12-year retrospective epidemiological and morphological study. Placenta 1985;6:93–106.

7. Jeffers MD, O'Dwyer P, Curran B, Leader M, Gillan JE: Partial hydatidiform mole: A common but underdiagnosed condition. A 3-year retrospective clinicopathological and DNA flow cytometric analysis. Int J Gynecol Pathol 1993;12:315–323.

8. Bracken MB, Brinton LA, Hayashi K: Epidemiology of hydatidiform mole and choriocarcinoma. Epidemiol Rev 1984;6:52–75.

9. Grimes DA: Epidemiology of gestational trophoblastic disease. Am J Obstet Gynecol 1984;150: 309–318.

10. Czernobilsky B, Barash A, Lancet M: Partial moles: A clinicopathologic study of 25 cases. Obstet Gynecol 1982;59:75–77.

11. Szulman AE, Surti U: The clinicopathologic profile of the partial hydatidiform mole. Obstet Gynecol 1982;59:597–602.

12. Szulman AE, Surti U: The syndromes of hydatidiform mole. I. Cytogenetic and morphologic correlations. Am J Obstet Gynecol 1978;131: 665–671.

13. Szulman AE, Surti U: The syndromes of hydatidiform mole. II. Morphologic evolution of the complete and partial mole. Am J Obstet Gynecol 1978;132:20–27.

14. Romero R, Horgan JG, Kohorn EI, Kadar N, Taylor KJW, et al: New criteria for the diagnosis of gestational trophoblastic disease. Obstet Gynecol 1985;66:553–558.

15. Bagshawe KD, Wilson H, Dublon P, Smith A, Baldwin M, et al: Follow-up after hydatidiform mole: Studies using radioimmunoassay for urinary human chorionic gonadotrophin (hCG). J Obstet Gynaecol Br Commonw 1973;80:461–468.

16. Curry SL, Hammond CB, Tyrey L, Creasman WT, Parker RT: Hydatidiform mole: Diagnosis, management, and long-term follow-up of 347 patients. Obstet Gynecol 1975;45:1–8.

17. Lurain JR, Brewer JI, Torok EE, Halpern B: Natural history of hydatidiform mole after primary evacuation. Am J Obstet Gynecol 1983;145: 591–595.

18. Goto S, Yamada A, Ishizuka T, Tomoda Y: Development of postmolar trophoblastic disease after partial molar pregnancy. Gynecol Oncol 1993; 48:165–170.

19. Berkowitz RS, Goldstein DP, Bernstein MR: Natural history of partial molar pregnancy. Obstet Gynecol 1983;66:677–681.

20. Rice LW, Berkowitz RS, Lage JM, Goldstein DP, Bernstein MR: Persistent gestational trophoblastic tumor after partial hydatidiform mole. Gynecol Oncol 1990;36:358–362.

21. Gardner HAR, Lage JM: Choriocarcinoma following a partial hydatidiform mole—A case report. Hum Pathol 1992;23:468–471.

22. Kajii T, Ohama K: Androgenetic origin of hydatidiform mole. Nature (London) 1977;268:633–634.

23. Wake N, Takagi N, Sasaki M: Androgenesis as a cause of hydatidiform mole. J Natl Cancer Inst 1978;60:51–57.

24. Kajii T, Kurashige H, Ohama K, Uchino F: XY and XX complete moles: Clinical and morphologic correlations. Am J Obstet Gynecol 1984; 150:57–64.

25. Vassilakos P, Riotton G, Kajii T: Hydatidiform mole: Two entities. A morphologic and cytogenetic study with some clinical considerations. Am J Obstet Gynecol 1977;127:167–170.

26. Surti U, Szulman AE, O'Brien S: Dispermic origin and clinical outcome of three complete hydatidiform moles with 46,XY karyotype. Am J Obstet Gynecol 1982;144:84–87.

27. Surti U: Genetic concepts and techniques. In: Gestational Trophoblastic Disease. Szulman AE, Buchsbaum HJ, eds. New York: Springer-Verlag, 1987;111–121.

28. Jacobs PA, Szulman AE, Funkhouser J, Matsuura JS, Wilson CC: Human triploidy: Relationship between parental origin of the additional haploid complement and development of partial hydatidiform mole. Ann Hum Genet 1982;46: 223–231.

29. Hemming JD, Quirke P, Womack C, Wells M, Elston CW, et al: Diagnosis of molar pregnancy and persistent trophoblastic disease by flow cytometry. J Clin Pathol 1987;40:615–620.

30. Davis JR, Kerrigan DP, Way DL, Weiner SA: Partial hydatidiform moles: Deoxyribonucleic acid content and course. Am J Obstet Gynecol 1987;157:969–973.

31. Lage JM, Berkowitz RS, Rice LW, Goldstein DP, Bernstein MR, et al: Flow cytometric analysis of DNA content in partial hydatidiform moles with persistent gestational trophoblastic tumor. Obstet Gynecol 1991;77:111–115.

32. Lage JM, Mark SD, Roberts DJ, Goldstein DP, Bernstein MR, et al: A flow cytometric study of 137 fresh hydropic placentas: Correlation between types of hydatidiform moles and nuclear DNA ploidy. Obstet Gynecol 1992;79:403–410.

33. Lawler SD, Fisher RA, Dent J: A prospective genetic study of complete and partial hydatidiform moles. Am J Obstet Gynecol 1991;164:1270–1277.

34. Martin DA, Sutton GP, Ulbright TM, Sledge GW, Stehman FB, et al: DNA content as a prognostic index in gestational trophoblastic neoplasia. Gynecol Oncol 1989;34:383–388.

35. Lage JM, Weinberg DS, Yavner DL, Bieber FR: The biology of tetraploid hydatidiform moles: Histopathology, cytogenetics, and flow cytometry. Hum Pathol 1989;20:419–425.

36. Fukunaga M, Ushigome S, Sugishita M: Application of flow cytometry in diagnosis of hydatidiform moles. Mod Pathol 1993;6:353–359.

37. Conran RM, Hitchcock CL, Popek EJ, Norris HJ, Griffin JL, et al: Diagnostic considerations in molar gestations. Hum Pathol 1993;24:41–48.

38. Genest DR, Laborde O, Berkowitz RS, Goldstein DP, Bernstein MR, et al: A clinicopathologic study of 153 cases of complete hydatidiform mole (1980–1990)—Histologic grade lacks prognostic significance. Obstet Gynecol 1991;78:402–409.

39. Iyengar V, Roberts D, Lage J: Histopathologic study of triploid partial moles. Mod Pathol 1993;6:74A. (Abstract)

40. Kurman RJ: The morphology, biology, and pathology of intermediate trophoblast—A look back to the present. Hum Pathol 1991;22:847–855.

41. Vejerslev LD, Dueholm M, Hassing N: Hydatidiform mole: Cytogenetic marker analysis in twin gestation. Report of two cases. Am J Obstet Gynecol 1986;155:614.

42. Lage JM, Driscoll SG, Yavner DL, Olivier AP, Mark SD, et al: Hydatidiform moles. Application of flow cytometry in diagnosis. Am J Clin Pathol 1988;89;596–600.

43. Messerli ML, Parmley T, Woodruff JD, et al: Inter- and intra-pathologist variability in the diagnosis of gestational trophoblastic neoplasia. Obstet Gynecol 1987;69:622–626.

44. Javey H, Borazjani G, Behmard S, Langley FA: Discrepancies in the histological diagnosis of hydatidiform mole. Br J Obstet Gynaecol 1979; 86:480–483.

45. Koenig C, Demopoulos RI, Vamvakas EC, Mittal KR, Feiner HD, et al: Flow cytometric DNA ploidy and quantitative histopathology in partial moles. Int J Gynecol Pathol 1993;12:235–240.

46. Schlaerth JB, Morrow CP, Rodriguez M: Diagnostic and therapeutic curettage in gestational trophoblastic disease. Am J Obstet Gynecol 1990;162: 1465–1471.

47. Berkowitz RS, Desai U, Goldstein DP, Driscoll SG, Marean AR, et al: Pretreatment curettage— A predictor of chemotherapy response in gestational trophoblastic disease. Gynecol Oncol 1980;10:39–43.

48. Berkowitz RS, Birnholz J, Goldstein DP, Bernstein MR: Pelvic ultrasonography and the management of gestational trophoblastic disease. Gynecol Oncol 1983;15:403–412.

49. Elston CW, Bagshawe KD: The diagnosis of trophoblastic tumours from uterine curettings. J Clin Pathol 1972;25:111–118.

50. Takeuchi S: Nature of invasive mole and its rational treatment. Semin Oncol 1982;9:181–186.

51. Silva EG, Tornos C, Lage J, Ordonez NG, Morris M, et al: Multiple nodules of intermediate trophoblast following hydatidiform moles. Int J Gynecol Pathol 1993;12:324–332.

52. Mazur MT: Metastatic gestational choriocarcinoma. Unusual pathologic variant following therapy. Cancer 1989;63:1370–1377.

53. Savage J, Subby W, Okagaki T: Adenocarcinoma of the endometrium with trophoblastic differentiation and metastases as choriocarcinoma: A case report. Gynecol Oncol 1987;26:257–262.

54. Pesce C, Merino MJ, Chambers JT, Nogales F: Endometrial carcinoma with trophoblastic differentiation. An aggressive form of uterine cancer. Cancer 1991;68:1799–1802.

55. Eckstein RP, Paradinas FJ, Bagshawe KD: Placental site trophoblastic tumour (trophoblastic pseudotumour): A study of four cases requiring hysterectomy, including one fatal case. Histopathology 1982;6:211–226.

56. Kurman RJ, Scully RE, Norris HJ: Trophoblastic pseudotumor of the uterus. An exaggerated form of "syncytial endometritis" simulating a malignant tumor. Cancer 1976;38:1214–1226.

57. Young RH, Scully RE: Placental site trophoblastic tumor: Current status. Clin Obstet Gynecol 1984;27:248–258.

58. Young RE, Kurman RJ, Scully RE: Proliferations and tumors of intermediate trophoblast of the placental site. Semin Diagn Pathol 1988;5:223–237.

59. Gloor E, Dialdas J, Hurlimann J, Ribolzi J, Barrelet L: Placental site trophoblastic tumor (trophoblastic pseudotumor) of the uterus with metastases and fatal outcome. An J Surg Pathol 1983;7:483–486.

60. Fukunaga M, Ushigome S: Metastasizing placental site trophoblastic tumor: An immunohistochemical and flow cytometric study of two cases. Am J Surg Pathol 1993;17:1003–1010.

5
Dysfunctional Uterine Bleeding

This chapter specifically addresses uterine bleeding due to alterations in the normal cyclical hormonal stimulation of the endometrium. This type of bleeding is commonly referred to as dysfunctional uterine bleeding (DUB).[1–4] Clinically, DUB indicates ovulatory dysfunction. By definition, DUB excludes postmenopausal bleeding or bleeding due to the presence of specific pathologic processes such as inflammation, polyps, hyperplasia, carcinoma, exogenous hormones, and complications of pregnancy. The endometrial changes associated with DUB are important to recognize, because they may be confused with more serious lesions such as hyperplasia.

Although DUB denotes abnormal bleeding with no underlying organic disorder, one common morphologic finding in these biopsies is the morphologic changes of endometrial glandular and stromal breakdown. The changes of glandular and stromal breakdown are not unique to DUB; they may be found in a variety of organic disorders, too. Conversely, not all biopsies of patients with a history of bleeding show evidence of breakdown. Nonetheless, endometrial breakdown and bleeding is commonly encountered, and the morphologic features of bleeding should be recognized in order to allow clear separation of these nonspecific artifacts and degenerative/regenerative changes from other, more specific histologic changes such as hyperplasia or carcinoma.

Because glandular and stromal breakdown is most extensive when associated with DUB, the morphologic features of this peculiar form of early tissue breakdown are first presented. It is important to recognize that glandular and stromal breakdown by itself is a nonspecific finding; changes in the intact, nonbleeding endometrial glands allow the assessment of the presence or absence of other specific organic abnormalities.

Morphologic Features of Glandular and Stromal Breakdown

Breakdown and bleeding patterns have been given a number of different descriptive terms, such as "lytic," "shedding," "slough," or even "menstrual" endometrium. These patterns of bleeding are somewhat different from the changes seen in menstrual endometrium, however, since they largely occur on a nonsecretory background and they are focal rather than diffuse abnormal-

TABLE 5.1. Features of endometrial breakdown and bleeding.

Stromal "collapse"
Stromal cell clusters
Fibrin thrombi
Nuclear debris at base of gland cells
Nuclear debris in stroma
Eosinophilic syncytial change
Hemosiderin
Foam cells
Stromal fibrosis and hyalinization

ities. "Glandular and stromal breakdown" is the best term to describe the morphologic features without attempting to assign an etiology or a prognosis.

Irregular endometrial glandular and stromal breakdown, the "breakdown and bleeding pattern," has certain unique features (Table 5.1) that should be recognized, since it commonly occurs with dysfunctional bleeding, especially anovulatory cycles. These changes also occur with organic lesions such as inflammation, polyps, hyperplasia, and carcinoma, where the pattern typically is focal. Regardless of whether the changes are more extensive or are relatively focal in the sections, abnormal glandular and stromal breakdown usually does not occur uniformly throughout the uterine cavity. As a result, abnormal bleeding usually leads to a heterogeneous pattern with fragments of intact, nonshedding endometrium admixed with endometrium showing the morphologic changes of abnormal bleeding. Menstrual endometrium also shows breakdown, but the changes affect all the tissue and occur on a background of late secretory phase glands (Chapter 2). Furthermore, in menstrual endometrium

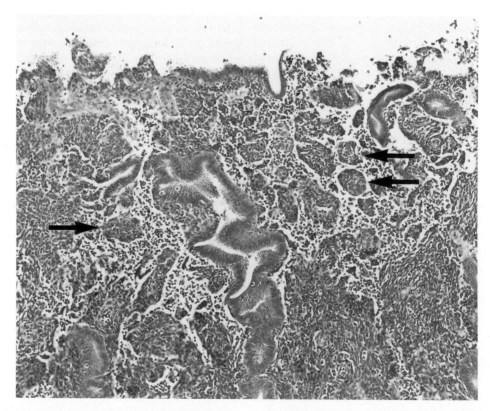

FIGURE 5.1. Glandular and stromal breakdown. Abnormal bleeding pattern associated with chronic inflammation secondary to retained placental site shows extensive glandular and stromal breakdown. Stromal cells are aggregated into rounded clusters (*arrows*) and are surrounded by blood. The glands show poorly developed secretory changes in this specimen. Other fields showed a residual placental site.

the breakdown is acute and lacks the changes of chronic bleeding, such as hemosiderin deposition or foam cell accumulation, seen in abnormal bleeding patterns.

Two factors complicate identification of breakdown and bleeding in endometrial biopsies. First, the operative procedure itself causes tissue fragmentation and hemorrhage. Second, when breakdown does occur, the pattern of tissue necrosis is unlike that seen in other organs. This unique morphologic expression of necrosis is due to the rapid expulsion of tissue into the uterine cavity. Consequently, extensive necrosis and autolysis often do not occur, and the tissue shows only early signs of degeneration.

Among the distinctive features of acute breakdown and bleeding is a particular pattern of hemorrhage in the stroma. This process is characterized by collapse of the stroma and coalescence of stromal cells into small aggregates and clusters separated by lakes of blood (Fig. 5.1). As stromal condensation becomes more advanced, small, rounded clusters of stromal cells, sometimes called "stromal blue balls," become detached from the surrounding tissue. These cellular clusters are characterized by tightly packed aggregates of hyperchromatic small nuclei with scant cytoplasm mixed with karyorrhectic debris (Fig. 5.2). They often are capped by attenuated surface epithelium or by eosinophilic cells forming a syncytium (see below). Sometimes these clusters of condensed cells form small polypoid extrusions along the endometrial surface (Fig. 5.3) as they detach from the intact stroma below. These are not true polyps.

Another characteristic feature of early breakdown, occurring before actual stromal collapse, is the accumulation of nuclear debris in the basal

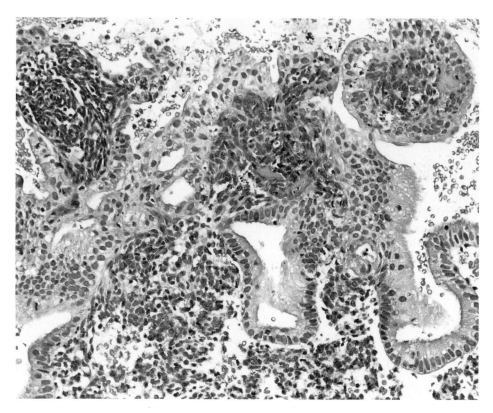

FIGURE 5.2. Glandular and stromal breakdown. Focus of glandular and stromal breakdown in proliferative endometrium due to anovulatory cycles. Collapse of the tissue results in distortion of the glands and condensation of stromal cells into tight clusters, so-called "stromal blue balls" (right upper corner). Nuclear dust is present at the base of glandular cells.

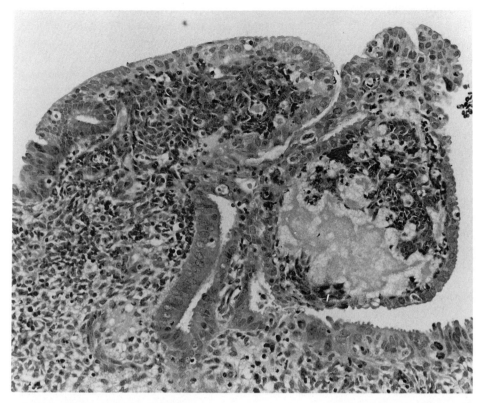

FIGURE 5.3. Glandular and stromal breakdown. A focus of breakdown just beneath the surface with collapsed stroma that is beginning to form characteristic clusters.

cytoplasm of glandular cells. This feature is prominent in premenstrual and menstrual endometrium but also occurs, to a lesser degree, with abnormal bleeding patterns (Fig. 5.2). The debris appears to represent nuclear karyorrhexis from individual cells within the glands.

Along with stromal collapse, fibrin thrombi typically form in small vessels and are another sentinel of chronic abnormal bleeding.[5] The thrombi form either in superficial portions of the spiral arteries or in ectatic venules in the stroma beneath the surface epithelium (Fig. 5.4). These ectatic vessels develop in association with any condition that results in prolonged endometrial growth that is not followed by physiologic shedding. Examples include anovulatory cycles, hyperplasia, polyps, and progestin effect. With loss of integrity of the vessel wall, the thrombi extend into the stroma. Sometimes thrombi partially organize, resulting in focal stromal fibrosis.

Fibrin by itself does not always signify true bleeding; some fibrin may be a result of the mechanical disruption of the biopsy procedure.

Another feature of active bleeding is eosinophilic syncytial change of the surface epithelium. This lesion, previously termed "papillary syncytial metaplasia,"[6] "papillary syncytial change,"[7] or "surface syncytial change,"[8] is a result of focal, irregular breakdown.[7] Because of its consistent association with breakdown, eosinophilic syncytial change appears to be a degenerative/regenerative alteration and is not a metaplastic transformation.[6,7] In eosinophilic syncytial change, portions of the surface epithelium coalesce into syncytial aggregates of eosinophilic cells (Figs. 5.5–5.7). The cells often randomly pile up into small papillae infiltrated by neutrophils, and these may contain microcystic spaces (Figs. 5.5 and 5.6). In this change the pink cells have sparsely vacuolated cytoplasm and indistinct cell

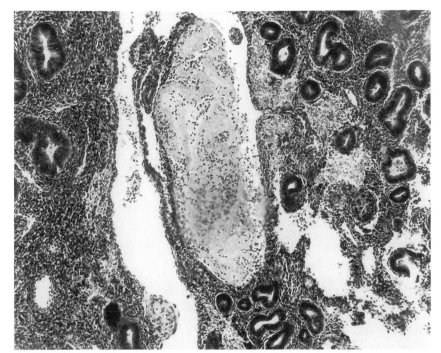

FIGURE 5.4. Fibrin thrombus with glandular and stromal breakdown. Proliferative endometrium with an ectatic venule that contains a fibrin thrombus. There is early associated glandular and stromal breakdown.

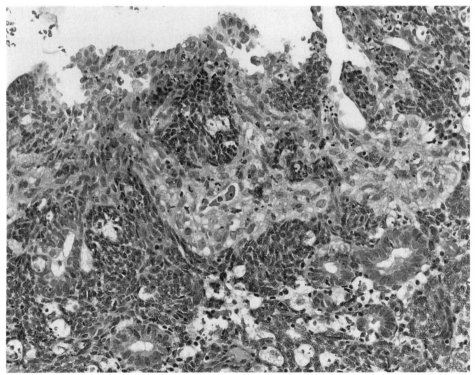

FIGURE 5.5. Glandular and stromal breakdown with eosinophilic syncytial change. A focus of prominent eosinophilic syncytial change in an area of breakdown in proliferative endometrium. The surface epithelium is heaped into a syncytium of eosinophilic cells with indistinct cell borders. A few clusters of stromal cells are entrapped in the syncytium.

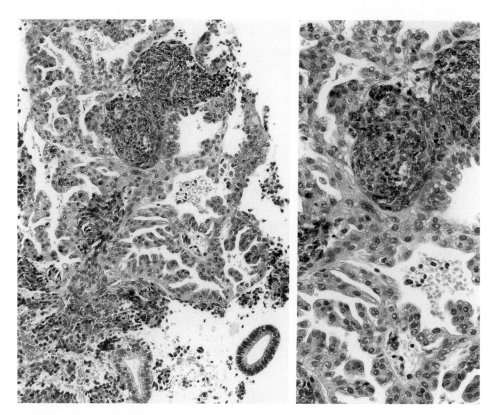

FIGURE 5.6. Glandular and stromal breakdown with eosinophilic syncytial change. *Left:* Proliferative endometrium with breakdown shows prominent eosinophilic syncytial change in a papillary configuration. The eosinophilic epithelium overlies several clusters of condensed stromal cells. *Right:* The eosinophilic cells in the papillae show little atypia.

borders, leading to the appearance of a syncytium (Fig. 5.7). Nuclei vary from oval to rounded and enlarged but have a uniform chromatin distribution (Figs. 5.6 and 5.7). At times the nuclei may be hyperchromatic with irregular borders. Occasional nucleoli and mitotic figures are present. These changes should not be interpreted as showing atypia.

Because of stromal collapse and tissue fragmentation associated with bleeding, the endometrial glands and surface epithelium become disrupted and crowded, yielding a pattern that can mimic complex hyperplasia or even adenocarcinoma (Fig. 5.8). It is important to recognize this distinctive pattern of breakdown and bleeding in order to avoid confusion of this nonspecific pattern with significant organic lesions. Glandular and stromal breakdown are recognized by the pattern of stromal collapse as well as the disrupted

glands. With breakdown and bleeding, these fragmented glands lose the stroma that should be present between intact glands. Even in hyperplasia where glands show marked crowding, the intervening stroma is attenuated but intact.

Other epithelial changes associated with breakdown are highly variable. As bleeding becomes chronic, variable amounts of hemosiderin deposits[9] and foam cells[10] appear in the stroma. Neither hemosiderin nor foam cells occur in normal cycling endometrium during the reproductive years, apparently because the tissue sloughs during menstruation. Foam cells are currently regarded as endometrial stromal cells that become distended with lipid following erythrocyte breakdown in areas of nonphysiologic hemorrhage.[10] These cells have abundant pale, faintly granular cytoplasm and small oval nuclei. Foam cells usually are associated with endometrial carci-

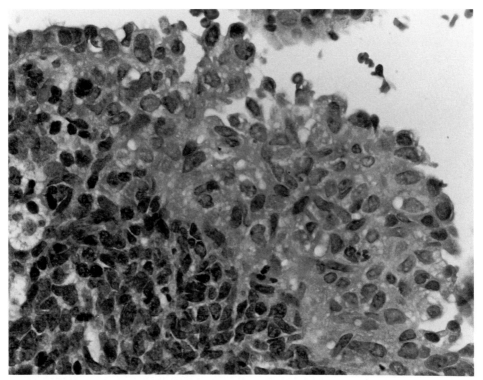

FIGURE 5.7. Glandular and stromal breakdown with eosinophilic syncytial change. A syncytium of surface epithelial cells overlying a focus of glandular and stromal breakdown shows haphazard nuclei and pale, sparsely vacuolated cytoplasm.

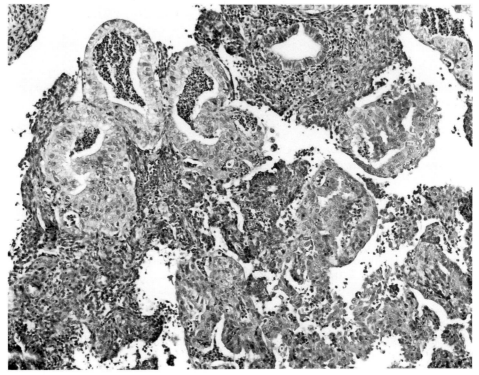

FIGURE 5.8. Glandular and stromal breakdown with artifactual crowding. Nonmenstrual secretory phase endometrium undergoing extensive breakdown shows artifactual crowding of the glands. The discontinuous, collapsed stroma around the glands helps to identify this pattern as an artifact.

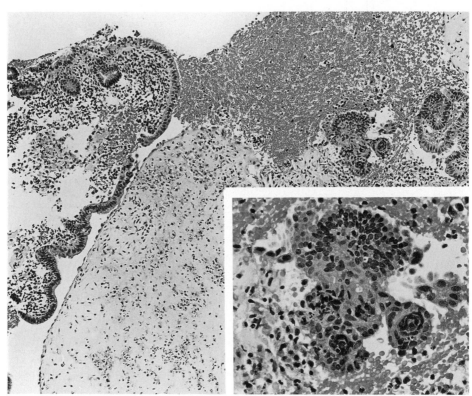

FIGURE 5.9. Hyalinized stroma secondary to glandular and stromal breakdown. A focus of hyalinized stroma in a sample that showed proliferative endometrium with glandular and stromal breakdown. This appearance is due to extravasation of fibrin into the stroma. *Inset:* Focus of breakdown with detached stromal clusters capped by eosinophilic epithelium.

noma (Chapter 10), but they can occur in hyperplasia or other benign pathologic conditions and therefore are a nonspecific finding. The architecture of the glands and the cytologic features of the epithelial cells, not the foam cells, are features that determine the pathologic diagnosis. Chronic bleeding occasionally results in patches of stromal hyalinization and fibrosis when bleeding is more severe and prolonged, and this appears to be related to fibrin deposition (Fig. 5.9).

Necrotic debris or old blood is sometimes present in the lumens of otherwise normal endometrial glands (Fig. 5.10). This debris seems to result from abnormal breakdown with entrapment of the debris within glands. The association with abnormal endometrial breakdown and bleeding is poorly defined, however, and often no definite abnormalities are present. Unless other morphologic abnormalities are found, luminal debris is a nonspecific finding with no known clinical significance. It should not be interpreted as endometritis.

Dysfunctional Uterine Bleeding

Dysfunctional abnormalities are frequent causes of uterine bleeding in perimenopausal and perimenarcheal women, and they occur to a lesser extent in women of reproductive age.[1,2,11–13] DUB occurs either because of lack of ovulation following follicular development (anovulatory cycles) or because of luteal phase abnormalities. The latter include luteal phase defect (LPD) and abnormal persistence of the corpus luteum (irregular shedding). Often, before a biopsy is done, DUB is managed by hormonal therapy. When bleeding persists, curettage often becomes necessary to control bleeding and exclude organic lesions. Clinicopathologic correlations of the full

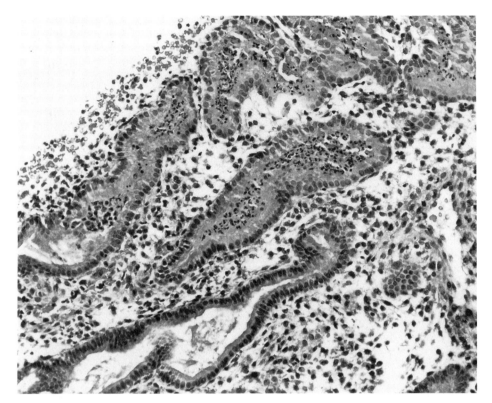

FIGURE 5.10. Debris in glandular lumens. Several glands in mid secretory phase endometrium contain cellular debris in their lumen. By itself, this finding has no known significance.

spectrum of morphologic changes associated with DUB are not known and may never be known. Nonetheless, there are certain endometrial alterations that can be correlated with abnormalities in the pattern of sex steroid hormone production.

Anovulatory cycles are, by far, the most common cause of DUB, and in some classifications DUB refers only to anovulatory bleeding. The prevalence of postovulatory luteal phase disorders as etiologies for DUB is not known. Ovarian dysfunction with anovulatory cycles or luteal phase abnormalities also may present with infertility (Chapter 3) rather than DUB.

To place dysfunctional abnormalities in the appropriate pathophysiologic context, these disorders can be placed into two broad categories, *estrogen-related* and *progesterone-related* bleeding. The more common is estrogen-related DUB, which refers to episodes of bleeding that are related to lack of ovulation with alterations in endogenous estrogen levels. Although not really a manifestation of DUB, atrophy is included as a form of estrogen-related bleeding because it occurs when the endometrium is deprived of estrogen for a relatively long period of time. In clinical classifications of bleeding disorders, atrophy is not regarded as a form of dysfunctional uterine bleeding, yet it is a significant cause of abnormal bleeding. The second, less frequent category of DUB is progesterone-related and reflects abnormal endogenous progesterone levels.

All these disorders, classified here as DUB, reflect variations in ovarian hormone production. Exogenous hormones may give endometrial patterns that are indistinguishable from the patterns seen in DUB due to endogenous hormone fluctuation. Whereas this chapter specifically addresses DUB, similar morphologic changes may be due to exogenous hormones; these effects are discussed further in Chapter 6.

Estrogen-Related Bleeding

Proliferative with Glandular and Stromal Breakdown

This term describes the endometrial changes resulting from anovulatory cycles. It is probably the most common change found in biopsies performed for abnormal bleeding in perimenopausal women. Anovulatory cycles with bleeding also occur in perimenarcheal adolescents in whom regular ovulatory cycles are not established. Anovulatory bleeding even occurs sporadically in women throughout the reproductive years. Usually, this bleeding does not lead to biopsy in younger patients, since the risk of other lesions, especially hyperplasia and carcinoma, is remote in these patients.[11,12] An exception to this occurs in women with chronic anovulation associated with the Stein–Leventhal syndrome (polycystic ovarian disease). In these cases, chronic anovulation leads to increased risk of development of hyperplasia or carcinoma, and biopsy is more frequent to rule out these abnormalities.

Anovulatory cycles result when a cohort of ovarian follicles begins to develop but ovulation does not occur. Chronic anovulation may be the result of a variety of disorders, including hypothalamic dysfunction and obesity, as well as increased androgen production by the adrenal glands or the ovaries.[1,2] The causes of absence of ovulation following recruitment of follicles are complex. They include defects in the hypothalamic-pituitary-ovarian axis such as hyperprolactinemia, abnormal feedback mechanisms of hormonal control, and local ovarian factors that interfere with ap-

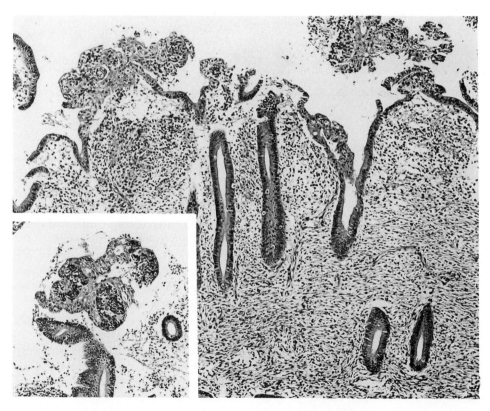

FIGURE 5.11. Proliferative with glandular and stromal breakdown. Anovulatory bleeding pattern in perimenopausal woman shows proliferative phase pattern with foci of breakdown along surface. This patient was not on hormones, but estrogen replacement therapy can present a similar appearance. *Inset:* Area of fragmentation in biopsy shows clusters of collapsed endometrium with stromal condensation and eosinophilic syncytial change on surface adjacent to detached proliferative glands.

propriate follicular development.[1] Whatever the pathogenesis, if ovulation does not occur, a corpus luteum does not develop and progesterone is not produced. The follicles produce estradiol, which stimulates endometrial growth. The developing follicles may persist for variable periods of time before undergoing atresia. As long as the follicles persist, estradiol is produced and the endometrium displays a proliferative pattern.

Bleeding associated with anovulatory cycles is of either the estrogen "withdrawal" or the estrogen "breakthrough" type. With estrogen withdrawal bleeding, the follicles recruited during the cycle undergo atresia and estradiol production falls precipitously. In this instance, the loss of estrogenic support of endometrial proliferation results in destabilization of lysosome membranes and vasoconstriction with bleeding. In contrast, estrogen breakthrough bleeding results from persisting follicles that produce estradiol; the proliferating endometrium becomes thicker but essentially outgrows its structural support. Focal vasoconstriction and thrombosis of dilated capillaries follow. In either event, the result is irregular breakdown and bleeding of the endometrium.

Although the terms "withdrawal" and "breakthrough" help to describe the mechanisms for estrogen-related bleeding, these terms have had different definitions among other authors. The lack of uniform usage of these terms limits their usefulness for reporting the pathologic changes associated with endometrial bleeding.

In most cases of anovulatory DUB, the endometrium shows a proliferative phase pattern with glandular and stromal breakdown (Fig. 5.11) (see also Figs. 5.2–5.6). The amount of tissue and the

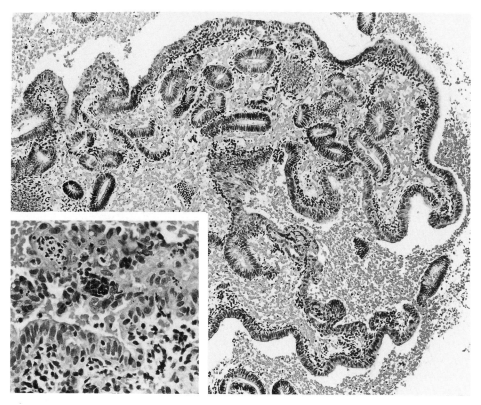

FIGURE 5.12. Weakly proliferative with glandular and stromal breakdown. Fragmented endometrium with isolated glands, extensive blood, and scant stroma from perimenopausal patient with anovulatory bleeding. The glandular epithelium is minimally stratified and shows only rare mitotic activity; it is therefore designated weakly proliferative. *Inset:* Focus of glandular and stromal breakdown with stromal cluster, nuclear debris, and eosinophilic syncytial change.

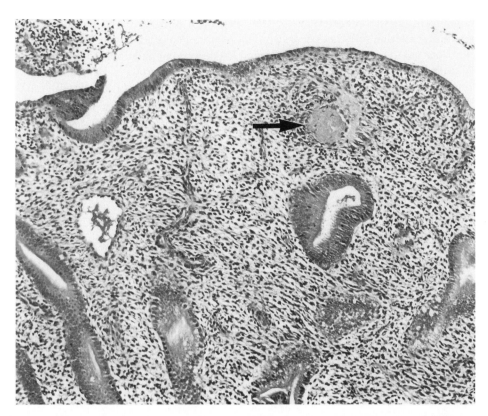

FIGURE 5.13. Ectatic venules with thrombi. Specimen from a perimenopausal patient with DUB due to apparent anovulatory cycles shows proliferative endometrium with a thrombus in superficial ectatic venule (*arrow*) and another dilated venule to the left of center. Glandular and stromal breakdown was present in other areas.

architectural pattern of the glands depend on the duration of unopposed estrogenic stimulation, not necessarily the dose of estrogen. Sporadic anovulation often results in rapid atresia of follicles with estrogen withdrawal bleeding. This results in minimal endometrial proliferation. A small amount of endometrium with poorly developed, weakly proliferative glands and stroma develops (Fig. 5.12). Chronic anovulation results in persistence of follicles and sustained unopposed estrogen stimulation. A greater quantity of endometrial tissue develops with actively proliferating glands and augmented glandular tortuosity. Dilated venules occur in the subepithelial stroma, and these often are thrombosed (Fig. 5.13). Because of continuous estrogenic stimulation, the tissue often shows estrogen-induced epithelial changes ("metaplasia"), especially ciliated cell and eosinophilic cell change (Chapter 8). The glands also may show focal subnuclear vacuoliza-

tion as a response to estrogen stimulation, but the extent and uniformity of the vacuolization are less than that seen in normal early secretory glands. The cytoplasmic changes and subnuclear vacuoles complicate the interpretation of the histologic pattern but do not change the diagnosis. Prolonged unopposed estrogenic stimulation also can lead to the development of varying degrees of hyperplasia and atypical hyperaplasia and even well-differentiated adenocarcinoma, but these organic lesions are not functional disorders and, as such, are not considered causes of DUB.

The most characteristic feature of bleeding associated with anovulatory cycles is endometrial glandular and stromal breakdown. As described earlier, these changes include nuclear dust at the base of glands, fibrin thrombi in small vessels, and stromal and glandular collapse (Figs. 5.2 and 5.3). One prominent feature is the "stromal blue balls" composed of small, dense spherical clusters of

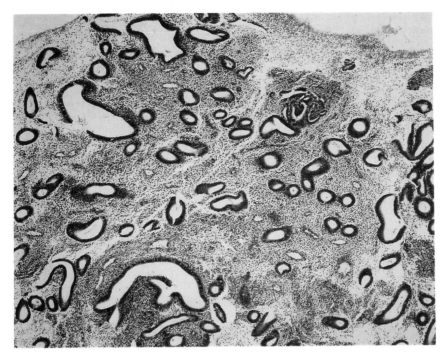

FIGURE 5.14. Disordered proliferative phase pattern. Portion of endometrium from a patient with apparent anovulatory bleeding shows disorganized proliferative phase glands with focal branching and glandular dilatation.

shedding endometrial stromal cells. Eosinophilic syncytial change of surface epithelium also often accompanies the breakdown pattern and can be prominent (Figs. 5.5 and 5.6).

When proliferative endometrium shows breakdown and bleeding, the pattern strongly suggests anovulatory cycles. Similar patterns can be caused by exogenous estrogens, and therefore a complete clinical history is needed to be certain that the bleeding pattern is truly due to anovulation. The differential diagnosis of proliferative phase endometrium with glandular and stromal breakdown also includes inflammation, polyps, and leiomyomas. In such cases, the presence of other features, such as plasma cells in chronic endometritis or the dense stroma and thick-walled vessels of polyps, establishes the proper diagnosis.

Disordered Proliferative Phase and Persistent Proliferative Phase

When chronic anovulatory cycles result in abundant proliferative tissue, mild degrees of disorganization characterized by focal glandular dilatation may occur. Usually these are regarded as variants of normal proliferative endometrium. Sometimes more sustained estrogen stimulation may result in the focal branching and some dilatation of glands, yielding a proliferative phase pattern that is neither normal nor hyperplastic (Fig. 5.14). The terms "disordered proliferative phase pattern" and "persistent proliferative phase" have been applied to describe this pattern of proliferative endometrium with tortuous and mildly disorganized glands. These descriptive diagnoses should be used in cases showing this pattern of mildly irregular and dilated proliferative glands. A designation of a disordered or persistent proliferative phase has utility in correlating the morphologic findings with the apparent pathophysiology. When used, these terms should be clarified in a note so that the clinical significance of the change is appreciated by the gynecologist.

In our experience, "disordered proliferative" often is inappropriately applied to a variety of patterns, including normal proliferative endometrium, proliferative endometrium with breakdown, artifactual crowding, basalis, and simple hyperplasia. The diagnosis of disordered proliferative phase should be reserved for cases in which assessment is based on intact, well-oriented fragments of tissue. In these areas the abnormal glands should be focal. These glands are qualitatively similar to those seen in hyperplasia, but they are limited in extent and interspersed among glands with a normal proliferative phase pattern. This criterion helps to separate the focal disordered proliferative phase pattern from simple hyperplasia, a more diffuse abnormality. If the tissue is extensively fragmented or disrupted by the procedure and contains mainly detached proliferative glands, it is best to diagnose the change only as proliferative. Extensive breakdown in proliferative endometrium can also display a disorganized appearance to the glands because of fragmentation, but again this change is not that of a true disordered proliferative phase pattern.

Atrophy

As previously noted, atrophy is an important cause of abnormal uterine bleeding in postmenopausal patients, being found in 25% or more of cases coming to biopsy. The percentage of patients with atrophy varies greatly among studies, probably reflecting different patient populations as well as variations in indication for biopsy and criteria for diagnosis of atrophy among various institutions.[14-19] In many laboratories, atrophy is found in up to 50% of biopsies taken for postmenopausal bleeding, and in one study 82% of cases of postmenopausal bleeding were due to atrophy.[16] Besides being common in postmenopausal patients, atrophic endometrium can occur in reproductive-age patients with premature ovarian failure, either idiopathic or due to radiation or chemotheraphy for malignancies.

With atrophy, tissue obtained at biopsy is typically scant, often consisting only of a small

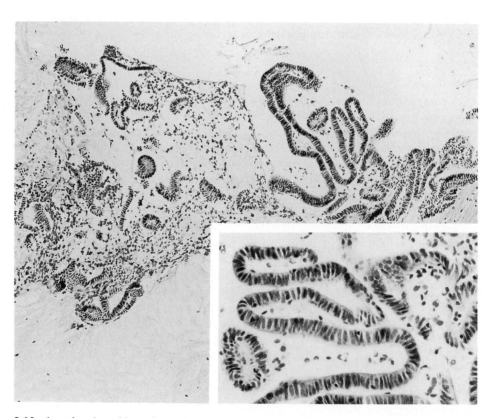

FIGURE 5.15. Atrophy. Atrophic endometrium consists of scant tissue that shows extensive fragmentation. The specimen consists largely of detached wisps and strips of epithelium with almost no stroma. *Inset:* The epithelial cells have small, dark nuclei, scant cytoplasm, and no mitotic activity.

amount of mucoid material. Characteristically, atrophic endometrium is composed of tiny strips and wisps of surface endometrium and detached, fragmented endometrial glands (Fig. 5.15). The epithelium is low columnar to cuboidal with small, dark nuclei and minimal cytoplasm. Stroma is scant or absent, consisting of a few clusters of small spindle cells. Mitotic activity is absent. The cystic change seen in atrophic glands in hysterectomy specimens is not observed in biopsies because tissue fragmentation from the procedure disrupts the glands. Breakdown and bleeding may be superimposed on the features of atrophy, although often, even when there is a history of abnormal uterine bleeding, the sections show no evidence of glandular and stromal breakdown.

Because of the paucity of tissue in biopsies of atrophic endometrium, specimens are often classified as insufficient or inadequate. This is not appropriate, because the scant tissue may be all that is present and therefore is completely representative of the lining of the uterine cavity. The minimal quantity of tissue should serve as a clue to the diagnosis; it does not represent an insufficient specimen (see below, Clinical Queries and Reporting).

Progesterone-Related Bleeding

Biopsies from reproductive-age and perimenopausal women occasionally show abnormal secretory phase patterns with associated nonmenstrual breakdown and bleeding. In such cases the pattern is secretory due to ovarian progesterone production, but the glandular and stromal changes usually are less advanced than those seen in normal late secretory endometrium.[20-24] The endometrial pattern does not correlate with any date of

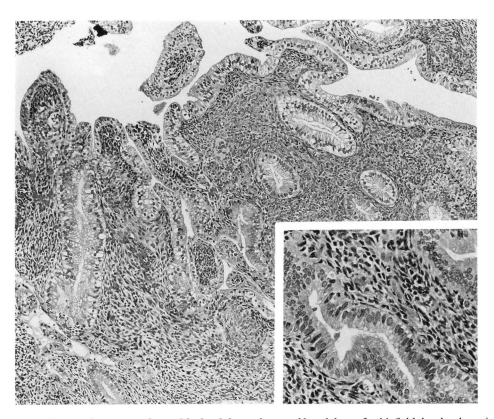

FIGURE 5.16. Abnormal secretory phase with glandular and stromal breakdown. In this field the glands are intact. The stroma shows evidence of breakdown with early collapse. *Inset*: the glands are tortuous with vacuolated cytoplasm and basally oriented nuclei corresponding to secretory day 18–19.

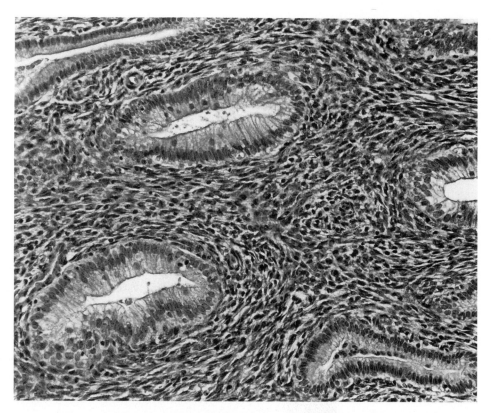

FIGURE 5.17. Abnormal secretory phase. The glands show secretory changes with basal nuclei and vacuolated cytoplasm but are small and tubular rather than tortuous. The stroma is dense. Other areas in the section showed glandular and stromal breakdown.

the normal luteal phase. The glands may show secretory changes yet lack marked tortuosity and secretory exhaustion, while the stroma lacks extensive predecidual change (Figs. 5.16 and 5.17). In other cases the glands appear to show a "hypersecretory" pattern, with vacuolated cytoplasm, marked tortuosity, and luminal secretion, while the stroma lacks predecidual change. In addition, the tissue shows foci of breakdown with characteristic changes such as nuclear dust, fibrin thrombi, and dense cell clusters, similar to that which occurs in the proliferative endometrium with glandular and stromal breakdown (Figs. 5.1–5.3). Often in abnormal secretory bleeding patterns, the glands show stellate shapes as they involute (Fig. 5.18). This latter pattern of collapsing, star-shaped secretory glands is nonspecific, however, and simply shows secretory gland regression that could be due to a variety of factors.

These changes may reflect DUB due to luteal phase abnormalities that include luteal phase defect (LPD) and irregular shedding. The etiology and frequency of dysfunctional bleeding due to luteal phase abnormalities are not known, however, since these disorders appear to be sporadic and do not persist long enough to permit clinicopathologic correlations. Alterations in the morphology of the endometrium due to changes in the absolute or relative levels of estrogen and progesterone have been well established in experimental systems,[25] so it is likely that abnormal secretory bleeding patterns are, at least in part, due to ovulatory abnormalities that involve the luteal phase. Nonetheless, the secretory patterns with nonmenstrual bleeding are not well characterized. Consequently, when a pattern of nonmenstrual phase secretory endometrium with breakdown is present, the abnormality may be due to defined or undefined luteal phase abnor-

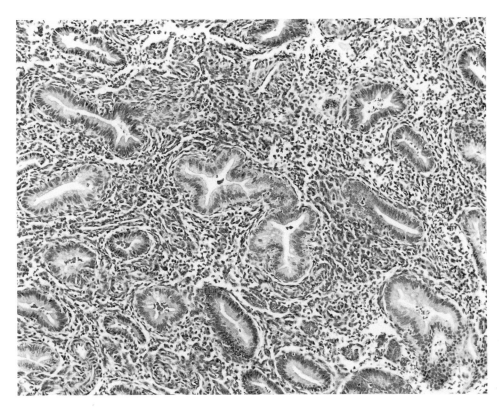

FIGURE 5.18. Abnormal secretory phase with glandular and stromal breakdown. Early collapse of endometrium with a poorly developed secretory phase pattern shows involuting, star-shaped glands. This pattern of gland involution is often seen focally in secretory phase endometrium that is undergoing nonmenstrual glandular and stromal breakdown.

malities or other causes that are not evident from the sections.

Luteal Phase Defect

Of the two defined luteal phase abnormalities that may cause abnormal bleeding, LPD probably occurs more frequently. As discussed in Chapter 2, in LPD the corpus luteum is "insufficient," either regressing prematurely or failing to produce an adequate amount of progesterone to sustain normal secretory phase development. This is a sporadic disorder of the reproductive and perimenopausal years. With LPD, ovulation occurs, so secretory changes develop. If abnormal bleeding is the result, the appearance is that of breakdown and bleeding in a nonmenstrual secretory phase pattern. The pattern is characterized by glands with secretory changes, including basally ori-ented nuclei and vacuolated cytoplasm, but lacking the tortuosity of late secretory phase glands. Focal breakdown is present with "stromal blue balls" and karyorrhectic debris. This pattern is nonspecific and may be due to other factors discussed below.

Irregular Shedding

Irregular shedding is attributed to a persistent corpus luteum with prolonged progesterone production.[12,20,22,23] This is the least studied and consequently the most poorly understood form of dysfunctional pattern. Some authors have used this term to refer to irregular secretory phase bleeding due to a variety of causes, including early pregnancy, inflammation, and exogenous hormone effects, but we prefer to restrict this term to bleeding due to true ovulatory dysfunc-

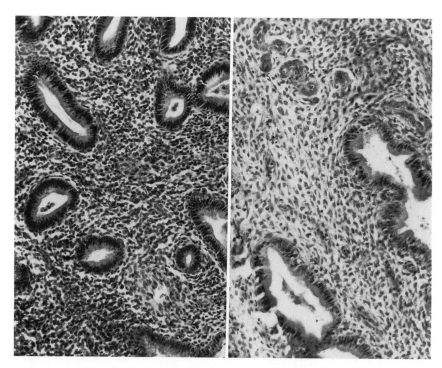

FIGURE 5.19. Irregular shedding with mixed phase pattern. Two fields from the same sample show a mixed phase pattern with proliferative (*left*) and secretory (*right*) changes. This mixed phase pattern may be due to a persistent corpus luteum, but the etiology cannot be determined by morphology alone, and clinical correlation is required.

tion. One pattern of irregular shedding yields a mixed phase pattern composed of secretory and proliferative endometrium (Fig. 5.19). The diagnosis is reserved for those specimens in which there is a mixed pattern of secretory and proliferative glands at least 5 days after the onset of bleeding. Irregular shedding is also manifested by irregular secretory phase development in which different foci show more than 4 day difference in the morphologic date. Focal breakdown and bleeding with glandular and stromal collapse is present, usually focally, but occasionally in a diffuse pattern. Although the frequency of irregular shedding as a cause of DUB is not known, it is an unusual event in our experience.

Abnormal Secretory Endometrium with Breakdown of Unknown Etiology

Some examples of secretory endometrium with abnormal, nonmenstrual bleeding patterns presumably reflect the specific luteal phase abnormalities described above. A variety of other fac-

tors may also be associated with a pattern of aberrant secretory phase development with superimposed bleeding (Table 5.2). For example, endometrial changes associated with abortions or ectopic pregnancies, response to exogenous progestins, tissue near a polyp, endometrium overlying leiomyomas, and endometrium involved with inflammation or adhesions all can show patterns of abnormal secretory development and bleeding. Other poorly understood ovarian disorders, such as a luteinized unrup-

TABLE 5.2. Possible causes of nonmenstrual secretory phase bleeding.

Luteal phase defects
Persistent corpus luteum (irregular shedding)
Organic lesions
Submucosal leiomyomas
Intrauterine adhesions
Inflammation
Complications of pregnancy[a]
Progestin effects

[a] See Chapter 3, Table 3.1.

tured follicle, presumably can result in abnormal secretory endometrial changes. With this latter entity, developing follicles are believed to undergo luteinization of the granulosa and theca cells with progesterone production in the absence of ovulation. In addition to these considerations, management of DUB often involves progestational therapy. If bleeding is not controlled, a curettage is performed. Accordingly, the histology may be complicated by progestin effects superimposed on the underlying abnormality.

These patterns show glands with secretory changes such as basally oriented nuclei and diffuse cytoplasmic vacuolization and absence of mitotic activity (Figs. 5.16–5.18). The glands may be tortuous. Often the stroma is dense, lacking edema or predecidua. The endometrium in such cases cannot be assigned to any histologic day of the normal secretory phase of the menstrual cycle. The changes of glandular and stromal breakdown are similar to those found in any bleeding phase endometrium with glandular and stromal collapse, " stromal blue balls," and eosinophilic syncytial change. With early breakdown, tortuous secretory glands often show star-shaped outlines (Fig. 5.18).

There are no clear-cut clinical correlations for many abnormal secretory phase patterns with breakdown, so the alterations at times defy precise pathologic diagnosis. Nonetheless, recognition of the general category of abnormal secretory bleeding patterns helps to exclude other specific organic lesions and suggests the possibility of a luteal phase dysfunctional abnormality if no other pathologic condition is clinically manifest.

Clinical Queries and Reporting

When a biopsy is done for DUB, the report should address the presence or absence of morphologic changes of breakdown and bleeding as well as any specific lesions. If the pattern is that of proliferative endometrium with breakdown and if the clinical history is appropriate, the changes can accurately be attributed to anovulatory cycles. A descriptive diagnosis such as "proliferative endometrium with glandular and stromal breakdown" offers a precise morphologic interpretation of the

anovulatory bleeding pattern that often is sufficient for clinical management. An additional comment indicating that the change is compatible with anovulatory cycles helps to clarify the diagnosis. If the changes show nonmenstrual secretory endometrium with breakdown but these are not diagnostic of a defined luteal phase abnormality, descriptive terms such as "abnormal secretory phase pattern with breakdown" communicate the observation of an abnormal yet benign appearance while not assigning definite morphologic etiology. In general, a comment regarding the absence of other possible causes of bleeding, such as hyperplasia, inflammation, pregnancy, or polyps, is useful in addressing specific clinical concerns.

Since atrophy is one of the most frequent causes of abnormal bleeding in postmenopausal patients, it is important to recognize the morphologic features of atrophy and correctly report the findings. A scant amount of endometrium consisting of detached strips of atrophic endometrial epithelium with little stroma should be regarded as consistent with atrophy and not "insufficient for diagnosis." A brief comment or description of the findings helps the clinician understand the basis of the diagnosis while giving reassurance that the endometrium has, in fact, been sampled.

Occasional biopsies show extensive breakdown and bleeding that largely obscures the cytologic details of the glands and stroma. Although it is usually possible to exclude neoplastic processes in such cases, detailed assessment of the endometrium to determine the underlying pathologic process becomes difficult. Unless the breakdown is clearly menstrual, i.e., reflecting the shedding at the end of a normal ovulatory cycle, breakdown patterns should not be diagnosed as "menstrual." Instead, it is better to use descriptive diagnoses that reflect the morphologic changes. On rare occasions endometrial biopsy in a postmenopausal patient may show only evidence of abnormal bleeding such as foam cells. In such cases the subtle evidence of abnormal bleeding should be recognized and reported; further sampling may be needed to determine the cause, since endometrial carcinoma becomes a more likely cause of abnormal bleeding in this age group.

It is imperative that the terms used in descriptive pathologic diagnoses be clearly understood by the clinician. The terms employed can be self-explanatory, especially when a brief microscopic description accompanies the report to clarify the histologic finding and to exclude more specific organic lesions. The diagnosis of "proliferative endometrium with glandular and stromal breakdown" is an example of a clinically relevant term that can be applied to apparent anovulatory bleeding. Diagnoses such as "disordered proliferative phase pattern" or "persistent proliferative phase" applied to the proliferative endometrium of anovulatory cycles are most useful when there is a clear understanding of the microscopic findings and the physiologic and clinical significance of the pattern. Therefore an explanatory note added to the diagnosis is helpful to describe the changes and indicate that the lesion lacks atypia or clear-cut criteria for hyperplasia. The terms "withdrawal" and "breakthrough" should be avoided in pathologic diagnoses because they lack clear definitions in the clinical literature regarding endometrial bleeding.

References

1. Speroff L, Glass RH, Kase NG: Clinical Gynecologic Endocrinology and Infertility. 4th ed. Baltimore: Williams & Wilkins, 1989.

2. Bayer SR, DeCherney AH: Clinical manifestations and treatment of dysfunctional uterine bleeding. JAMA 1993;269:1823–1828.

3. Galle PC, McRae MA: Abnormal uterine bleeding. Finding and treating the cause. Postgrad Med 1993;93:73–81.

4. Mishell DR, Jr: Abnormal uterine bleeding. In: Comprehensive Gynecology. Herbst AL, Mishell DR, Jr, Stenchever MA, Droegemueller W, eds. St. Louis: Mosby-Year Book, 1992;1079–1099.

5. Picoff RC, Luginbuhl WH: Fibrin in the endometrial stroma: Its relation to uterine bleeding. Am J Obstet Gynecol 1964;88:642–646.

6. Clement PB: Pathology of the uterine corpus. Hum Pathol 1991;22:776–791.

7. Zaman SS, Mazur MT: Endometrial papillary syncytial change. A nonspecific alteration associated with active breakdown. Am J Clin Pathol 1993; 99:741–745.

8. Silverberg SG, Kurman RJ: Tumors of the uterine corpus and gestational trophoblastic disease. Atlas of Tumor Pathology, 3rd series, Fascicle 3. Washington, DC: Armed Forces Institute of Pathology, 1992.

9. Reeves G, Sommers SC: Endometrial hemosiderin as evidence of metrorrhagia. Obstet Gynecol 1962;19:790–792.

10. Fechner RE, Bossart MI, Spjut HJ: Ultrastructure of endometrial stromal foam cells. Am J Clin Pathol 1979;72:628–633.

11. Altchek A: Dysfunctional uterine bleeding in adolescence. Clin Obstet Gynecol 1977;20:633–650.

12. Scommegna A, Dmowski WP: Dysfunctional uterine bleeding. Clin Obstet Gynecol 1973;16:221–254.

13. Aksel S, Jones GS: Etiology and treatment of dysfunctional uterine bleeding. J Obstet Gynecol 1974;44:1–13.

14. Rubin SC: Postmenopausal bleeding: Etiology, evaluation, and management. Med Clin N Am 1987;71:59–69.

15. Schindler AE, Schmidt G: Post-menopausal bleeding: A study of more than 1000 cases. Maturitas 1980;2:269–274.

16. Choo YC, Mak KC, Hsu C, Wong TS, Ma HK: Postmenopausal uterine bleeding of nonorganic cause. Obstet Gynecol 1985;66:225–228.

17. Meyer WC, Malkasian GD, Dockery MB, Decker DG: Postmenopausal bleeding from atrophic endometrium. Obstet Gynecol 1971; 38:731–738.

18. Gambrell RD: Postmenopausal bleeding. J Am Geriatr Soc 1974;22:337–343.

19. Lidor A, Ismajovich B, Confino E, David MP: Histopathological findings in 226 women with post-menopausal uterine bleeding. Acta Obstet Gynecol Scand 1983;65:41–43.

20. Kurman RJ, Mazur MT: Benign diseases of the endometrium. In: Blaustein's Pathology of the Female Genital Tract. 4th ed. Kurman RJ, ed. New York: Springer-Verlag, 1994;367–409.

21. Dallenbach-Hellweg G: The endometrium of infertility. A review. Pathol Res Pract 1984; 78:527–537.

22. Dallenbach-Hellweg G: Histopathology of the Endometrium. 4th ed. New York: Springer-Verlag, 1987.

23. Hendrickson MR, Kempson RL: Surgical Pathology of the Uterine Corpus (Major Problems in Pathology Series). Volume 12. Philadelphia: W.B. Saunders, 1980.

24. Buckley CH, Fox H: Biopsy Pathology of the Endometrium. New York: Raven Press, 1989;234–247.

25. Good RG, Moyer DL: Estrogen-progesterone relationships in the development of secretory endometrium. Fertil Steril 1968;19:37–45.

6
Effects of Hormones

Women receive hormone preparations for a variety of reasons, including birth control, dysfunctional uterine bleeding, perimenopausal and postmenopausal symptoms, endometriosis, endometrial hyperplasia and carcinoma, breast carcinoma, and certain types of infertility. Usually the exogenous hormone is some form of progestin, but estrogenic and even androgenic hormones are used for some disorders. The endometrium shows the effects of these hormones.

An endometrial biopsy or curettage may be done when abnormal bleeding occurs or when hormone therapy does not correct abnormal bleeding that is thought to be dysfunctional. Sometimes, however, the biopsy is intended to evaluate the status of the endometrium following hormonal therapy, as in the case of hyperplasia managed with progestin therapy or routine follow-up of patients on hormone replacement therapy. In other circumstances the endometrial sampling is coincidental with another procedure, such as tubal ligation. The hormone, the dosage, and the duration of therapy influence the appearance of the endometrium in biopsy specimens. Clinical information regarding hormone use helps in the pathologic interpretation, but this history sometimes is incomplete when the specimen comes to the pathology laboratory. Consequently, the possibility of exogenous hormonal effects should always be kept in mind.

This chapter reviews the different types of hormones affecting the endometrium: 1) hormones used in reproductive-age women that clearly have estrogenic or progestogenic effects, such as oral contraceptives; 2) estrogen–progestin hormone replacement therapy in postmenopausal women; and 3) other hormones with less well-established effects on the endometrium.

Estrogenic Hormones

Estrogen therapy is largely used in perimenopausal or postmenopausal women to treat symptoms of the menopause, such as vasomotor instability, atrophic vaginitis, and osteoporosis.[1,2]

Postmenopausal estrogen replacement also significantly reduces morbidity and mortality from cardiovascular disease.[3] Estrogenic substances include conjugated estrogens, such as Premarin (Wyeth-Ayerst Laboratories, Philadelphia, PA), and other synthetic estrogens, such as ethinyl estradiol or diethylstilbestrol (DES). Use of estrogenic hormones by themselves is associated with an increased risk of developing endometrial adenocarcinoma in some studies, however, so the use of these hormones without a progestin is now unusual in patients with a uterus. Consequently, the effects of unopposed exogenous estrogen in biopsy specimens are seen less frequently than the effects of combined estrogen–progestin compounds. Nonetheless, some patients do receive estrogen replacement only.

Unopposed use of estrogenic hormones causes the endometrium to grow and proliferate. The result is variable, depending on the dose and duration of use. Often the pattern is that of proliferative phase endometrium, showing tubular to tortuous glands and abundant stroma. The patterns can be identical to those seen with anovulatory cycles and may have superimposed breakdown and bleeding. Continued, prolonged estrogenic stimulation can lead to disordered proliferative phase patterns and hyperplasia. Estrogen-related epithelial cytoplasmic changes, especially squamous differentiation and ciliated cell change, also often occur.

In some patients continued estrogen use leads to atypical hyperplasia and adenocarcinoma.[3,4] The risk of malignancy increases with the duration of therapy. Usually unopposed estrogen use for at least 2 to 3 years is found in patients who develop adenocarcinoma, and the highest risk is in patients who have taken estrogens for 10 or more years. The duration of therapy generally is more important than the dose of the estrogen. When carcinoma develops, it usually is low grade and superficially invasive, but high-grade lesions may occur.

All of the estrogen-related changes are reviewed elsewhere in the text, including normal proliferative phase patterns (Chapter 2), proliferative with glandular and stromal breakdown (Chapter 5), hyperplasia and cytoplasmic change (Chapter 8), and carcinoma (Chapter 9). The reader should refer to those chapters for detailed morphologic descriptions of the specific entities.

Progestins and Oral Contraceptives

Although progestin effects are common, the subject of progestin-related changes is complex. Various forms of these synthetic analogues of progesterone, also termed "progestogens" or "progestagens," are widely used, either alone or in combination with an estrogen. Progestin-only therapy is useful in the empirical medical management of abnormal uterine bleeding that clinically appears to be dysfunctional. These hormones, such as medroxyprogesterone acetate or norethindrone acetate (Table 6.1), suppress ovulation and endometrial growth. They also lead to secretory maturation and progesterone withdrawal bleeding, effecting a medical curettage. Consequently, progestins are especially helpful in managing ovulatory disorders where irregular, noncyclical endometrial growth results in abnormal bleeding. Often a trial of progestin is given in an attempt to alleviate apparent dysfunctional bleeding, and if the bleeding does not resolve, biopsy or curettage follows to exclude other organic pathology. Other progestins, such as oral or injectable medroxyprogesterone acetate, are used to treat neoplasia of the breast or endometrium. Still others, such as norgestrel, are used for contraception. Progestins, especially oral contraceptives, also are used to treat endometriosis.

Progestins, usually given in combination with estrogens, are the basis for the oral contraceptive

TABLE 6.1. Product trade name and generic name of commonly prescribed progestins.

Product name	Generic name
Agestin (Wyeth-Ayerst Laboratories, Philadelphia, PA)	Norethindrone acetate
Depo-Provera (Upjohn, Kalamazoo, MI)	Medroxyprogesterone acetate
Norlutate (Parke-Davis, Morris Plains, NJ)	Norethindrone acetate
Norlutin (Parke-Davis)	Norethindrone
Megace (Bristol-Myers Oncology, Evansville, IN)	Megestrol acetate
Micronor (Ortho Pharmaceutical Corp., Raritan, NJ)	Norethindrone
Ovrette (Wyeth-Ayerst)	Norgestrel
Provera (Upjohn)	Medroxyprogesterone acetate

or "birth control pill." Most of the oral contraceptives are used in a fixed-dose formulation, with small doses of both the estrogen and the progestin daily. Some oral contraceptives use a "phasic" combination with increasing amounts of progestin over a 21-day medication period. In either case the combination estrogen and progestin is administered over 3 weeks, and no medication is given in the 4th week to allow withdrawal bleeding to occur. Some oral contraceptives contain only progestin. The dose of progestin and estrogen used in modern oral contraceptives is much lower than that used in the initial formulations of oral contraceptives 20 to 30 years ago. Consequently, the pharmacologic effects of these steroid contraceptives are somewhat different from those originally described.

The morphologic appearance of the endometrium following progestin therapy is variable and depends on the underlying status of the endometrium as well as the dose and duration of progestin therapy.[4–10,10a] Progestin effects also can persist for several weeks to months following cessation of their use. To help simplify this complex subject, the effects of the progestins can be placed into three general morphologic patterns that form the basis for understanding the entire spectrum of progestin-mediated changes. These patterns include: 1) decidual (pregnancy-like) changes, 2) secretory changes, and 3) atrophic changes (Table 6.2). The pattern encountered depends on the degree of estrogen "priming" of the endometrium and the dose and duration of administration of the progestin. In reality, there often is

TABLE 6.2. Morphologic features of progestin effects.

Decidual (pregnancy-like) effects
   Abundant tissue, often polypoid
   Glands show marked secretory activity
   Stroma appears decidualized with lymphoid infiltrate
   Vascular ectasia
Secretory effects
   Moderate to sparse amount of tissue
   Mildly tortuous secretory glands lined by columnar cells
   Stromal cells plump, oval
   Vascular ectasia
Atrophic effects
   Sparse tissue
   Glands small and atrophic, not coiled
   Variable amount of stroma with plump to spindle-shaped
      cells

overlap between the various patterns of progestin effect in the endometrium.

Decidual Pattern

The decidual or pregnancy-like pattern, as the term implies, features differentiation of endometrial glands and stroma to a point where they resemble the endometrium in pregnancy with decidual transformation of the stroma. Although the term "decidua" applies most strictly to the endometrium of pregnancy, this term also is useful for describing this progestin-induced pattern. This exaggerated effect typically occurs in endometrium that is influenced by high estrogen levels and therefore is actively growing and proliferating. This morphology is most common following high-dose progestin therapy for anovulatory cycles or for hyperplasia. In these cases the amount of tissue can be copious, and the biopsy or curettage can yield large polypoid tissue fragments (Fig. 6.1). Although the tissue is polypoid, these do not represent true polyps. With marked progestin effect, the stromal cells become enlarged and show abundant cytoplasm and prominent cell borders, resembling the decidua of pregnancy. The stroma can show occasional mitotic figures. In this form of marked progestin effect, the glands develop a hypersecretory pattern with vacuolated cytoplasm and abundant luminal secretions. Some glands are dilated. The Arias-Stella reaction with nuclear enlargement and hyperchromasia may occur in glands, but this is very rare. The spiral arteries also can show marked thickening. The venules in the superficial portion of the endometrium become ectatic (Fig. 6.2). Occasional cases of decidua-like progestin effect show prominent squamous change (metaplasia) within glands. This change is usually seen in cases where the biopsy that led to therapy demonstrates hyperplasia, often with no squamous differentiation.[9]

Cases with advanced decidual changes often show areas of breakdown and bleeding, especially as the dilated venules thrombose (Fig. 6.3). As a result, many of the features of breakdown and bleeding described in Chapter 5 are superimposed on the progestin effect. With breakdown, the collapse of the stroma and glands significantly alters their appearance, partially masking the patterns of development. In these areas of break-

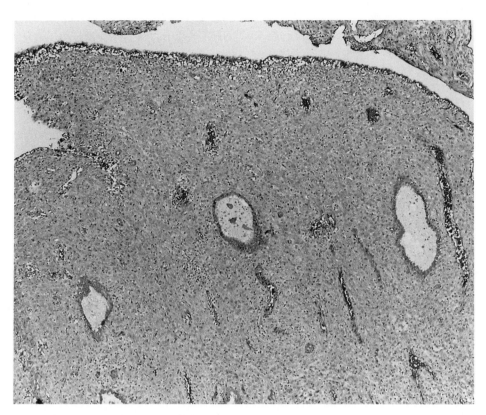

Figure 6.1. Progestin effect, decidua pattern. Marked decidual reaction following progestin therapy of anovulatory bleeding. The changes resemble the endometrial decidual transformation in pregnancy. Glands with secretory exhaustion are surrounded by abundant decidualized stroma. Small ectatic vessels are present in the superficial portions of the endometrium.

down, the decidua-like character of the stromal cells is lost as the cells degenerate and lose cytoplasm. The glands fragment and become haphazardly oriented. Consequently, it remains important to avoid areas of active bleeding and find intact tissue in order to accurately assess the changes associated with progestin effect.

Secretory Pattern

The secretory pattern of progestin effect mimics the glandular and stromal changes seen in the luteal (secretory) phase of the menstrual cycle. This pattern is closely related to the pregnancy-like changes described above, but neither the glands nor the stroma show such an exaggerated response. With the secretory pattern, the glands are tortuous and the glandular cells have basally oriented nuclei (Figs. 6.4 and 6.5). These low columnar cells typically have a small amount of pale-staining supranuclear cytoplasm. The stromal cells show predecidual change as they gain cytoplasm and become mildly enlarged. Although the glandular and stromal changes superficially resemble the secretory phase endometrium of a menstrual cycle, neither the glands nor the stroma are appropriately developed for any day of the normal cycle (Fig. 6.6). Usually the glands appear to be underdeveloped, lacking tortuosity. Stromal predecidual change tends to be confluent, lacking the intermittent edema that characterizes most of the normal secretory phase. Scattered mitotic figures can be found in the stroma. As with other progestin-related patterns, the superficial stroma contains ectatic venules.

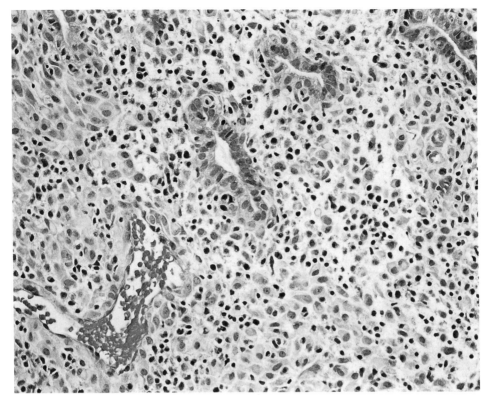

Figure 6.2. Progestin effect, decidua pattern. Marked decidual change in the stroma and small inactive glands lined by a single layer of epithelium characterize the decidual pattern of progestin effect. An ectatic venule is present in the lower left part of the field.

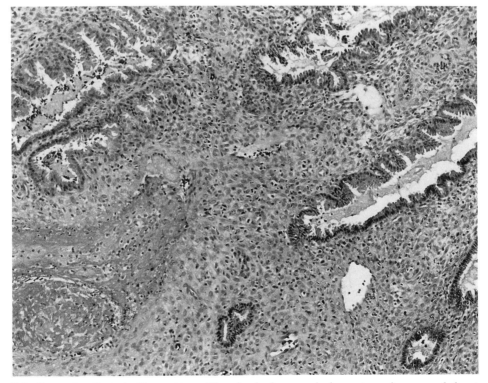

Figure 6.3. Progestin effect, decidua pattern. The glands show marked secretory changes and the stroma is transformed into decidua-like cells. A fibrin thrombus fills a dilated venule in the left lower corner. Thrombi such as this result in bleeding that frequently leads to biopsy.

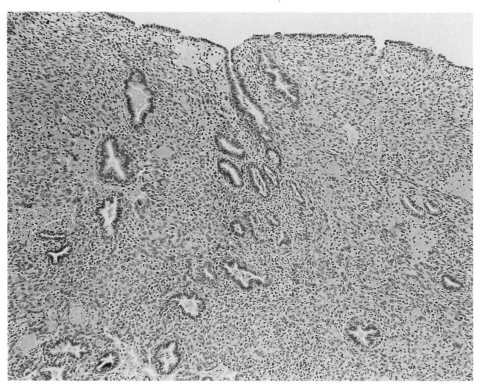

Figure 6.4. Progestin effect, secretory pattern. The endometrium has some resemblance to secretory endometrium of the normal luteal phase with tortuous glands and abundant, predecidualized stroma. The amount of stroma is increased relative to the normal secretory phase and lacks edema. The glands, while slightly tortuous, are markedly underdeveloped relative to glands in the normal luteal phase.

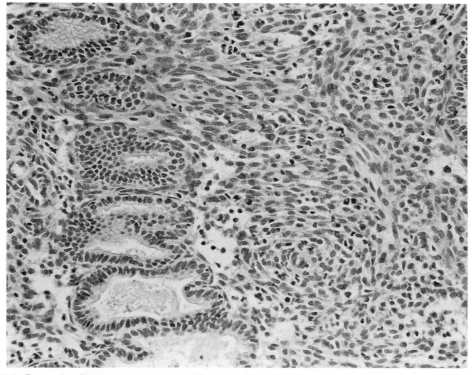

Figure 6.5. Progestin effect, secretory pattern. High magnification of pattern resembling secretory phase endometrium shows a tortuous gland with secretions. The stromal cells are plump, having a moderate amount of cytoplasm.

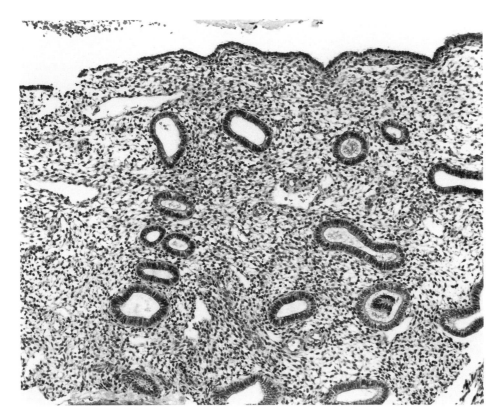

Figure 6.6. Progestin effect, secretory pattern. Under-developed secretory glands in abundant stroma that does not show decidual change. Several ectatic venules are present in the superficial stroma. Neither the glands nor the stroma are appropriately developed for a normal postovulatory secretory phase. This patient was taking oral contraceptives.

Atrophic Pattern

The atrophic pattern represents the other end of the spectrum of progestin effect, in which the endometrium is hypoplastic. This pattern evolves following prolonged progestin therapy or with continued use of contraceptive hormones. The glands atrophy, although they continue to show weak secretory changes. The glands lose their tortuosity and are small and tubular with scant to absent luminal secretions (Fig. 6.7). The epithelium is low columnar with basal nuclei and a small amount of pale cytoplasm.

When the progestin dose is low, the stromal cells remain enlarged but lose their decidua-like appearance. Instead, they are plump and ovoid with only a moderate amount of cytoplasm. Cell borders become indistinct, and stromal mitoses are not found. Vascular channels beneath the surface epithelium become ectatic. In contrast to the physiologic atrophy pattern of the postmenopausal endometrium, progestin-induced atrophy often has more abundant stroma while the glands become tiny and indistinct.

Other Stromal Changes

Whereas the glands atrophy with prolonged progestin effect, with high doses of progestin the stroma retains a decidua-like appearance. In such cases the stroma can show alterations that can be confusing or alarming. For instance, the stroma can appear hyperplastic and pseudosarcomatous with increased cellularity as well as nuclear hyperchromasia, enlarged nucleoli, and variation in cell and nuclear size.[11,12] This pseudosarcomatous change is rare with modern progestin therapy, however, and is infrequent in our

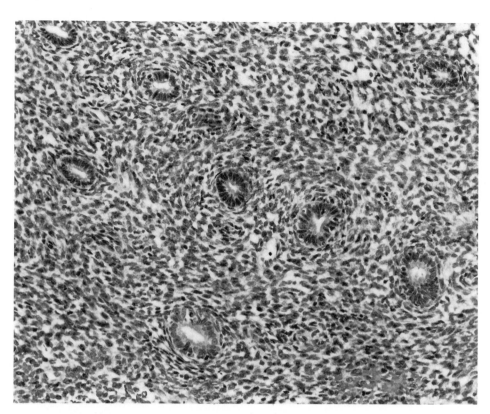

Figure 6.7. Progestin effect, atrophic pattern. Small atrophic glands in spindle-cell stroma show scant secretory changes. The abundant stroma composed of plump cells with a moderate amount of cytoplasm dis- tinguishes this pattern from atrophy due to lack of estrogen. This pattern is commonly seen in women on continous oral contraceptives.

experience. The stroma can show other peculiar alterations. One change occasionally seen is clustering of groups of enlarged stromal cells with intervening areas of myxoid change or edema (Fig. 6.8). This change can impart an epithelioid appearance to some of the decidualized cells, especially when the cells are enlarged with prominent cell borders. The decidualized stromal cells can develop other epithelioid features such as eccentric nuclei and vacuolated cytoplasm (Fig. 6.9).[13,13a] In such cases the decidualized stroma can mimic signet-ring cells of metastatic carcinoma.

In some cases of progestin effect, infiltrates of lymphocytes or neutrophils yield patterns that can suggest endometritis. For instance, with prolonged progestin effect the stroma often contains a moderate infiltrate of stromal granular lymphocytes and mononuclear cells (Fig. 6.10). These are the normal lymphoid cells of the endometrium that appear exaggerated due to the relative atrophy of the other components. This striking infiltrate can mimic chronic inflammation. An absence of plasma cells and no evidence of gland infiltration by inflammatory cells are helpful features to separate this progestin effect from true inflammation (Chapter 7). Also, especially in pregnancy-like patterns of progestin effect, multiple small foci of breakdown are accompanied by a neutrophilic response. These neutrophils, however, are a localized response to tissue necrosis and do not represent an infectious process.

Often there is overlap between the various patterns of progestin effect that depend on the duration of progestin use, the dose of the progestin, and underlying endogenous estrogen levels. In some cases different fields from the same specimen show different patterns of progestin effect that can range from decidualized stroma to a secretory or atrophic change. Consequently, mor-

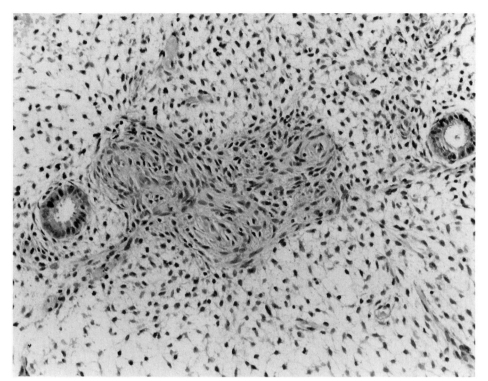

Figure 6.8. Progestin effect, atrophic pattern. An aggregate of tightly packed, plump stromal cells in an edematous, myxoid background. Clustering of stromal cells such as this is occasionally seen with progestin effect. The two glands present are atrophic. The patient was on long-term oral contraceptives.

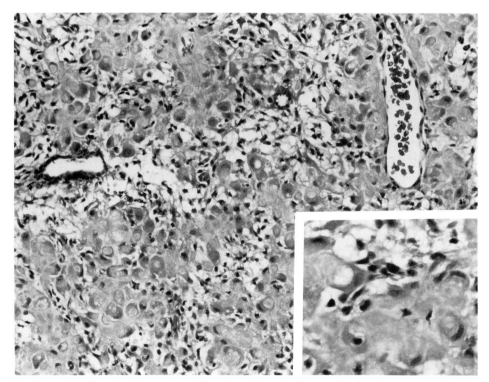

Figure 6.9. Progestin effect, decidua pattern. The decidual cells have vacuolated cytoplasm and eccentric nuclei resulting in a signet-ring cell appearance (*inset*). The cells are clustered with intervening myxoid zones. A markedly atrophic gland is present to the left of center and a dilated venule is seen to the right. The patient was on high-dose megestrol acetate for breast cancer.

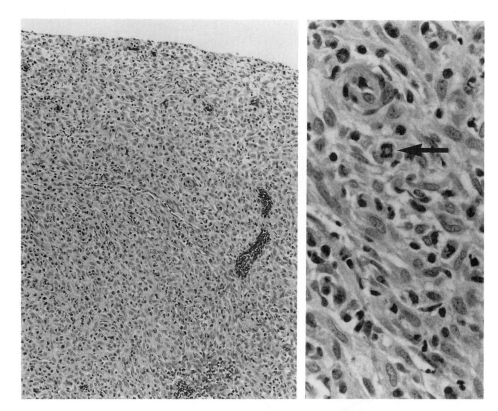

Figure 6.10. Progestin effect, decidua pattern. *Left:* Abundant stroma containing a rich infiltrate of stromal granular lymphocytes mimicking chronic inflammation. No glands are present in this field. *Right:* High magnification shows decidualized stroma and numerous granular lymphocytes but no plasma cells. A stromal mitosis (*arrow*) is present.

phologic identification of progestin effects requires recognition of the spectrum of changes that may be found. Furthermore, some patients on progestins, especially those on oral contraceptives, can even show proliferative phase patterns when the estrogenic influence is present but the progestin influence is temporarily decreased or absent. Long-term use of oral contraceptives rarely may result in permanent endometrial atrophy after the agent is discontinued.[14]

Combined Estrogen and Progestin As Replacement Therapy for Menopausal Women

Because of the possible deleterious consequences of unopposed estrogen therapy on the endometrium, estrogen replacement is nearly always given with a progestin in perimenopausal and postmenopausal patients with a uterus. Combined estrogen–progestin hormonal replacement can be given either sequentially or in combination.[15,16] Sequential medication uses daily estrogen for the first 21 to 25 days of the month and daily progestin added for the last 10 to 13 days. This regimen results in withdrawal bleeding. The continuous regimen uses both estrogen and progestin daily. Breakthrough bleeding may occur during the first 6 months with the continuous regimen, but then bleeding usually stops. Patients receiving either the sequential or the combined regimen may undergo biopsy as part of the routine surveillance to ensure that no neoplasm develops.

With the sequential estrogen–progestin regimen, the endometrium often shows a weakly proliferative pattern with small, tubular glands in scant stroma. The epithelium can have occasional mitotic figures. The pattern is identical to the weakly proliferative phase pattern seen in association with anovulatory dysfunctional bleeding due to estrogen withdrawal (Chapter 5). Sometimes the tissue shows a superimposed progestin effect with poorly developed secretory changes in the glands (Fig. 6.11).[17] This latter pattern of secretory changes is especially likely to be seen if the biopsy is taken during the period of progestin administration. In these cases the glandular cells show mild tortuosity, basal nuclei, some cytoplasmic vacuoles, and scant luminal secretions. In biopsy material, focal glandular and stromal breakdown also may be seen (Fig. 6.12). With the combination regimens, the endometrium usually is atrophic,[9,18,19] and often an atrophic pattern is seen with sequential therapy, too.[17] Secretory changes can be seen, however, especially if higher doses of estrogen and progestin are used.[10a] Occasionally a patient receiving either the sequential or the combination regimen

may have a more significant lesion in the biopsy specimen. Polyps, hyperplasia, and carcinoma are lesions that have been found in a few cases. In general, however, estrogen–progestin replacement therapy controls endometrial growth, and significant organic lesions are less common than in women not receiving this therapy.

Progestin-Like Effects with No Hormone Use

On rare occasions endometrial tissue will show morphologic features of a progestin effect even though there is clearly no history of exogenous hormone use. These changes may be seen in both premenopausal and postmenopausal women, and their etiology is poorly understood. In premenopausal women these patterns can be decidua-like[20] or can resemble "pill effect" changes,

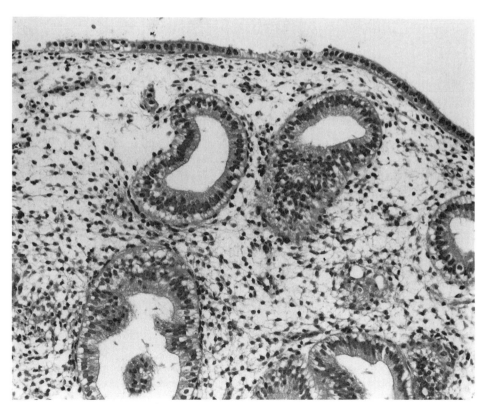

Figure 6.11. Estrogen–progestin therapy. Endometrium from a postmenopausal woman receiving estrogen–progestin replacement therapy shows small secretory glands with extensive subnuclear vacuoles. This progestin effect resembles days 16–17 of the secretory phase of the normal cycle.

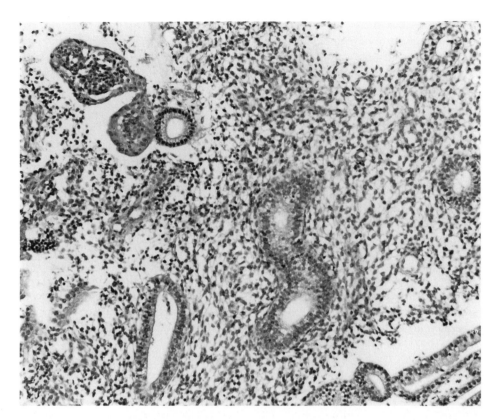

Figure 6.12. Estrogen–progestin therapy. Fragmented endometrial sample from a postmenopausal woman on estrogen–progestin replacement therapy. Small glands show secretory changes with vacuolated cytoplasm and basally oriented nuclei. Focal glandular and stromal breakdown is seen in the left upper corner.

with hypoplastic secretory glands and plump stromal cells (Fig. 6.13). It is possible that this alteration is due either to abnormal persistence of a functioning corpus luteum or to the so-called luteinized unruptured follicle. This latter entity, as the name implies, occurs when a follicle develops, does not rupture (ovulate), and persists with luteinization of the granulosa and theca cells. If progesterone is produced by the unruptured follicle, then the result could be a progestin effect from the endogenous source.

There have been a few examples of idiopathic endometrial decidual reaction in postmenopausal women who are not on hormones (Fig. 6.14).[13] These patients have tended to present with abundant polypoid tissue. The etiology of the change is not known, but it may be due to local mechanical factors rather than a response to progesterone-like hormones. Mechanical stimulation, including biopsy, can cause increased decidual changes

in the progesterone-primed endometrium.[6,21] Also, an intrauterine device (IUD) may lead to an enhanced decidual reaction in the endometrium.[6,22,23]

Effects of Other Hormones

Tamoxifen

Tamoxifen is a nonsteroidal antiestrogen that is widely used in the hormonal therapy of breast carcinoma. The effect of tamoxifen on the endometrium is not completely understood, however, and appears to depend on the menopausal status and the dose and duration of tamoxifen use. Current data suggest it can act as both an estrogen antagonist and an agonist. Most normally cycling premenopausal patients taking tamoxifen continue to have regular menstrual cycles, but some develop amenorrhea. With use, serum estrogen

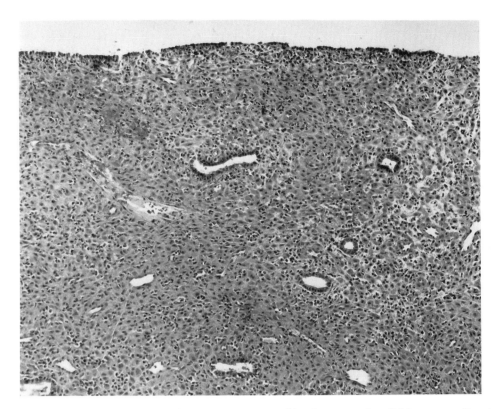

Figure 6.13. Progestin-like effect with no hormone use. Endometrium from premenopausal woman shows small, atrophic glands in abundant predecidualized stroma resembling progestin effect. This patient was not taking hormones but did have a small, palpable ovarian cyst that may have been a source of endogenous progesterone production, such as a persistent corpus luteum or a luteinized unruptured follicle.

and progesterone levels often are increased to two or three times the normal levels. In postmenopausal women, tamoxifen has estrogenic effects on vaginal epithelium.

There are a few examples of endometrial hyperplasia and carcinoma occurring in patients on tamoxifen, and some studies suggest an increased incidence of endometrial carcinoma in patients receiving tamoxifen.[24–29a] The relative risk of developing endometrial carcinoma appears to be within the same range as reported with unopposed estrogen use.[24] The apparent increase may be due to increased rate of detection of otherwise asymptomatic, "silent" tumors, however. Some patients receiving tamoxifen develop high-grade carcinomas, but in general those carcinomas associated with tamoxifen use do not differ in grade from carcinomas that occur in patients not receiving this hormone.[26,29a]

Endometrial polyps also may arise in patients on tamoxifen.[30–33] These patients are postmenopausal and have received long-term tamoxifen therapy for metastatic breast carcinoma. In our experience, most of these polyps show mildly hyperplastic changes and resemble hyperplastic polyps seen in patients who are not on hormone therapy (Fig. 6.15) (Chapter 8). These polyps may show focal glands with vacuolated cytoplasm consistent with partial secretory change. In at least one reported polyp, the stroma also showed decidual changes that could not be attributed to any exogenous progestin use.[31] Some polyps, however, show markedly hyperplastic glands, and others show cystic glands with focal "adenomatous" change or atypia.[30,31] Occasionally endometrial polyps in patients receiving tamoxifen show foci of secretory changes in the glands with clear to vacuolated cytoplasm (Fig. 6.16). The mechanism of the secretory effects is not known.

The current data are partially anecdotal and

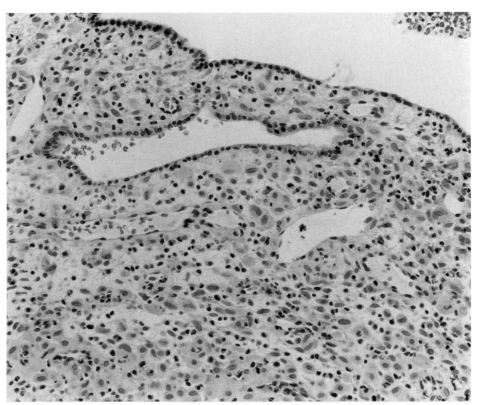

Figure 6.14. Decidua-like stroma in an 82-year-old. Endometrium shows decidua-like stroma, dilated atrophic glands, and ectatic venules beneath surface epithelium. The patient presented with postmenopausal bleeding and had not been on hormones. The specimen also showed fragments of a large, benign polyp.

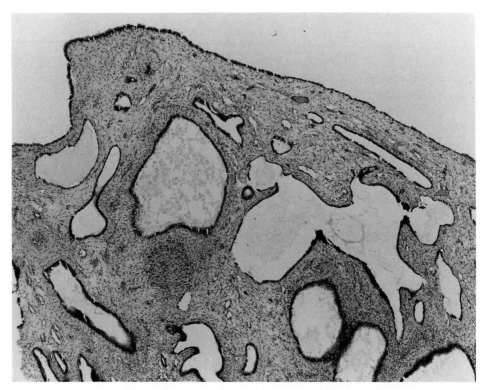

Figure 6.15. Tamoxifen-related polyp. Portion of a large polyp removed by curette in a postmenopausal patient on tamoxifen for breast carcinoma. The polyp showed weak proliferative activity.

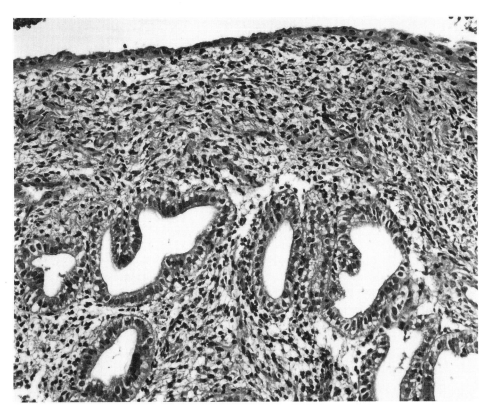

Figure 6.16. Tamoxifen effect with secretory change. Endometrial biopsy from woman with breast cancer shows weak secretory effect manifested by small subnuclear vacuoles. The patient had undergone bilateral oophorectomy several years previously. Subsequent curettage showed a polyp with focal secretory changes.

inconclusive regarding the long-term effects of tamoxifen on endometrial growth and histology. With the expanding role of tamoxifen in the treatment and possible prevention of breast carcinoma, more clinical information will be accumulated regarding this drug's influence on the endometrium.

Clomiphene Citrate

Clomiphene citrate is another antiestrogen that is used to induce ovulation in the treatment of infertile patients who are anovulatory.[1] It also may be used to treat luteal phase defects. This hormone stimulates multiple follicles to develop, and ovulation follows. It is thought to act by competitively binding to estrogen receptors in the hypothalamus, causing increased levels of follicle-stimulating hormone (FSH) and luteinizing hormone (LH) that induce ovulation. Like tamox-

ifen, clomiphene citrate has been found to have estrogenic as well as antiestrogenic activity.

Morphologic effects of clomiphene on the endometrium are difficult to assess. Biopsies often are taken in the luteal phase of clomiphene-induced cycles to assess the endometrial development. Usually the pattern is that of normally developing secretory phase endometrium that can be histologically dated, and this has been our experience. Often the histologic date correlates with the chronological postovulatory date, but sometimes the endometrium shows a significant lag in development. It is postulated that clomiphene citrate may cause luteal phase defects (LPDs) (Chapter 2).[34–38] Some investigators do not find a significant association of LPDs with clomiphene citrate use, however.[39,40]

One recent study of the morphologic effects of clomiphene citrate on the endometrium suggested that the drug causes significant alterations in secretory phase development.[41] Decreased gland tortuosity with scant secretions in clomiphene-treated cases were described. The gland-to-stroma ratio was reportedly decreased relative to secretory endometrium in nontreated cases. In early secretory endometrium, the subnuclear vacuoles appeared to be larger and more sharply defined, and later in the secretory phase, the luminal secretions appeared to be hyalinized and inspissated. The stroma also showed decreased predecidual change compared to nontreated endometrium. This report suggests that clomiphene may cause reproducible morphologic changes in secretory phase endometrium. Another study reported advanced secretory activity in clomiphene citrate-induced cycles.[42] Other investigators have found no changes in endometrial morphology following clomiphene citrate administration.[43,44] Further evaluation, including double-blinded studies, is necessary to establish whether or not clomiphene citrate yields consistent abnormalities in gland and stromal development.

Danazol

Danazol is structurally related to testosterone and is a weak androgen.[45] Its main metabolite, ethisterone, is a weak progestin, however.[46] This steroid is used for the treatment of endometriosis.[1] Because it suppresses endometrial growth, it also may be used to treat endometrial hyperplasia.[47]

The few studies of the effects of danazol on the endometrium show changes similar to those with progestins (Fig. 6.17).[46,48,49] Within a few months of use, the amount of tissue is reduced.[50] Glands show weak and irregular secretory changes with mild tortuosity, basal nuclei, and some cytoplasmic vacuolization. The stroma is hypercellular. With prolonged therapy, the glands show atro-

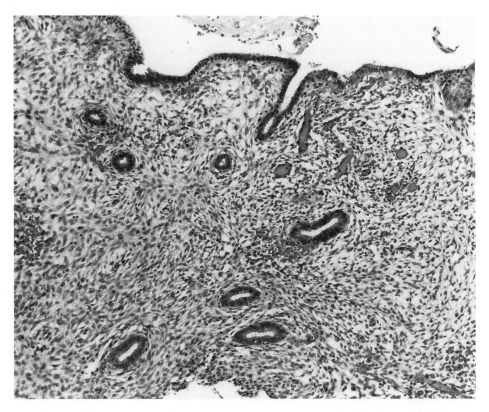

Figure 6.17. Danazol effect. Small glands in abundant stroma resemble progestin effect. The patient was on danazol therapy for endometriosis.

phy with scant to no secretory activity.[45,49,50] Vascular ectasia also can occur.[51] Occasional patients will show some proliferative activity with stromal and glandular mitoses.

Human Menopausal Gonadotropins/ Human Chorionic Gonadotropin

Human menopausal gonadotropins (hMG) (Pergonal, Serono Laboratories, Inc. Norwell, MA) are extracted from the urine of postmenopausal women and consist of FSH and LH. They are used to induce ovulation in the treatment of infertility due to anovulation, such as polycystic ovarian disease. Human chorionic gonadotropin (hCG) has structural and biologic similarities to LH and is used to simulate and improve upon the midcycle LH surge associated with ovulation. This hormone is used in conjunction with hMG and also can be used along with clomiphene citrate-induced ovulation.

The effects of hMG and hCG on endometrial morphology are difficult to define. Some studies suggest that the main change caused by administration of hMG/hCG is endometrial "inadequacy" with retarded development of more than 2 days when the histologic date is compared to the chronologic date.[52–55] These changes are similar to those commonly found in LPD (Chapter 2). In one study, 27% of patients treated with hMG/hCG showed inadequacy in development with out-of-phase histologic dates.[52] Other studies, however, have reported "advanced" histology with more highly developed secretory changes than expected for the cycle day, gland-stromal dyssynchrony, or normal glandular development.[56–57b] Despite the apparent discrepancies in the findings between studies, there are no specific morphologic alterations that can be definitely correlated with the effects of these hormones. For the pathologist interpreting biopsies from women who receive these hormones, accurate histologic dating is the most important consideration.

Gonadotropin-Releasing Hormone Agonists

Gonadotropin-releasing hormone (GnRH) agonists include leuprolide acetate, buserlin acetate,

and goserelin acetate. They are also referred to as "luteinizing hormone-releasing hormone agonists." These preparations are used to suppress the endometrium prior to resectoscopic ablation and to decrease the size of leiomyomas before surgical removal.[58] They are also used to prevent spontaneous LH surges before oocyte retrieval and to improve follicular development for ovulation induction during in vitro fertilization (IVF) and gamete intrafallopian transfer (GIFT).[1,57b] These compounds may also have utility in conjunction with progestins for contraception. When used to suppress endometrial growth, GnRH agonists cause marked atrophy of the endometrium.[51] When they are used in conjunction with a progestin, the endometrium shows apparent secretory changes consistent with progestin effect.[59]

Antiprogestin RU 486

The synthetic progestogenic steroid RU 486, or mifepristone, has high affinity for progesterone receptors in the endometrium, which causes its antiprogesterone action.[60] Its main use is for spontaneous termination of early pregnancy, although currently it is not available for this purpose in the United States. This drug has been assessed for possible contraceptive use, and preliminary studies suggest that it retards the secretory phase.[60–63] It results in inhibition of glandular secretory activity with degenerative and vascular changes. Stromal mitotic activity increases. In postmenopausal women receiving estrogen alone, this drug has effects similar to progesterone, suggesting it acts as a progesterone agonist.[60–62,64]

Clinical Queries and Reporting

A wide variety of indications for hormone use all influence the reasons for biopsy and the clinical questions posed to the pathologist. Most biopsies that show hormone effects are done for one of the following reasons: 1) surveillance during postmenopausal hormone replacement therapy, 2) evaluating abnormal uterine bleeding related to hormone therapy, 3) assessing treatment of hyperplasia, and 4) evaluating the status of the endometrium following hormone manipulation of ovulation or endometrial growth in infertility therapy. For each of these indications, there are specific considerations in interpretation and reporting.

Postmenopausal Hormone Replacement

Surveillance biopsy of asymptomatic postmenopausal patients receiving estrogen or estrogen–progestin replacement therapy usually is an office-based procedure intended to provide a small representative sample. The primary concern is whether or not the endometrium shows evidence of hyperplasia or neoplasia that would require cessation or change of the hormone therapy. The presence or absence of these changes should be explicitly stated in the report. This information can appear either in the diagnosis or as a comment. In these cases accurate reporting of the degree of proliferative activity, if any, also is important.

Abnormal Uterine Bleeding

There are several situations in which hormone therapy is related to abnormal bleeding. Sometimes patients on oral contraceptives or other progestins experience "breakthrough bleeding," which indicates bleeding of a noncyclical type. This may occur as irregular bleeding during the first few months of oral contraceptive use or later after many months of oral contraceptive use. Often the bleeding is due to atrophy and increased "fragility" of the tissue with focal glandular and stromal breakdown. In other situations, hormone therapy may be used as primary therapy for abnormal bleeding, especially dysfunctional bleeding (Chapter 5). Usually these patients have anovulatory cycles, and a progestin is given to suppress proliferation. If the bleeding is not controlled by progestin, then biopsy is done.

Other hormone therapies, too, may lead to abnormal bleeding. For example, tamoxifen therapy for breast cancer, or estrogen or estrogen-replacement therapy for menopausal symptoms, may be associated with bleeding. Biopsy in such cases is done to rule out significant organic lesions. Also, megestrol acetate (Megace) therapy for breast cancer may lead to decidual transforma-tion of the endometrium with focal glandular and stromal breakdown.

In any of these cases in which hormone therapy is associated with abnormal bleeding, the biopsy is done to assess the status of the endometrium and to rule out possible underlying organic disorders such as polyps, inflammation, hyperplasia, or neoplasia. In addition, the biopsy may be therapeutic, removing the abnormal tissue that is bleeding. Most of these biopsies show progestin effects that range from decidual patterns to atrophic patterns. When the patient has received unopposed estrogen, however, the pattern usually is proliferative. A specific diagnosis should be rendered. If this is not possible, a descriptive diagnosis should be made. When glandular and stromal breakdown also is present, this should be reported. In all these cases it is important to exclude other lesions such as hyperplasia or carcinoma, so a comment regarding the absence of these lesions is generally indicated.

Treatment of Hyperplasia

Hyperplasia, either with or without atypia, may be managed by progestin therapy to suppress gland growth and then rebiopsied to determine the efficacy of the therapy. In these cases it is important to note whether or not there is evidence of continued gland growth and hyperplasia, and whether or not atypia is found. In progestin-treated hyperplasia, the underlying pattern of gland growth and cellular differentiation often becomes distorted. Frequently the tissue resembles that seen in early pregnancy. When there is a well-developed decidua-like response, it is difficult to fully assess the degree of gland complexity, and the secretory changes of the glands make evaluation of cytologic atypia difficult or impossible. In such cases it is important to state clearly that progestin effect is present and that it may not be possible to fully assess the degree of the glandular abnormality. An effort also should be made to review the previous material to assess the effect of the therapy on the hyperplasia.

Infertility Therapy

When biopsy is done during hormone therapy in the infertile patient, the clinical questions depend on the hormone used and the indication for biopsy. Often during treatment with a drug such as clomiphene citrate the gynecologist wishes to know whether secretory phase development is normal and, if so, the precise histologic date (Chapter 2). When ovulation-inducing medication is used, one obvious question is whether the endometrium shows secretory changes that reflect ovulation or if the pattern is proliferative. The gynecologist also is concerned with the possibility of an LPD that will be reflected in retarded maturation when compared to the time of ovulation. Usually this determination requires only accurate histologic dating of secretory endometrium. However, on occasion abnormalities in secretory phase development are found, and these should be clearly noted. For example, when a disparity between the glands and stroma is seen, the pathologist should clearly indicate that irregular maturation is present. A comment regarding the approximate histologic date for both the glands and the stroma further clarifies the pathologic findings.

In addition to the specific situations for hormone use given above, hormone effects, especially progestin-related changes, can be found in other biopsy specimens when the hormone use is incidental. These cases include biopsies done during evaluation of pelvic pain, prehysterectomy sampling, or curettage at the time of tubal ligation. Furthermore, progestin effects can persist for a variable period of one or more months after the drug is discontinued. In addition, some of these cases may represent an endogenous progestin effect with no exogenous hormone use. Consequently, the finding of the histologic changes of apparent progestin effect is not negated by the clinical history. When the biopsy clearly shows progestin effect, we recommend using the term "progestin effect" as the diagnosis with an accompanying brief description of the changes.

In some cases the glands and stroma show some changes that suggest progestin effect but the features are not diagnostic. Usually these cases show glands with poorly developed secretory changes and plump stromal cells that appear to be partly decidualized. If the clinical history does not establish progestin use and the changes by themselves are not diagnostic of progestin effect, then it is best to give a descriptive diagnosis. This diagnosis can reflect the fact that irregular secretory changes are present and suggest the possibility of progestin effect. A descriptive diagnosis would serve to indicate that the changes are benign and due to an imbalance in the amounts of sex steroid hormones, regardless of their source.

References

1. Speroff L, Glass RH, Kase NG: Clinical Gynecologic Endocrinology and Infertility. 4th ed. Baltimore: Williams & Wilkins, 1989.
2. Schiff I: Menopause. In: Gynecology: Principles and Practice. Kistner RW, ed. Chicago: Year Book Medical Publishers, 1986;565–582.
3. Grady D, Rubin SM, Petitti DB, Fox CS, Black D, et al: Hormone therapy to prevent disease and prolong life in postmenopausal women. Ann Intern Med 1992;117:1016–1037.
4. Whitehead MI, Fraser D: The effects of estrogens and progestogens on the endometrium. Obstet Gynecol Clin North Am 1987;14:299–320.
5. Ober W: Effects of oral and intrauterine administration of contraceptives on the uterus. Hum Pathol 1977;8:513–527.
6. Dallenbach-Hellweg G: Histopathology of the Endometrium. 4th ed. New York: Springer-Verlag, 1987.
7. Kurman RJ, Mazur MT: Benign diseases of the endometrium. In: Blaustein's Pathology of the Female Genital Tract. 4th ed. Kurman RJ, ed. New York: Springer-Verlag, 1994;367–409.
8. Hendrickson MR, Kempson RL: Surgical Pathology of the Uterine Corpus (Major Problems in Pathology series). Volume 12. Philadelphia: W.B. Saunders, 1980.
9. Deligdisch L: Effects of hormone therapy on the endometrium. Mod Pathol 1993;6:94–106.
10. Hesla, J. Kurman R, Rock J: Histologic effects of oral contraceptives on the uterine corpus and cervix. Semin Reprod Endocrinol 1989;7:213–219.
10a. Moyer DL, deLignieres B, Driguez P, Pez JP: Prevention of endometrial hyperplasia by progesterone during long-term estradiol replacement: Influence of bleeding pattern and secretory changes. Fertil Steril 1993;59:992–997.
11. Dockerty MB, Smith RA, Symmonds RE: Pseudomalignant endometrial changes induced by administration of new synthetic progestins. Staff Meetings of the Mayo Clinic 1959;34:321–328.
12. Cruz-Aquino M, Shenker L, Blaustein A: Pseudosarcoma of the endometrium. Obstet Gynecol 1967;29:93–96.

13. Clement PB, Scully RE: Idiopathic postmeno-pausal decidual reaction of the endometrium. Int J Gynecol Pathol 1988;7:152–161.

13a. Iezzoni: JC, Mills SE: Predecidualized signet-ring stromal cells mimicking adenocarcinoma in endometrial biopsy specimens. Mod Pathol 1994;70: 90A (abstract).

14. Bernardini L, Araujo FE, Balmaceda JP: A case of permanent endometrial hypotrophy after long-term use of oral contraceptives. Hum Reprod 1993;8:543–546.

15. Gelfand MM, Ferenczy A: A prospective 1-year study of estrogen and progestin in postmenopausal women: Effects on the endometrium. Obstet Gynecol 1989;74:398–402.

16. Mishell DR, Jr: Menopause. In: Comprehensive Gynecology. Herbst AL, Mishell DR, Jr, Stenchever MA, Droegemueller W, eds. St. Louis: Mosby Year Book, 1992;1245–1280.

17. Byrjalsen I, Thormann L, Meinecke B, Riis BJ, Christiansen C: Sequential estrogen and progestogen therapy—Assessment of progestational effects on the postmenopausal endometrium. Obstet Gynecol 1992;79:523–528.

18. Magos AL, Brewster E, Singh R, O'Dowd T, Brincat M: Amenorrhea and endometrial atrophy with continuous oral estrogens and progestogen therapy in post-menopausal women. Obstet Gynecol 1985; 65:496–499.

19. Hillard TC, Siddle NC, Whitehead MI, Fraser DI, Pryse-Davies J: Continuous combined conjugated equine estrogen-progestogen therapy—effects of medroxyprogesterone acetate and norethindrone acetate on bleeding patterns and endometrial histologic diagnosis. Am J Obstet Gynecol 1992; 167:1–7.

20. Te Linde RW, Henriksen E: Decidualike changes in the endometrium without pregnancy. Am J Obstet Gynecol 1940;39:733-749.

21. Dallenbach-Hellweg G, Hohagen F: On the problem of premature decidualization induced by the embryo transfer. Lab Invest 1985;52: 17A. (Abstract)

22. Tamada T, Okagaki T, Maruyama M, Matsumoto S: Endometrial histology associated with an intrauterine contraceptive device. Am J Obstet Gynecol 1967;98:811-817.

23. Bonney WA, Glasser SR, Clewe TH, Noyes RW, Cooper CL: Endometrial response to the intrauterine device. Am J Obstet Gynecol 1966;96: 101–113.

24. Andersson M, Storm HH, Mouridsen HT: Incidence of new primary cancers after adjuvant therapy and radiotherapy for early breast cancer. J Natl Cancer Inst 1991;83:1013–1017.

25. Segna RA, Dottino RR, Deligdisch L, Cohen CJ: Tamoxifen and endometrial cancer. Mt Sinai J Med 1992;59:416–418.

26. Magriples U, Naftolin F, Schwartz PE, Carcangiu ML: High-grade endometrial carcinoma in tamoxifen-treated breast cancer patients. J Clin Oncol 1993;11:485–490.

27. Gusberg SB: Tamoxifen for breast cancer: Associated endometrial cancer. Cancer 1990;65: 1463–1464.

28. Fornander T, Cedermark B, Mattsson A, Skoog L, Theve T, et al: Adjuvant tamoxifen in early breast cancer: Occurrence of new primary cancers. Lancet 1989;1:117–120.

29. Seoud Ma-F, Johns J, Weed JC, Jr: Gynecologic tumors in tamoxifen-treated women with breast cancer. Obstet Gynecol 1993;82:165–169.

29a. Fisher B, Costantino JP, Redmond CK, Fisher ER, Wickerham DL, et al: Endometrial cancer in tamoxifen-treated breast cancer patients: findings from the National Surgical Adjuvant Breast and Bowel Project (NSABP) B-14, J Natl Cancer Inst 1994;86:527–537.

30. Nuovo MA, Nuovo GJ, McCaffrey FM, Levine RU, Barron B, et al: Endometrial polyps in postmenopausal patients receiving tamoxifen. Int J Gynecol Pathol 1989;8:125–131.

31. Corley D, Rowe J, Curtis MT, Hogan WM, Noumoff JS, et al: Postmenopausal bleeding from unusual endometrial polyps in women on chronic tamoxifen therapy. Obstet Gynecol 1992;79:111-116.

32. Cohen I, Shapira J, Altaras M, Cordoba M, Rosen D, et al: Endometrial decidual changes in a postmenopausal woman treated with tamoxifen and megestrol acetate. Br J Obstet Gynaecol 1992; 99:773–774.

33. Lahti E, Blanco G, Kauppila A, Apajasarkkinen M, Taskinen PJ, et al: Endometrial changes in postmenopausal breast cancer patients receiving tamoxifen. Obstet Gynecol 1993;81:660-664.

34. Wentz AC: Endometrial biopsy in the evaluation of infertility. Fertil Steril 1980;33:121–124.

35. Keenan JA, Herbert CM, Bush JR, Wentz AC: Diagnosis and management of out-of-phase endometrial biopsies among patients receiving clomiphene citrate for ovulation induction. Fertil Steril 1989;51:964–967.

36. Cook CL, Schroeder JA, Yussman MA, Sanfilippo JS: Induction of luteal phase defect with clomiphene citrate. Am J Obstet Gynecol 1984;149: 613–616.

37. Van Hall EV, Mastboom JL: Luteal phase insufficiency in patients treated with clomiphene. Am J Obstet Gynecol 1969;103:165–171.

38. Yeko TR, Bardawil WA, Nicosia SM, Dawood MY, Maroulis GB: Histology of midluteal corpus luteum and endometrium from clomiphene citrate-induced cycles. Fertil Steril 1992;57:28–32.

39. Hecht BR, Bardawil WA, Khan-Dawood FS, Dawood MY: Luteal insufficiency: Correlation between endometrial dating and integrated progesterone output in clomiphene citrate-induced cycles. Am J Obstet Gynecol 1990;163:1986–1991.

40. Lamb EJ, Colliflower WW, Williams JW: Endometrial histology and conception rates after clomiphene citrate. Obstet Gynecol 1972;39:389–396.

41. Benda JA: Clomiphene's effect on endometrium in infertility. Int J Gynecol Pathol 1992;11:273–282.

42. Birkenfeld A, Navot D, Levij IS, Laufer N, Beier-Hellwig K, et al: Advanced secretory changes in the proliferative human endometrial epithelium following clomiphene citrate treatment. Fertil Steril 1986;45:462–468.

43. Thatcher SS, Donachie KM, Glasier A, Hillier SG, Baird DT: The effects of clomiphene citrate on the histology of human endometrium in regularly cycling women undergoing in vitro fertilization. Fertil Steril 1988;49:296–301.

44. Li TC, Warren MA, Murphy C, Sargeant S, Cooke ID: A prospective, randomised, cross-over study comparing the effects of clomiphene citrate and cyclofenil on endometrial morphology in the luteal phase of normal, fertile women. Br J Obstet Gynaecol 1992;99:1008–1013.

45. Floyd WS: Danazol: Endocrine and endometrial effects. Int J Fertil 1980;25:75–80.

46. Fedele L, Marchini M, Bianchi S, Baglioni A, Bocciolone L, et al: Endometrial patterns during danazol and buserelin therapy for endometriosis: Comparative structural and ultrastructural study. Obstet Gynecol 1990:76:79–84.

47. Soh E, Sato K: Clinical effects of danazol on endometrial hyperplasia in menopausal and postmenopausal women. Cancer 1990;66:983–988.

48. Wentz AC, Jones GS, Sapp KC, King TM: Progestational activity of danazol in the human female subject. Am J Obstet Gynecol 1976; 126:378–384.

49. Marchini M, Fedele L, Bianchi S, Dinola G, Nava S, et al: Endometrial patterns during therapy with danazol or gestrinone for endometriosis—Structural and ultrastructural study. Hum Pathol 1992;23:51–56.

50. Jeppsson S, Mellquist P, Rannevik G: Short-term effects of danazol on endometrial histology. Acta Obstet Gynecol Scand Suppl 1984;123:41–44.

51. Brooks PG, Serden SP, Davos I: Hormonal inhibition of the endometrium for resectoscopic endometrial ablation. Am J Obstet Gynecol 1991; 164:1601–1608.

52. Reshef E, Segars JH, Hill GA, Pridham DD, Yussman MA, et al: Endometrial inadequacy after treatment with human menopausal gonadotropin/human chorionic gonadotropin. Fertil Steril 1990;54:1012–1016.

53. Bonhoff A, Naether O, Johannisson E, Bohnet HG: Morphometric characteristics of endometrial biopsies after different types of ovarian stimulation for infertility treatment. Fertil Steril 1993;59:560–566.

54. Campbell BF, Phipps WR, Nagel TC: Endometrial biopsies during treatment with subcutaneous pulsatile gonadotropin releasing hormone and luteal phase human chorinonic gonadotropins. Int J Fertil 1988;33:329.

55. Sterzik K, Dallenbach C, Schneider V, Sasse V, Dallenbach-Hellweg G: In vitro fertilization: The degree of endometrial insufficiency varies with the type of ovarian stimulation. Fertil Steril 1988;50:457–462.

56. Garcia JE, Acosta AA, Hsiu J-G, Jones HW, Jr: Advanced endometrial maturation after ovulation induction with human menopausal gonadotropin/human chorionic gonadotropin for in vitro fertilization. Fertil Steril 1984;41:31–35.

57. Sharma V, Whitehead M, Mason B, Pryse-Davies J, Ryder T, et al: Influence of superovulation on endometrial and embryonic development. Fertil Steril 1990;53:822–829.

57a. Benadiva CA, Metzger DA: Superovulation with human menopausal gonadotropins is associated with endometrial gland-stroma dyssynchrony. Fertil Steril 1994;61:700–704.

57b. Macrow PJ, Li T-C, Seif MW, Buckley CH, Elstein M: Endometrial structure after superovulation: A prospective controlled study. Fertil Steril 1994; 61:696–699.

58. Casper RF: Clinical uses of gonadotropin-releasing hormone analogues. Can Med Assoc J 1991; 144:153–158.

59. Lemay A, Jean C, Faure N: Endometrial histology during intermittent intranasal luteinizing hormone-releasing hormone (LH-RH) agonist sequentially combined with an oral progestogen as an antiovulatory contraceptive approach. Fertil Steril 1987;48:775–782.

60. Spitz IM, Bardin CW: Mifepristone (RU 486)—A modulator of progestin and glucocorticoid action. N Engl J Med 1993;329:404–412.

61. Swahn ML, Bygdeman M, Cekan S, Xing S, Masironi B, et al: The effect of RU 486 administered during the early luteal phase on bleeding pattern,

hormonal parameters and endometrium. Hum Reprod 1990;5:402–408.

62. Li T-C, Dockery P, Thomas P, Rogers AW, Lenton EA, et al: The effects of progesterone receptor blockade in the luteal phase of normal fertile women. Fertil Steril 1988;50:732–742.

63. Batista MC, Cartledge TP, Zellmer AW, Merino MJ, Axiotis C, et al: Delayed endometrial matura-

tion induced by daily administration of the anti-progestin RU-486—A potential new contra-ceptive strategy. Am J Obstet Gynecol 1992;167: 60–65.

64. Koering MJ, Healy DL, Hodgen GD: Morpho-logic response of endometrium to a progesterone receptor antagonist, RU486, in monkeys. Fertil Steril 1986;45:280–287.

7
Endometritis

Endometritis usually is a disorder of the reproductive years, although it may occur in postmenopausal patients. Endometrial inflammation typically accompanies pelvic inflammatory disease of the upper genital tract.[1,2] It may also be associated with a recent pregnancy, either an abortion or a term pregnancy.[3-5] Other possible causes include instrumentation, such as a prior biopsy, an intrauterine contraceptive device, cervical stenosis, or the presence of an organic lesion such as a polyp, leiomyoma, hyperplasia, or carcinoma.[5] Endometritis typically presents with intermenstrual vaginal bleeding, and sometimes it causes menorrhagia. Since this disorder also may be associated with infertility, it is important to recognize it, both for the therapy and for the prognosis of the infertile patient.[6,7] In one study, 8% of outpatient endometrial biopsies showed endometritis.[8]

Endometrial inflammation often is nonspecific and rarely has morphologic features that indicate a definite etiology. The nonspecific forms of endometritis have traditionally been separated into chronic and acute forms, depending on the type of inflammatory infiltrate; most are referred to as chronic nonspecific endometritis. The inflammatory infiltrate often is a mixed acute and chronic inflammatory process, however, and neutrophils as well as plasma cells and lymphocytes can be present. Rigorous separation of the type of inflammatory process is less important than recognition of the presence of inflammation. Acute endometrial inflammation is relatively infrequent except for puerperal-related infections, and these latter cases rarely come to biopsy or curettage.

Nonspecific Endometritis

Endometritis may be diffuse or focal and can range from a subtle inflammatory infiltrate to a pronounced inflammatory reaction. Endometritis typically shows a pattern of a mixed inflammatory infiltrate containing plasma cells and lymphocytes, and, not infrequently, neutrophils (polymorphonuclear leukocytes) and eosinophils. In addition to inflammatory cells, there is a constellation of histologic findings that facilitate recognition of endometrial inflammation (Table 7.1).[8] The other morphologic changes include reactive stroma, epithelial changes, abnormal glandular development, and evidence of glandular and stromal breakdown.[8,9]

TABLE 7.1. Morphologic features of nonspecific endometritis.

Plasma cell infiltrate
Increased number of lymphocytes and lymphoid follicles
Variable presence of neutrophils in surface epithelium and glands
Reactive stromal response
Altered gland development
Breakdown and bleeding

Inflammatory Cells

Plasma cells are the most important histologic feature for the diagnosis of endometritis.[4,5,10,11] Their presence is required to establish the diagnosis of chronic endometritis, because, in contrast to lymphocytes, they are not present in normal endometrium. Plasma cells may be diffuse and easily recognizable but more commonly are focal and widely dispersed. Plasma cells generally are most numerous in the periglandular and subepithelial stroma and around lymphoid aggregates (Fig. 7.1). Plasma cells should be readily identifiable and numerous before establishing a diagnosis of chronic endometritis unless associated features of inflammation are clearly present (see below).[8] The diagnosis of endometritis should not rest on the finding of an apparent plasma cell, however, in endometrium that otherwise appears normal. In cases where the plasma cell infiltrate appears subtle or equivocal, the background pattern is as important as the quantity of plasma cells for establishing the diagnosis of endometritis. The number of plasma cells does not appear to correlate with the severity of the lesion.[3,8]

Normal endometrial stromal cells, especially predecidualized cells in the late secretory phase, can resemble plasma cells, having eccentric nuclei and a pale perinuclear zone. The plasma cell, however, is identified by its distinctive, clumped

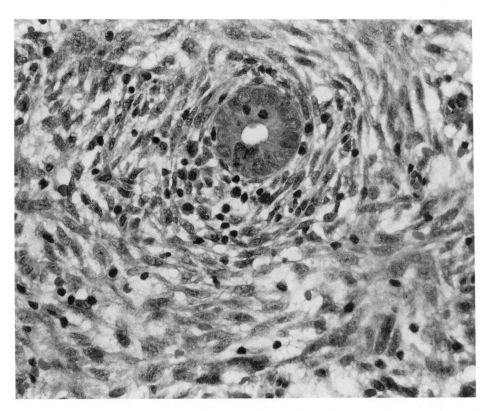

FIGURE 7.1. Nonspecific chronic endometritis. Scattered plasma cells and lymphocytes surround a small proliferative gland. The stromal cells are reactive, with elongated, spindle-shaped nuclei, and they swirl around the gland.

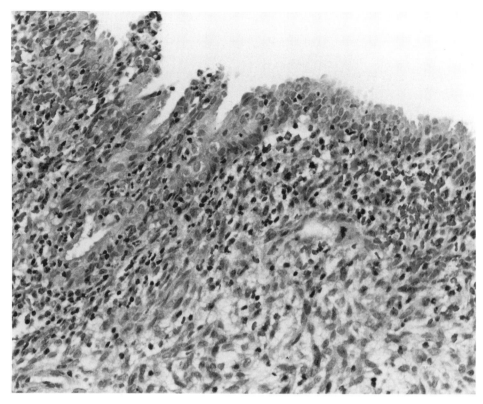

FIGURE 7.2. Nonspecific acute and chronic endometritis. A dense inflammatory infiltrate composed of plasma cells, lymphocytes, and a few neutrophils forms a bandlike infiltrate in the subepithelial stroma. The stroma has a reactive pattern, with spindle-shaped cells.

chromatin arrangement yielding a clock-face pattern. A methyl green pyronin histochemical stain[4] or immunohistochemistry for immunoglobulin G can help demonstrate plasma cells[12] when the cytologic features by routine histology are not diagnostic.

Whereas plasma cells may be the predominant inflammatory component of endometritis, more severe inflammation commonly shows a mixed inflammatory infiltrate. Often the inflammatory infiltrate includes numerous lymphocytes that tend to concentrate in the subepithelial stroma (Fig. 7.2). Lymphoid follicles become prominent (Fig. 7.3) and may show germinal centers; larger transformed lymphocytes and immunoblasts also may be interspersed (Fig. 7.4).[13-15]

Neutrophils as a part of the inflammatory infiltrate indicate an acute process (Figs. 7.2 and 7.5). This neutrophilic inflammatory infiltrate typically involves the surface epithelium and

gland lumen, sometimes forming microabscesses in the glands.[8-11] Neutrophils, however, also can be present in menstrual endometrium as well as in foci of glandular and stromal breakdown without signifying an infectious process. Like lymphocytes, the presence of neutrophils alone is not sufficient to indicate inflammation. The distribution of these cells in the endometrium and the accompanying cellular infiltrates must be considered before making the diagnosis of endometritis.

Acute endometritis without a chronic (plasma cell) component is extremely unusual and occurs most frequently in the postpartum or postabortal patient. Patients with pregnancy-related acute inflammation rarely come to biopsy or curettage, however. When acute endometritis is present, there is a neutrophilic infiltrate in the glands with microabscess formation and infiltration of neutrophils into the surface epithelium. Marked inflammation also will result in formation of gran-

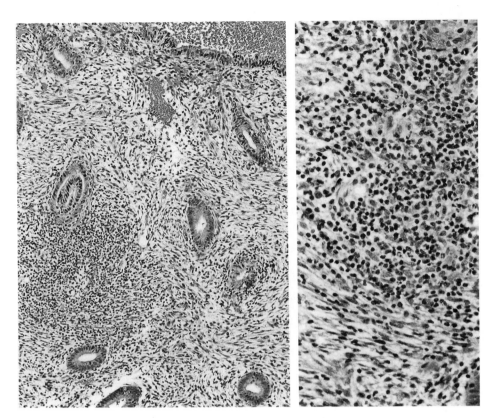

FIGURE 7.3. Nonspecific chronic endometritis. *Left*: Proliferative glands surrounded by spindle-shaped cells. A lymphoid follicle is present. *Right*: The lymphoid follicle is composed predominantly of lymphocytes, but scattered plasma cells also are present. The presence of plasma cells distinguishes inflammatory lymphoid follicles from normal lymphoid follicles that occur in noninflamed endometrium.

ulation tissue with a network of small vessels in a fibroblastic stroma (Fig. 7.6).

On occasion eosinophils may be present as a part of the inflammatory infiltrate.[8] They are not normally present in the endometrium. Like lymphocytes or neutrophils, eosinophils should be present in a background of inflammatory changes to be a component of endometritis. Eosinophilic infiltrates also can occur following curettage, apparently as a result of the instrumentation,[16] and in this case they represent a nonspecific response to the procedure.

Endometritis also can have a component of histiocytes. Usually these cells are widely distributed in a mixed inflammatory infiltrate. Hemosiderin-laden stromal cells and histiocytes often are interspersed.[3,5] Sometimes histiocytes can be prominent, with large aggregates of these cells in the stroma surrounded by plasma cells and lymphocytes. When the histiocytes develop abundant, foamy cytoplasm, the process becomes xanthogranulomatous.[11,17–20]

Stromal Changes

With endometritis the stroma typically shows reactive changes.[3,8,11] Stromal cells become spindle-shaped, resembling fibroblasts, and are elongate and bipolar, in contrast to the rounded, ovoid shape of the nonreactive stromal cell (Figs. 7.1 and 7.3). The reactive process is also characterized by a swirling, interlacing pattern of the spindle cells, which may form "pinwheel" arrangements (Fig. 7.7). Plasma cells usually are interspersed in the reactive stroma. Superficial stroma may become edematous.[8]

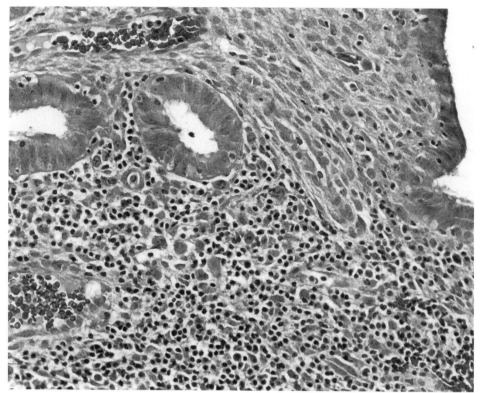

FIGURE 7.4. Nonspecific chronic endometritis. A mixed inflammatory infiltrate with scattered transformed lymphocytes and immunoblasts. Transformed lymphocytes are often associated with chlamydia infection.

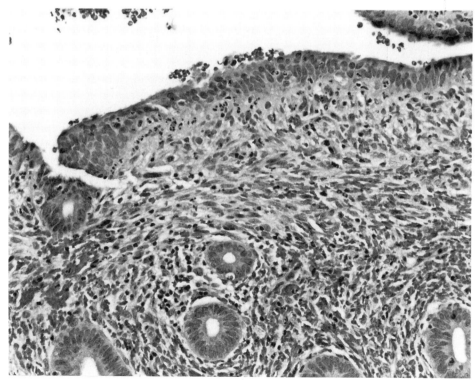

FIGURE 7.5. Nonspecific acute and chronic endometritis. Neutrophils infiltrate the surface epithelium, and the deeper stroma contains numerous lymphocytes and plasma cells.

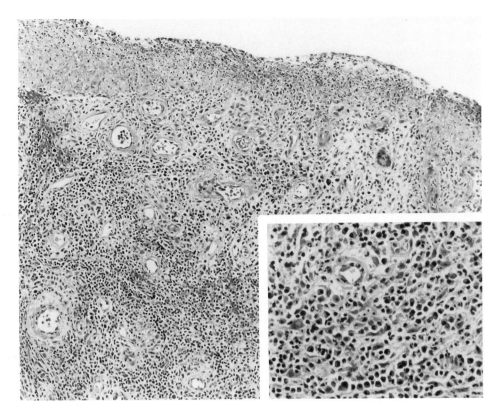

FIGURE 7.6. Acute endometritis with granulation tissue. Normal endometrium is replaced by granulation tissue composed of numerous capillaries in a dense background of inflammatory cells. The surface is ulcerated. *Inset*: The inflammation is characterized by numerous plasma cells, neutrophils, and lymphocytes.

Epithelial Changes

Reactive cellular changes also affect the endometrial surface and glandular epithelium. The epithelium may show squamous and eosinophilic cell change (Chapter 9), especially when the inflammation is long-standing and intense.[8,9] The cells may become stratified, with prominent nucleoli, cleared chromatin, and increased mitotic activity (Fig. 7.8).

Abnormal Glandular Development

In cycling patients the endometrial response to hormones is often diminished. Usually the endometrium has proliferative phase characteristics, with tubular glands showing mitotic activity. In the secretory phase the glands may lose their normal pattern of reactivity. Secretory changes occur in ovulating women, but they often show abnormal development with less gland tortuosity and distension than is seen in a normal, noninflamed secretory phase. The changes can include irregular or retarded maturation of secretory phase endometrium. Glands may appear underdeveloped, lacking tortuosity and luminal secretions.

Glandular and Stromal Breakdown

Endometritis also results in focal glandular and stromal breakdown. With severe and prolonged chronic inflammation, the changes of irregular bleeding with glandular and stromal breakdown and regeneration become prominent. Irregular breakdown leads to a corrugated surface with foci of regenerating and shedding endometrium interspersed. The inflamed stroma becomes dense and less responsive to hormonal changes. Because of the irregular growth, the tissue may become polypoid, and the resemblance to a

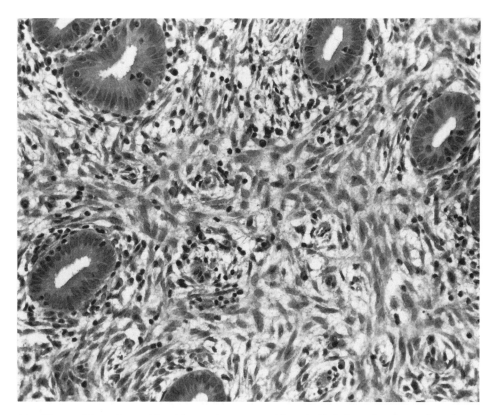

FIGURE 7.7. Nonspecific endometritis with reactive stroma. Chronically inflamed endometrium shows reactive stroma with interlacing, elongate spindle cells that resemble fibroblasts. Plasma cells and lymphocytes are interspersed.

polyp is accentuated by the dense stroma that accompanies the inflammation. Recent and chronic bleeding patterns also may be present, with areas of stromal collapse, glandular breakdown, stromal fibrosis, macrophages, and hemosiderin deposition (Chapter 5).

Specific Infections

Although the etiology of chronic endometritis usually is not apparent in biopsy specimens, some morphologic changes may occur that offer clues to the etiology. For example, the endometrium may harbor other changes, such as a retained subinvoluted implantation site following a pregnancy or abortion, a placental site nodule from a remote pregnancy, or other lesions, such as a polyp.

The inflammatory response associated with

Chlamydia trachomatis infection is usually marked. The inflammatory infiltrate tends to be diffuse, with plasma cells, lymphocytes, and lymphoid follicles with transformed lymphocytes.[1,9,21] The inflammatory response to chlamydia also may be mixed, with an infiltrate of acute as well as chronic inflammatory cells. Stromal necrosis and reactive atypia of the epithelium also may be present.[9] These marked inflammatory changes are not specific for chlamydia, however, but appear to reflect the presence of upper genital tract infection and acute salpingitis. One study has shown that neutrophils in the endometrial surface epithelium and in gland lumens, along with a dense subepithelial stromal lymphocytic infiltrate, plasma cells, and germinal centers containing transformed lymphocytes, are features that are predictive of a diagnosis of upper genital tract infection and acute salpingitis.[1] The finding of one or more plasma cells per × 120 field in the

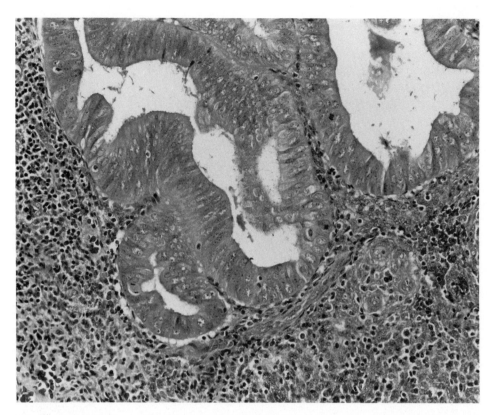

FIGURE 7.8. Nonspecific endometritis with reactive epithelial changes. Reactive epithelium in markedly inflamed endometrium secondary to actinomycosis. The reactive glandular cells have abundant, eosinophilic cytoplasm and enlarged nuclei. A dense chronic inflammatory infiltrate surrounds the glands. The patient was using an IUD.

stroma and five or more neutrophils per × 400 field in surface epithelium was strongly associated with upper genital tract infection and salpingitis. *Chlamydia trachomatis* or *Neisseria gonorrheae* are most frequently associated with these findings of a marked acute and chronic inflammatory infiltrate, although infections with *C. trachomatis* produce a greater concentration of plasma cells and more lymphoid follicles than *N. gonorrheae*.[1]

Granulomatous

Granulomatous inflammation of the endometrium is infrequent. Often the process is due to mycobacterium, especially *Mycobacterium tuberculosis*, and the infection usually indicates advanced disease. Although rare in the United States, in some countries tuberculous endometritis is more commonly encountered in endometrial biopsies undertaken during assessment of primary or sec-

ondary female infertility, since endometrial involvement is a reflection of more widespread disease that also affects the fallopian tubes in most cases.[22,23] Tuberculous endometritis also can cause abnormal uterine bleeding in postmenopausal patients.[24] In tuberculous infection the granulomatous response is variable. Often the granulomas are non-necrotizing.[23,23a] Well-formed granulomas may be difficult to identify unless the endometrium is biopsied in the late secretory phase when the granulomas have had sufficient time to develop.[5,10,25] The surrounding stroma can show a lymphocytic infiltrate. As with any form of inflammation, gland development may be altered, and the glands may lack an appropriate secretory response if the biopsy is taken in the luteal phase.[25] Acid-fast stains rarely demonstrate the characteristic organism in endometrial infections, and culture may be needed to establish the diagnosis.[23] Fungal infections, including cryptococcosis, coccidioidomycosis, and blastomycosis, rarely involve the endometrium resulting in granulomatous inflammation[4] Cytomegalovirus infection has been seen in association with poorly formed endometrial granulomas.[26] Sarcoidosis, too, may rarely lead to non-necrotizing granuloma formation in the endometrium.[27] Necrotizing granulomatous inflammation has been seen following endometrial hysteroscopic ablation therapy.[28,29]

Actinomycosis

Infection by *Actinomyces israelii* is another rare cause of endometritis. This organism typically is found in endometritis associated with use of the intrauterine device (IUD). Use of the IUD has decreased in the United States, so actinomycotic endometritis is also infrequent. When actinomycosis-associated inflammation is present, the inflammatory response usually is intense, with many plasma cells, lymphocytes, and neutrophils throughout the tissue (Fig. 7.8). The organisms show the typical sulfur granule morphology and can be stained by tissue Gram and methenamine-silver stains.[11]

Cytomegalovirus

Rarely, endometrial biopsy will show evidence of cytomegalovirus infection. This may occur in immunosuppressed patients or it may be found in women with no known underlying disorder.[30–33] Regardless of immunologic status, the tissue shows the characteristic nuclear and cytoplasmic inclusions in epithelial cells and occasional endothelial cells (Fig. 7.9). The stroma may show a sparse plasma cell infiltrate, but other changes associated with inflammation, such as a spindle-cell reactive stroma, may not be found. One reported case had small, ill-defined, non-necrotizing granulomas in the endometrium but no visible

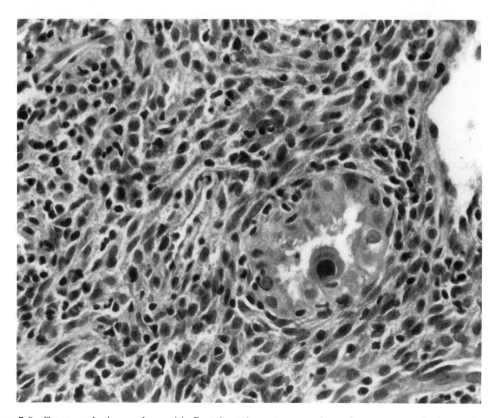

FIGURE 7.9. Cytomegalovirus endometritis. Postabortal curettage specimen shows cytomegalovirus endometritis. A single glandular cell contains a prominent dark nuclear inclusion and granular cytoplasmic inclusions.

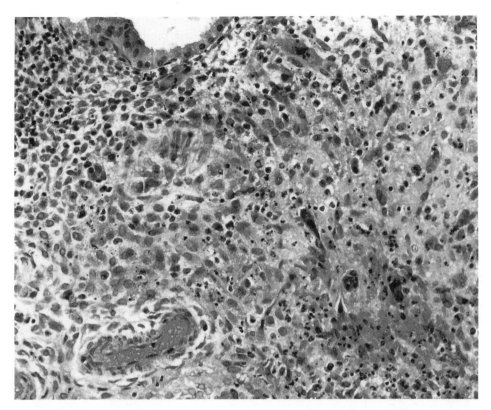

FIGURE 7.10. Herpesvirus endometritis. Area of necrosis in secretory endometrium due to herpesvirus infection. Multinucleate cells showing viral cytopathic effect are present. The patient was not immunocompromised, but herpesvirus was also present in the endocervix.

inclusions, although the presence of the virus was demonstrated by polymerase chain reaction for viral DNA.[26]

Herpesvirus

Herpesvirus rarely infects the endometrium, but it may occur, usually as an ascending process associated with cervical infection.[34-37] When present in the endometrium, it can cause patchy necrosis of the glands and stroma (Fig. 7.10).[37] The diagnosis is established by identifying cells that show typical herpesvirus cytopathic effect. Cowdry type A inclusion and multinucleate cells with molded ground glass nuclei can be found in the glandular epithelium or the stroma in areas of necrosis (Fig. 7.11). Several nonviral alterations, including optically clear nuclei associated with the presence of trophoblast[38] and cytoplasmic nuclear invaginations in the Arias-Stella reaction,[39]

may superficially resemble herpesvirus effect. Immunohistochemical stains for herpesvirus antigens can be helpful in documenting the presence of the virus.

Mycoplasma

The morphologic changes associated with mycoplasma, especially *Ureaplasma urealyticum*, have been described.[40,41] The inflammatory pattern, termed "subacute focal inflammation," is subtle but distinctive. In this condition the inflammatory infiltrate is patchy, focal, and difficult to discern. It is best seen in the mid secretory phase from days 20 to 23 when stromal edema accentuates the inflammatory foci (Fig. 7.12). The areas of inflammation consist mainly of lymphocytes with macrophages and only rare plasma cells or neutrophils.[40-42] These small inflammatory foci tend to be located beneath surface epithelium, around

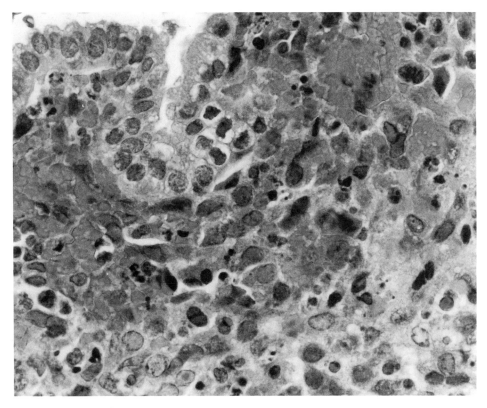

FIGURE 7.11. Herpesvirus endometritis. The nuclei of infected cells have a ground glass appearance and contain inclusions of herpesvirus.

spiral arterioles, or adjacent to glands.[40] Chronic lesions may appear granulomatous.[40] Biopsies that are not timed for the edematous portion of the secretory phase may miss these abnormalities because the inflammatory infiltrate cannot be distinguished from normal lymphoid tissue of the endometrium. Subacute focal inflammation also has been linked with the presence of pelvic adhesions.[41]

Differential Diagnosis

One of the most difficult problems in the differential diagnosis of endometritis is to decide whether apparent inflammatory cells represent true inflammation or whether they are a part of the normal cellular infiltrate of the endometrium. Normal stromal cells can resemble plasma cells, having the same size and an eccentric nucleus. The cytologic features of the nuclei distinguish stromal cells from plasma cells, since the latter have a characteristic clock-face chromatin pattern.

Normal lymphoid aggregates and stromal granular lymphocytes can be difficult to distinguish from an inflammatory infiltrate, especially if the tissue is poorly preserved. Normal lymphoid aggregates, however, are typically widely spaced and located near the basalis and do not include plasma cells. Stromal granular lymphocytes are uniformly distributed throughout the stroma and are most prominent in the late secretory phase. These cells have dark, irregular nuclei that often appear bilobed; their cytoplasm is faintly granular. Stromal granular lymphocytes normally occur in tissue that lacks other features of inflammation, including plasma cells, reactive stroma, and glands that appear out of phase. Granular lymphocytes become especially prominent in decidualized gestational endometrium or in endometrium that shows progestin effect, espe-

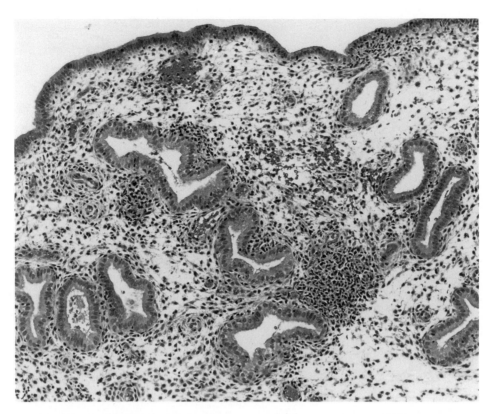

Figure 7.12. Subacute focal inflammation. Patchy chronic inflammatory infiltrate adjacent to glands and vessels in mid secretory endometrium. Plasma cells are sparse. This pattern is associated with mycoplasma infection.

cially when the stroma shows a decidua-like reaction (Chapter 6). In these cases the infiltrate can be so marked that at casual inspection it resembles the lymphoid response seen with endometritis. In such cases the absence of plasma cells is especially helpful in distinguishing this pattern from a true inflammatory response. The presence of decidualized stromal cells, usually containing atrophic glands showing faint secretory activity, indicates that the process is an effect of progesterone or a synthetic progestin.

Neutrophils, like lymphocytes, can be present without indicating an infectious process. They normally occur in areas of stromal necrosis associated with bleeding and in necrotic tissues such as decidua or degenerating polyps. Menstrual endometrium also shows neutrophilic infiltrates as part of the physiologic tissue breakdown. These neutrophilic infiltrates secondary to necrosis and breakdown do not represent infection. They are recognized and separated from infection-related

inflammation by their lack of infiltration into the epithelium as well as their association with glandular and stromal breakdown. On occasion neutrophils also may be found only in gland lumens but not infiltrating the epithelium. This phenomenon apparently is due to entrapment of cellular debris from a previous cycle and is a finding of no known significance.

Inflamed endocervix may also be sampled during endometrial biopsy or curettage. This tissue is a contaminant that has no relevance as long as the endometrium itelf is free of an inflammatory infiltrate. Foci of nonspecific cervical inflammation usually are a minor component of the tissue in endometrial samples. Endocervical epithelium that shows squamous metaplasia or microglandular hyperplasia often is present and helps to identify these foci (Chapter 2).

Another possible contaminant in biopsy specimens consists of aggregates of free-floating histiocytes that do not infiltrate endometrial glands or

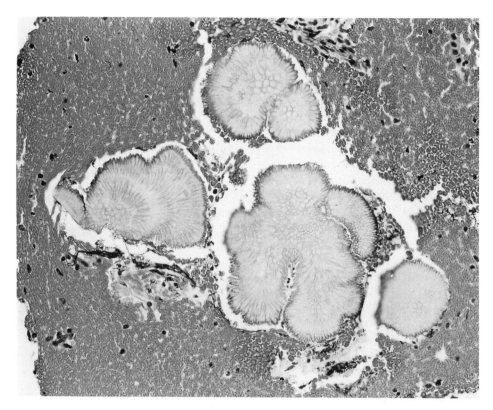

FIGURE 7.13. Pseudoactinomycotic radiate granules. These granular structures superficially resemble sulfur granules of actinomycosis. The filamentous structures are thicker than actinomycosis filaments, however, and do not stain for organisms with Gram or silver stains. The patient had an IUD in place at the time of the biopsy. The endometrium was not inflamed.

stroma. These histiocytes are a response to extracellular mucin in the endocervical canal or cellular debris in the cavity (Chapter 2). Large sheets of histiocytes may be found in curettings following cervical stenosis with obstruction of the os. In the absence of an inflammatory infiltrate in the endometrial stroma that includes plasma cells, these free-floating histiocytes do not indicate inflammation. Immunostains for histiocytes, such as lysozyme or HAM 56, can be very useful for demonstrating these cells.

Pseudosulfur granules, also known as "pseudoactinomycotic radiate granules," may occur in the lower female genital tract, especially in association with an IUD.[43,44] These radiate structurs mimic the appearance of true actinomycotic organisms but actually represent an unusual response (Splendore–Hoeppli phenomenon) to foreign bodies or bacteria (Fig. 7.13). Pseudosulfur granules do not stain with tissue Gram stains or with methenamine-silver, while true actinomyces do. These peculiar structures are not associated with other endometrial abnormalities, including endometritis, and should not be mistaken for actinomycetes.

Inflamed glands may show reactive changes, with nuclear enlargement and prominent nucleoli, and the cytologic features may suggest hyperplasia or neoplasia (Fig. 7.8). In addition, the spindle-shaped, reactive stromal cells of endometritis may be difficult to distinguish from the fibrous stroma of a polyp or from the desmoplasia of carcinoma. The architecture of tubular and uniform glands is usually preserved during inflammation, and it is important to evaluate glands in areas that do not show fragmentation or breakdown. Other underlying abnormalities, such as hyperplasia and neoplasms, may become secondarily inflamed, especially if the lesion or associated bleeding results in dilatation of the internal os with secondary infection. These lesions should retain the typical morphology of the glands and stroma that would allow their diagnosis in the absence of an inflammatory response. There are no data to suggest that chronic inflammation has a significant relationship to the genesis of either hyperplasia or carcinoma of the endometrium. Polyps should be localized abnormalities with at least a partial lining of surface epithelium, and these generally do not contain plasma cells.

Severe chronic endometritis can produce an intense lymphoid infiltrate with large lymphoid cells or immunoblasts that can resemble signs of malignant lymphoma or a leukemic infiltrate.[13-15] Usually with severe inflammation, the cellular infiltrate is mixed, with a combination of plasma cells, neutrophils, and lymphoid cells with follicle formation, whereas lymphoma or leukemic infiltrates usually are composed of a relatively monotonous cell population. Involvement of the endometrium by malignant lymphoma is rare in the absence of disseminated disease. The most common hematologic malignancy to involve the endometrium is non-Hodgkin lymphoma, usually the diffuse large-cell type, but this is a rare finding in biopsy specimens.

Clinical Queries and Reporting

Accurate diagnosis of endometritis is important, since the presence of inflammation can establish a cause for abnormal bleeding or unexplained infertility. Most cases of endometritis have no specific etiology that can be determined by histologic study of the biopsy specimens. When endometritis is present, however, a statement to indicate whether the sections also show a demonstrable cause of the inflammation, such as evidence of a recent pregnancy or an organic lesion, such as a polyp, may be helpful for subsequent clinical management. The presence of such lesions helps to establish the clinical cause and significance of the inflammation.

The intensity of the inflammation also should be noted, especially since severe inflammation with neutrophils in the surface epithelium, a dense subepithelial stromal lymphocytic infiltrate, and lymphoid follicles with transformed lymphocytes raises the possibility of upper genital tract inflammation and salpingitis.

Specific infections, such as tuberculosis or cytomegalovirus, should clearly be indicated when they are present. If special stains for organisms are performed the results should be given in the report.

References

1. Kiviat NB, Wolner-Hanssen P, Eschenbach DA, Wasserheirt JN, Paavonen JA, et al: Endometrial histopathology in patients with culture-proved upper genital tract infection and laparoscopically diagnosed acute salpingitis. Am J Surg Pathol 1990;14:167–175.
2. Paavonen J, Aine R, Teisala K, Heinonen PK, Punnonen R: Comparison of endometrial biopsy and peritoneal fluid cytologic testing with laparoscopy in the diagnosis of acute pelvic inflammatory disease. Am J Obstet Gynecol 1985;151:645–650.
3. Cadena D, Cavanzo FJ, Leone CL, Taylor HB: Chronic endometritis. A comparative clinicopathologic study. Obstet Gynecol 1973;41:733–738.
4. Dallenbach-Hellweg G: Histopathology of the Endometrium. 4th ed. New York: Springer-Verlag, 1987.
5. Rotterdam H: Chronic endometritis. A clinicopathologic study. Pathol Annu 1978;13:209–231.
6. Czernobilsky B: Endometritis and infertility. Fertil Steril 1978;30:119–130.
7. Wallach EE: The uterine factor in infertility. Fertil Steril 1972;23:138–158.
8. Greenwood SM, Moran JJ: Chronic endometritis. Morphologic and clinical observations. Obstet Gynecol 1981;58:176–184.
9. Winkler B, Reumann W, Mitao M, Gallo L, Richart RM, et al: Chlamydial endometritis. A histological and immunohistochemical analysis. Am J Surg Pathol 1984;8:771–778.
10. Buckley CH, Fox H: Biopsy Pathology of the Endometrium. New York: Raven Press, 1989.
11. Kurman RJ, Mazur MT: Benign diseases of the endometrium. In: Blaustein's Pathology of the Female Genital Tract. 4th ed. Kurman RJ, ed. News York: Springer-Verlag, 1994;367–409.
12. Crum CP, Egawa K, Fenoglio CM, Richart RM: Chronic endometritis. The role of immunohistochemistry in the detection of plasma cells. Am J Obstet Gynecol 1983;147:812–815.
13. Young RH, Harris NL, Scully RE: Lymphoma-like lesions of the lower female genital tract. A report of 16 cases. Int J Gynecol Pathol 1985; 4:289–299.

14. Ferry JA, Young RH: Malignant lymphoma, pseudolymphoma, and hematopoietic disorders of the female genital tract. Pathol Annu 1991;26:227–263.

15. Skensved H, Hansen A, Vetner M: Immunoreactive endometritis. Br J Obstet Gynaecol 1991;98:578–582.

16. Miko Tl, Lampe LG, Thomazy VA, Molnar P, Endes P: Eosinophilic endomyometritis associated with diagnostic curettage. Int J Gynecol Pathol 1988;7:162–172.

17. Ladefoged C, Lorentzen M: Xanthogranulomatous inflammation of the female genital tract. Histopathology 1988;13:541–551.

18. Russack V, Lammers RJ: Xanthogranulomatous endometritis. Arch Pathol Lab Med 1990;114:929–932.

19. Lopez JI, Nevado M: Exuberant xanthogranulomatous-like reaction following endometrial curettage. Histopathology 1989;15:315–322.

20. Shintaku M, Sasaki M, Baba Y: Ceroid-containing histiocytic granuloma of the endometrium. Histopathology 1991;18:169–172.

21. Paavonen J, Aine R, Teisala K, Heinonen PK, Punonen R, et al: Chlamydial endometritis. J Clin Pathol 1985;38:726–732.

22. Bazaz-Malik G, Maheshwari B, Lal N: Tuberculous endometritis. A clinicopathological study of 1000 cases. Br J Obstet Gynaecol 1983;90:84–86.

23. Nogales-Ortiz F, Tarancon I, Nogales FF: The pathology of female genital tuberculosis. A 31-year study of 1436 cases. Obstet Gynecol 1979;53:422–428.

23a. Shireman PK: Endometrial tuberculosis acquired by a health care worker in a clinical laboratory. Arch Pathol Lab Med 1992;116: 521–523.

24. Schaefer G, Marcus RS, Kramer EE: Postmenopausal endometrial tuberculosis. Am J Obstet Gynecol 1972;112:681-687.

25. Govan ADT: Tuberculous endometritis. J Pathol Bacteriol 1962;83:363–372.

26. Frank TS, Himebaugh KS, Wilson MD: Granulomatous endometritis associated with histologically occult cytomegalovirus in a healthy patient. Am J Surg Pathol 1992;16:716–720.

27. Ho K-L: Sarcoidosis of the uterus. Hum Pathol 1979;10:219–222.

28. Ferryman SR, Stephens M, Gough D: Necrotising granulomatous endometritis following endometrial ablation therapy. Br J Obstet Gynaecol 1992;99:928–930.

29. Ashworth MI, Moss CT, Kenyon WE: Granulomatous endometritis following hysteroscopic resection of the endometrium. Histopathology 1991;18:185–187.

30. Sayage L, Gunby R, Gonwa T, Husberg B, Goldstein R, et al: Cytomegalovirus endometritis after liver transplantation. Transplantation 1990;49:815–817.

31. Brodman M, Deligdisch L: Cytomegalovirus endometritis in a patient with AIDS. Mt Sinai J Med (NY) 1986;53:673–675.

32. Dehner LP, Askin FB: Cytomegalovirus endometritis: Report of a case associated with spontaneous abortion. Obstet Gynecol 1975;45:211–214.

33. McCracken AW, A'Agostino AN, Brucks AB, Kingsley WB: Acquired cytomegalovirus infection presenting as viral endometritis. Am J Clin Pathol 1974;61:556–560.

34. Goldman RL: Herpetic inclusions in the endometrium. Obstet Gynecol 1970;36:603–605.

35. Abraham AA: Herpes virus hominis endometritis in a young woman wearing an intrauterine contraceptive device. Am J Obstet Gynecol 1978;131:340–342.

36. Schneider V, Behm FG, Mumau VR: Ascending herpetic endometritis. Obstet Gynecol 1982;58:259–262.

37. Duncan DA, Varner RE, Mazur MT: Uterine herpes virus infection with mutifocal necrotizing endometritis. Hum Pathol 1989;20:1021–1024.

38. Mazur MT, Hendrickson MR, Kempson RL: Optically clear nuclei. An alteration of endometrial epithelium in the presence of trophoblast. Am J Surg Pathol 1983;7:415–423.

39. Dardi LE, Ariano L, Ariano MC, Gould VE: Arias-Stella reaction with prominent nuclear pseudoinclusions simulating herpetic endometritis. Diag Gynecol Obstet 1982;4:127–132.

40. Horne HW, Hertig AT, Kundsin RB, Kosasa TS: Sub-clinical endometrial inflammation and T-mycoplasma. A possible cause of human reproductive failure. Int J Fertil 1973;18:226–231.

41. Burke RK, Hertig AT, Miele CA: Prognostic value of subacute focal inflammation of the endometrium, with special reference to pelvic adhesions as observed on laparoscopic examination. An eight-year review. J Reprod Med 1985;30:646–650.

42. Khatamee MA, Sommers SC: Clinicopathologic diagnosis of mycoplasma endometritis. Int J Fertil 1989;34:52–59.

43. O'Brien PK, Roth-Moyo LA, Davis BA: Pseudo-sulfur granules associated with intrauterine contraceptive devices. Am J Clin Pathol 1981;75:822–825.

44. Bhagavan BS, Ruffier J, Shinn B: Pseudoactinomycotic radiate granules in the lower female genital tract. Relationship to the Splendore–Hoeppli phenomenon. Hum Pathol 1982;13:898–904.

8
Polyps

Most endometrial polyps appear to originate from localized hyperplasia of the basalis, although their pathogenesis is not well understood. Polyps occur over a wide age range, but are most common in women in the fourth and fifth decades, becoming less frequent after age 60.[1–3] Usually they present with abnormal uterine bleeding.[4] They have been implicated as a cause of abnormal bleeding in between 2% and 23% of patients coming to biopsy.[2,5–7] They also have been implicated as a possible cause of infertility, either by physically interfering with blastocyst implantation or by altering the development of secretory phase endometrium, making it less receptive to the implanting embryo.[8–11] A few endometrial polyps have been found in patients receiving tamoxifen therapy for breast carcinoma.[12,13] Large polyps that extend into the endocervix and dilate the internal os can cause endometritis. In general, polyps are benign growths with no malignant potential.[4] Occasional cases of carcinoma, including serous carcinoma and even mixed mesodermal tumors, can be confined to a polyp.[3,14–20] Furthermore, polyps have been associated with the occurrence of carcinoma in several studies.[3,21–23] Nonetheless, ployps are not regarded as a major risk factor for the development of carcinoma. Most lesions are successfully treated with curettage or hysteroscopic excision.

The large variation in the reported prevalence of polyps reflects the difficulties in establishing the histologic diagnosis. Polyps often are fragmented and removed piecemeal at curettage and therefore they can be difficult to recognize. Hysteroscopy can be useful to confirm the diagnosis of polyp,[5,24] although in one study as many as 13% of polyp-like structures seen by hysteroscopy were not confirmed histologically.[2]

Classification and Histologic Features

Polyps vary greatly in size, ranging from microscopic abnormalities that are only a few millimeters across to huge lesions that can fill the uterine cavity or prolapse through the endocervical canal. Usually polyps are small and solitary, but they can be large or multiple. They can be sessile or pedunculated. The glands and stroma of endometrial polyps can show diverse histologic patterns.[1,3,4,25–27] There are six morphologic forms of endometrial polyps: hyperplastic, atrophic, functional, mixed endometrial–endocervical, adenomyomatous, and the atypical polypoid adenomyoma (Table 8.1).[1] This classification has little clinical significance but is useful for correct iden-

TABLE 8.1. Classification of endometrial polyps.

Hyperplastic
Atrophic
Functional
Mixed endometrial–endocervical
Adenomyomatous
Atypical polypoid adenomyoma

TABLE 8.2. Histologic features of polyps.

Larger tissue fragments
   Polypoid shape
   Surface epithelium on three sides
Dense stroma
Thick-walled arteries
Glands dilated and more tortuous than normal glands
   Glands appear "out of phase" or hyperplastic
Separate fragments of normal endometrial tissue

tification of these lesions and separation of some polyps from hyperplasia.

Each type of polyp is identified by the changes that occur in the glands and stroma.[1,4] Despite their diverse growth patterns, all polyps show several histologic features that facilitate their diagnosis (Table 8.2). One important feature of polyps in biopsy specimens is the presence of large, polypoid tissue fragments (Fig. 8.1). These large fragments tend to be lined on three sides by surface epithelium. Often much smaller fragments of normal endometrium are admixed with the large fragments of a polyp. Polyps also commonly show dense stroma. In addition, they frequently contain thick-walled vessels, especially when they become large. Small veins in the superficial stroma become ectatic. The glands in polyps are irregular in shape and have a highly variable architecture. They may be focally crowded. The

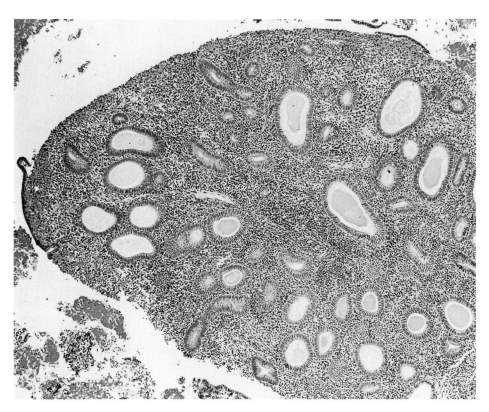

FIGURE 8.1. Hyperplastic polyp. The glands in the polyp are irregular and the stroma is dense. In contrast to the other tissue fragments that showed atrophic endometrium, this large polypoid fragment of tissue represents a polyp.

glands lack the uniform orientation of normal endometrial glands and may lose their perpendicular orientation to surface epithelium and course parallel to the surface. In secretory endometrium the irregularly shaped glands often lack normal development and appear to be "out of phase."[2] These irregular glands can also appear as focal hyperplasia in a background of proliferative or atrophic endometrium.

In addition to these characteristic features, polyps may show evidence of focal glandular and stromal breakdown, usually due to thrombosis of the dilated superficial veins (Chapter 5). Chronic bleeding leads to hemosiderin deposition in the stroma. Occasionally a larger polyp will show extensive ischemic necrosis of the distal portion. The specific features of each type of polyp that assist in the pathologic classification are given below.

Hyperplastic Polyps

Hyperplastic polyps are most common. They are highly variable in size, measuring up to several centimeters in greatest dimension (Fig. 8.1). They often are only diagnosed on microscopic examination. Regardless of size, they show irregular, proliferating glands with pseudostratified nuclei and mitotic activity (Figs. 8.2–8.4). The glands generally resemble those in hyperplasia without atypia, either simple or complex (Chapter 9). The surface and glandular epithelium in hyperplastic polyps often shows epithelial cytoplasmic changes. These include squamous, eosinophilic, and ciliated cell changes (Fig. 8.5). Cytoplasmic changes usually occur in the glands, but sometimes they occur along the surface where they can be focal or extensive.

Hyperplastic polyps usually have a moderate

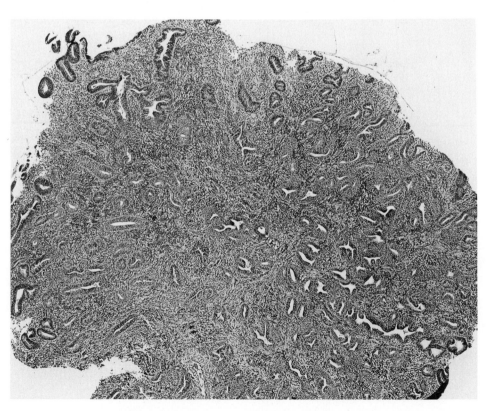

FIGURE 8.2. Hyperplastic polyp. The irregularly shaped glands resemble those in hyperplasia. In contrast to the diffuse process that characterizes hyperplasia, this was a focal abnormality. The remaining endometrium was proliferative.

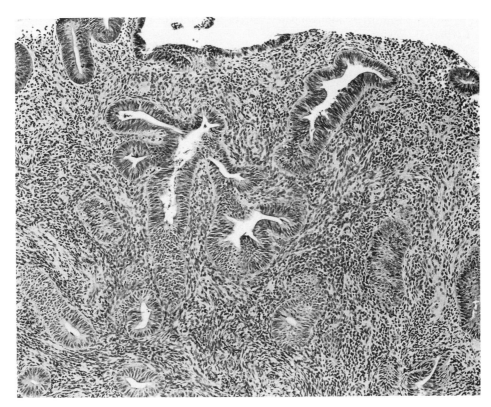

FIGURE 8.3. Hyperplastic polyp. Higher magnification of polyp in Fig. 8.2 shows irregular glands with pseudo-stratified nuclei. The dense stroma is a feature of polyps. The presence of proliferative endometrium elsewhere in the curettings distinguishes a polyp from hyperplasia, which tends to be diffuse.

amount of intervening stroma between the glands, but sometimes the glands are closely packed. The stroma is dense and compact but otherwise similar to the stroma of proliferative phase endometrium. Larger polyps typically have clusters of thick-walled arteries in dense stroma.

Identifying endometrium not involved by the polyp is especially helpful for accurate diagnosis of a hyperplastic polyp, since the polyp may resemble a diffuse hyperplasia. The endometrium that is not involved by the polyp is usually proliferative or atrophic, but sometimes it is secretory.

Atrophic Polyps

Atrophic polyps, also know as "inactive polyps," are usually seen in postmenopausal women. These polyps contain atrophic glands lined by low columnar epithelium showing no mitotic ac-tivity. The glands often are dilated with round contours, and the stroma appears dense and fibrotic (Fig. 8.6). Many of these polyps apparently represent hyperplastic polyps that no longer show proliferative activity.

Functional Polyps

These polyps, like the endometrium around them, are hormonally responsive and show proliferative or secretory changes. They occur in premenopausal patients and can be difficult to diagnose. Features such as a polypoid shape, dense stroma, and thick-walled vessels are helpful for their recognition (Fig. 8.7). Unlike normal glands, the glands in the functional polyp lose their orientation to surface epithelium and have a haphazard distribution. In well-oriented fragments, the glands may appear to branch toward the surface like veins on a leaf. The stroma in

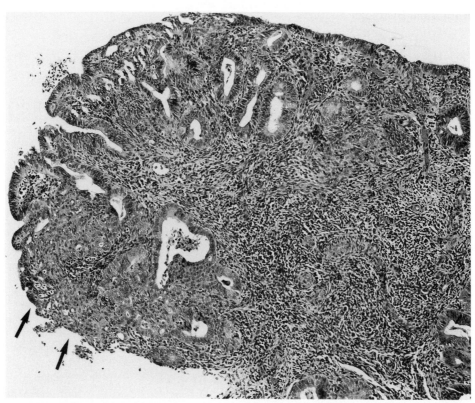

FIGURE 8.4. Hyperplastic polyp. Small polyp with irregular, crowded glands showing focal squamous change (*arrows*).

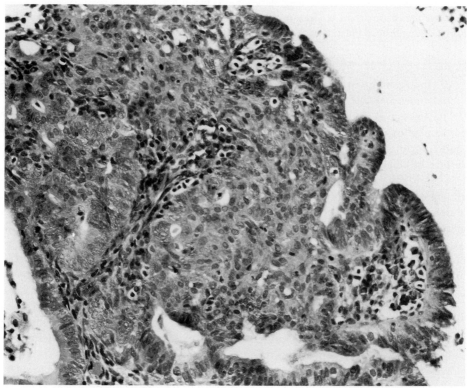

FIGURE 8.5. Squamous change in hyperplastic polyp. High magnification of area in a polyp shows nonkeratinizing squamous change. Same case as Fig. 8.4.

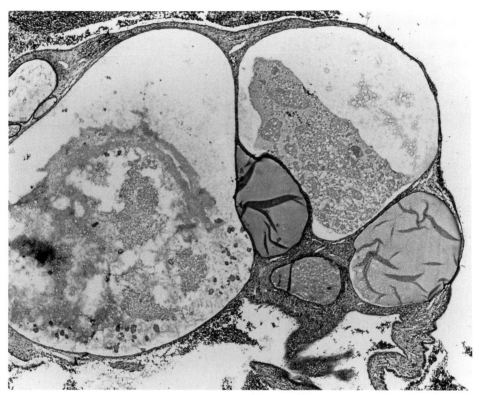

FIGURE 8.6. Atrophic polyp. Polyp with cystic glands lined by atrophic epithelium.

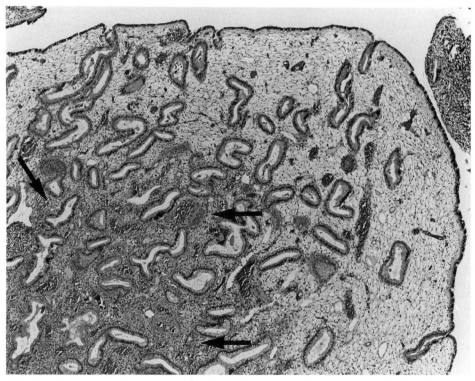

FIGURE 8.7. Functional polyp. Irregular glands with early secretory changes surrounded by edematous stroma. The stalk of the polyp has dense stroma and thick-walled vessels (*arrows*).

151

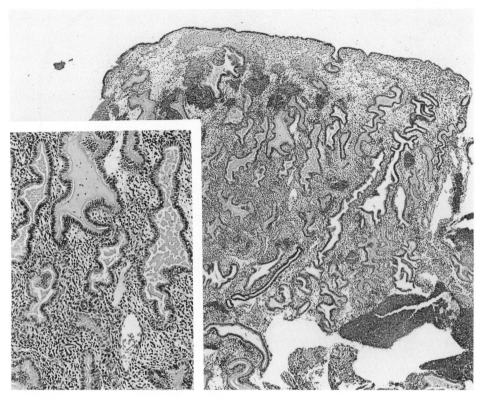

FIGURE 8.8. Functional polyp. Polypoid tissue fragment shows irregular secretory glands with dense central stroma and superficial edema. Endometrium elsewhere in the sections showed a normal mid secretory phase pattern. *Inset*: The glands show secretory exhaustion and the stroma is dense.

a polyp may show edema or predecidual change but often is dense and inactive. When polyps have secretory changes, the glands often are not as well developed as those in the surrounding endometrium (Fig. 8.8). The result is that they appear to be "out of phase" and the stroma shows decreased edema and predecidual formation. Some examples of "dyssynchronous" endometrium probably represent functional polyps that are too fragmented for accurate diagnosis.

Mixed Endometrial–Endocervical Polyps

Some polyps originate in the upper endocervix and lower uterine segment and show both endocervical and endometrial-type gland development (Fig. 8.9). These polyps tend to have a fibrous stroma resembling the stroma of the lower uterine segment.

Adenomyomatous Polyps

These polyps have smooth muscle in their stroma, usually as irregular bundles and strands in proximity to thick-walled vessels. Most often these are large hyperplastic polyps in which the stroma has undergone partial smooth muscle change. Although smooth muscle is present, the glands are invested by stroma.

Atypical Polypoid Adenomyoma

This is an unusual and distinctive polyp characterized by glands that are lined by atypical epithelium and surrounded by cellular smooth muscle (Fig. 8.10).[28,29] It typically occurs in premenopausal or perimenopausal women, with a mean age of about 40 years. We have seen these lesions in women as old as 56, however. A few cases have been associated with Turner syndrome and appear to be a complication of long-term estrogenic

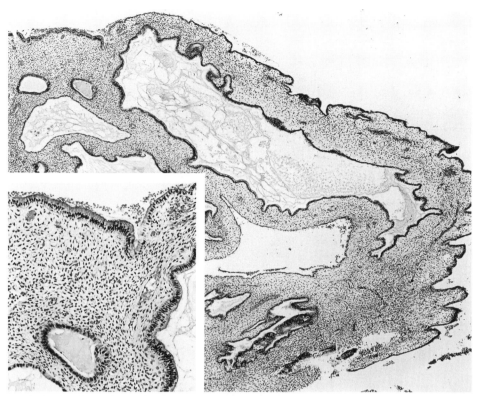

FIGURE 8.9. Mixed endometrial–endocervical polyp. This polyp occurred in a 60-year-old and is characterized by irregular, dilated glands in fibrous stroma. *Inset*: the epithelium is partially endocervical-type with columnar mucinous cells.

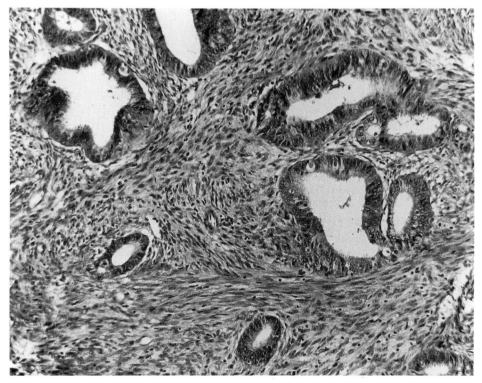

FIGURE 8.10. Atypical polypoid adenomyoma. Irregular, atypical glands are haphazardly distributed in smooth muscle. The smooth muscle has a characteristic pattern of short, interlacing fascicles.

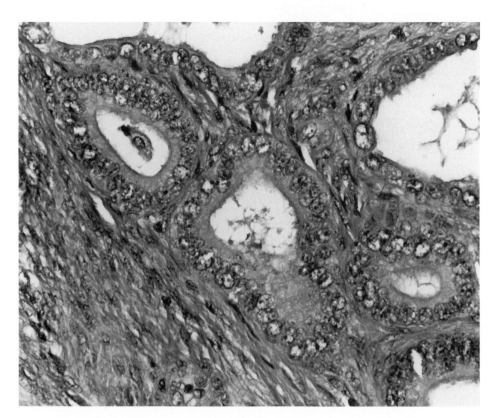

FIGURE 8.11. Atypical polypoid adenomyoma. The glandular epithelium is atypical with enlarged, stratified nuclei that have clumped chromatin and prominent nucleoli.

stimulation of the endometrium.[30] Often these lesions arise in the lower uterine segment, but they can also arise in the corpus.[29]

The glands of the atypical polypoid adenomyoma are haphazardly arranged but generally are not markedly crowded or back-to-back. They resemble the glands in simple atypical hyperplasia. The glandular cells have enlarged, stratified, and rounded nuclei with a vesicular chromatin pattern and prominent nucleoli (Fig. 8.11). The cytoplasm is eosinophilic and the glands resemble those found in atypical hyperplasia (Chapter 9). The glands often show squamous change (metaplasia), containing central nonkeratinizing nests of squamous cells (Fig. 8.12). Central necrosis may occur in the squamous nests.

Smooth muscle encompasses the glands, and endometrial stroma is largely absent. The smooth muscle is arranged in short interlacing fascicles that contrast with the elongate bundles of smooth muscle found in normal myometrium or in adenomyomatous polyps (Fig. 8.10). The smooth muscle component can show increased mitotic activity, with up to two mitoses per 10 high-power fields (HPFs), but there is no evidence of cytologic atypia. The smooth muscle is diffusely reactive for desmin.

As with any type of polyp, the endometrium not involved by the atypical polypoid adenomyoma can be highly variable and can show proliferative, secretory, gestational, or hyperplastic changes. The atypical polypoid adenomyoma often presents in curettings as large polypoid tissue fragments admixed with small fragments of noninvolved endometrium. There have been a few reports of endometrial adenocarcinoma in association with an atypical polypoid adenomyoma, and we have seen similar cases.[30a,30b] Usually this lesion does not show aggressive growth, however, and curettage may be curative.

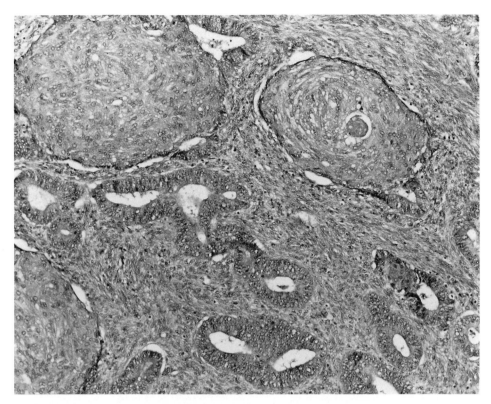

FIGURE 8.12. Atypical polypoid adenomyoma. Large nests of squamous cells fill several of the glands. Focal necrosis is present in the center of one of the squamous nests. This necrosis is a common finding in atypical polypoid adenomyomas and has no significance.

Differential Diagnosis

Endometrial polyps may be difficult to identify in curettings and are often missed. When the specimen is large and polypoid-shaped, has surface epithelium covering three sides, and contains dense stroma with thick-walled vessels, the diagnosis is straightforward. Often polyps are microscopic abnormalities or they are highly fragmented by the biopsy procedure. Because of fragmentation and lack of clear-cut diagnostic features, the differential diagnosis often includes normal proliferative or secretory endometrium. Subtle features, such as irregular gland shape and distribution and somewhat denser stroma, are helpful in the recognition of a small polyp that is admixed with normal proliferative or secretory endometrium.

Tangential sectioning of normal endometrium is a frequent consideration in the differential di-

agnosis of small and fragmented polyps. Basalis, especially, can resemble a polyp because it has irregular glands, dense stroma, and prominent arteries. Basalis, however, lacks a lining of surface epithelium and does not have a polypoid shape. The vessels in basalis consist of small aggregates of radial arteries, usually numbering six or more in cross section. Levels through the tissue block often show transitions to normal functionalis if the area in question represents basalis. Conversely, if the tissue represents a true polyp, the step sections often reveal surface epithelium, at least focally.

The fibroblastic spindle-cell stromal response that occurs in endometritis may resemble the fibrous stroma of a polyp. However, with inflammation, there is a plasma cell infiltrate in the stroma, and the epithelium also may be infiltrated by neutrophils.

Irregular polypoid tissue due to progestin effect

also may superficially resemble a polyp in a biopsy or curettage specimen. These specimens usually contain atrophic glands and a decidua-like stroma. The finding of normal endometrium admixed with polypoid tissue fragments is helpful for identifying polyps in questionable cases.

Diffuse hyperplasia (Chapter 9) is also included in the differential diagnosis of polyp, especially the hyperplastic polyp. Both polyps and hyperplasia have an irregular proliferation of glands with a variable amount of stroma. Hyperplasia, furthermore, often becomes polypoid. Hyperplasia is a diffuse process, however, usually affecting all or most of the endometrium, while polyps are focal and admixed with normal, nonhyperplastic endometrium. In small biopsies the distinction may not be possible, and the question of whether a small polypoid fragment of tissue represents a portion of a polyp or an area from a diffuse hyperplasia cannot be resolved. Dilatation and curet-

tage or hysteroscopy may be necessary to establish the correct diagnosis.

A large hyperplastic polyp also may resemble adenosarcoma (Chapter 11), since both lesions are polypoid with hyperplastic glands. Adenosarcoma typically has a leaflike pattern with broad-based papillae lined by surface epithelium. In contrast, a polyp has a smooth outline. In addition, adenosarcoma, unlike benign polyps, has a more cellular stroma with increased mitotic activity that aggregates in cuffs around the glands. Polyps have fibrous stroma that lacks prominent cellularity and has a low mitotic rate. Large polyps typically have thick-walled vessels, which are lacking in adenosarcoma.

The differential diagnosis for functional polyps includes changes due to ovulatory dysfunction, such as luteal phase defect (LPD) or exogenous hormone effects. These polyps show secretory changes that are out of phase with the surround-

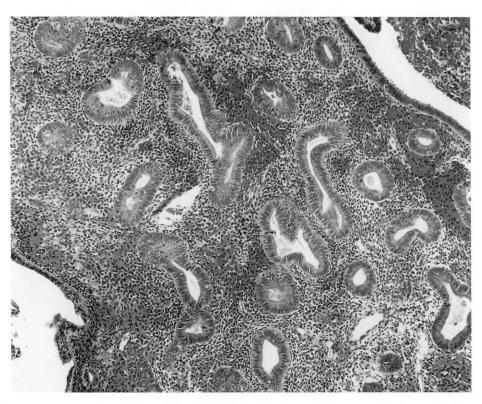

FIGURE 8.13. Adhesion. Intrauterine adhesion with irregular glands in dense stroma. This lesion was identified by hysteroscopy in a 23-year-old patient who was being evaluated for infertility. She had no known risk factors for the development of adhesions.

ing endometrium. Functional polyps are composed of polypoid tissue fragments covered with surface epithelium and containing dense stroma and thick-walled vessels. Surrounding fragments of endometrium that show normal secretory changes are especially helpful for establishing the diagnosis of a functional polyp.

The atypical polypoid adenomyoma may resemble carcinoma because it shows atypical glands in smooth muscle. The glands in the atypical polypoid adenomyoma, however, do not fulfill criteria for well-differentiated adenocarcinoma, lacking features of invasion such as cribriform or confluent growth (Chapter 9). It is extremely unusual to find well-differentiated or moderately differentiated adenocarcinoma invading myometrial smooth muscle in endometrial curettings. Accordingly, in curettings atypical glands surrounded by smooth muscle represent an atypical polypoid adenomyoma until proven otherwise. Squamous change is common in the atypical polypoid adenomyoma but also can occur in adenocarcinoma or hyperplasia. In atypical polypoid adenomyoma with squamous change, however, the affected glands are invested by smooth muscle, and this is an important feature that helps to identify the lesion (Fig. 8.11). The rare examples of adenocarcinoma occurring in association with atypical polypoid adenomyoma show typical endometrioid features without smooth muscle investing the malignant glands.[30a,30b]

Adhesions

Endometrial adhesions are bands of tissue that bridge the endometrial cavity. These may consist of fibrous tissue that forms as a result of inflammation associated with an abortion or pregnancy, and their presence is known as Asherman syndrome.[1,9,31,32] In these cases the endometrium is largely replaced by a proliferation of fibroblasts, but this is an extraordinarily rare finding in biopsy material.

We have observed, on occasion, another type of intrauterine adhesion formed by a band of endometrial tissue with dense stroma and small, nonreactive glands. This form of adhesion typically is found in premenopausal women and its etiology is

not known. Because such adhesions consist of dense stroma and poorly developed glands, they may be indistinguishable from fragments of a polyp (Fig. 8.13). Correlation of histologic features with other information, such as hysteroscopic findings, may be necessary to establish the diagnosis.

Clinical Queries and Reporting

Diagnosis of a polyp is important because its presence often offers an explanation for why a patient has abnormal bleeding. On the other hand, classification of polyps is of importance to the pathologist as an aid for recognition, but is of little relevance to the gynecologist for therapeutic decisions. In fact, subclassification of polyps may unnecessarily complicate the pathologic report. Usually it is only important to indicate that a benign polyp is present. Often a comment regarding the status of endometrium not involved by the polyp also can be helpful for the gynecologist. For instance, if curettings in a postmenopausal patient show a polyp and separate fragments of atrophic endometrium, a comment or diagnosis that reflects all of these observations is warranted, since it also indicates the status of the endometrium not involved by the primary lesion. This type of interpretive comment helps the gynecologist understand that the endometrial cavity has been sampled beyond the focal polyp.

When the atypical polypoid adenomyoma is diagnosed, a comment should be included to describe the lesion, because most gynecologists are not familiar with it. It is necessary to indicate that the lesion is benign and that it does not represent atypical hyperplasia or carcinoma.

At times endometrial sampling may yield tissue suggestive, but not diagnostic, of a polyp. Small samples and markedly fragmented tissue may show features suggestive of a polyp but can be especially difficult to accurately diagnose. In limited samples, small fragments of polypoid tissue with hyperplastic glands may represent portions of a hyperplastic polyp or they may represent a sample of a diffuse hyperplasia. In such cases, a descriptive diagnosis to indicate the presence of an abnormality, coupled with a microscopic description of the findings, is most helpful to the clinician. If the diagnosis is not straightforward, further evaluation, including a dilatation and curettage or hysteroscopy, may be necessary to establish the correct diagnosis.

References

1. Kurman RJ, Mazur MT: Benign diseases of the endometrium. In: Blaustein's Pathology of the Female Genital Tract. 4th ed. Kurman RJ, ed. New York: Springer-Verlag, 1994;367–409.

2. Van Bogaert L-J: Clinicopathologic findings in endometrial polyps. Obstet Gynecol 1988;71: 771–773.

3. Peterson WF, Novak ER: Endometrial polyps. Obstet Gynecol 1956;8:40–49.

4. Schlaen I, Bergeron C, Ferenczy A, Wong P, Naves A, et al: Endometrial polyps: A study of 204 cases. Surg Pathol 1988;1:375–382.

5. Loffer FD: Hysteroscopy with selective endometrial sampling compared with D&C for abnormal uterine bleeding. The value of a negative hysteroscopic view. Obstet Gynecol 1989;73:16–20.

6. Schindler AE, Schmidt G: Post-menopausal bleeding: A study of more than 1000 cases. Maturitas 1980;2:269–274.

7. Choo YC, Mak KC, Hsu C, Wong TS, Ma HK: Postmenopausal uterine bleeding of nonorganic cause. Obstet Gynecol 1985;66:225–228.

8. Dallenbach-Hellweg G: The endometrium of infertility. A review. Pathol Res Pract 1984;178: 527–537.

9. Wallach EE: The uterine factor in infertility. Fertil Steril 1972;23:138–158.

10. Foss BA, Horne HW, Hertig AT: The endometrium and sterility. Fertil Steril 1958;9:193–206.

11. Sillo-Seidl G: The analysis of the endometrium of 1,000 sterile women. Hormones 1971;2:70–75.

12. Nuovo MA, Nuovo GJ, McCaffrey FM, Levine RU, Barron B, et al: Endometrial polyps in postmenopausal patients receiving tamoxifen. Int J Gynecol Pathol 1989;8:125–131.

13. Corley D, Rowe J, Curtis MT, Hongan WM, Noumoff JS, et al: Postmenopausal bleeding from unusual endometrial polyps in women on chronic tamoxifen therapy. Obstet Gynecol 1992;79:111–116.

14. Dinh TV, Slavin RE, Bhagavan BS, Hannigan EV, Timason EM, et al: Mixed mullerian tumors of the uterus. A clinicopathologic study. Obstet Gynecol 1989;74:388-392.

15. Salm R: The incidence and significance of early carcinomas in endometrial polyps. J Pathol 1972; 108:47–53.

16. Wolfe SA, Mackles A: Malignant lesions arising from benign endometrial polyps. Obstet Gynecol 1962;20:542–550.

17. Silva EG, Jenkins R: Serous carcinoma in endometrial polyps. Mod Pathol 1990;3:120–128.

18. Kahner S, Ferenczy A, Richart RM: Homologous mixed mullerian tumors (carcinosarcoma) confined to endometrial polyps. Am J Obstet Gynecol 1975;121:278–279.

19. Barwick KW, Livolsi VA: Heterologous mixed mullerian tumor confined to an endometrial polyp. Obstet Gynecol 1979;53:512–514.

20. Silverberg SG, Major FJ, Blessing JA, Fetter B, Askin FB, et al: Carcinosarcoma (malignant mixed mesodermal tumor) of the uterus. A Gynecologic Oncology Group pathologic study of 203 cases. Int J Gynecol Pathol 1990;9:1–19.

21. Pettersson B, Adami H-O, Lindgren A, Hesselius I: Endometrial polyps and hyperplasia as risk factors for endometrial carcinoma. A case-control study of curettage specimens. Acta Obstet Gynecol Scand 1985;64:653–659.

22. Armenia CS: Sequential relationship between endometrial polyps and carcinoma of the endometrium. Obstet Gynecol 1967;30:524–529.

23. Gray LA, Robertson RW, Jr, Christopherson WM: Atypical endometrial changes associated with carcinoma. Gynecol Oncol 1974;2:93–100.

24. Fraser IS: Hysteroscopy and laparoscopy in women with menorrhagia. Am J Obstet Gynecol 1990;162:1264–1269.

25. Dallenbach-Hellweg G: Histopathology of the Endometrium. 4th ed. New York: Springer-Verlag, 1987.

26. Silverberg SG, Kurman RJ: Tumors of the uterine corpus and gestational trophoblastic disease. Atlas of Tumor Pathology, 3rd series, Fascicle 3. Washington, DC: Armed Forces Institute of Pathology, 1992.

27. Buckley CH, Fox H: Biopsy Pathology of the Endometrium. New York: Raven Press, 1989.

28. Mazur MT: Atypical polypoid adenomyomas of the endometrium. Am J Surg Pathol 1981;5: 473–482.

29. Young RH, Treger T, Scully RE: Atypical polypoid adenomyoma of the uterus. A report of 27 cases. Am J Clin Pathol 1986;86:139–145.

30. Clement PB, Young RH: Atypical polypoid adenomyoma of the uterus associated with Turner's syndrome. Int J Gynecol Pathol 1987;6:104–113.

30a. Lee KR: Atypical polypoid adenomyoma of the endometrium associated with adenomyomatosis and adenocarcinoma. Gynecol Oncol 1993;51: 416–418.

30b. Staros EB, Shilkitus WF: Atypical polypoid adenomyoma with carcinomatous transformation: A case report. Surg Pathol 1991;4:157–166.

31. Friedler S, Margalioth EJ, Kafka I, Yaffe H: Incidence of post-abortion intra-uterine adhesions evaluated by hysteroscopy. A prospective study. Hum Reprod 1993;8:442–444.

32. Schenker JG, Margalioth EJ: Intrauterine adhesions: An updated appraisal. Fertil Steril 1982; 37:593–610.

9
Endometrial Hyperplasia and Epithelial Cytoplasmic Change

Endometrial hyperplasia is a nonphysiologic, noninvasive proliferation of the endometrium that results in a morphologic pattern of glands with irregular shapes and varying size.[1-6] This disorder results from sustained, unopposed estrogen stimulation and presents clinically as abnormal uterine bleeding. Sometimes hyperplasia is encountered incidentally in biopsies done for other reasons, such as an infertility workup or prior to or during hormone replacement therapy. Hyperplasia can mimic a wide variety of normal physiologic changes, artifacts resulting from tissue sampling and processing, benign organic disorders, and well-differentiated adenocarcinoma. Since management of these conditions and the different forms of hyperplasia can range from no treatment to hysterectomy, correct diagnosis is essential.

Hyperplasia occurs most frequently in perimenopausal women, since they frequently have anovulatory cycles, but also occurs in postmenopausal women who either have excess endogenous estrogen levels or are receiving exogenous estrogen.[1,3] Hyperplasia may arise on occasion in young women, including teenagers, since sporadic anovulation occurs in the reproductive ages and anovulatory cycles are frequent in adolescents.[7-9] In the reproductive years, women with chronic anovulation associated with the Stein–Leventhal syndrome (polycystic ovaries) are especially prone to develop hyperplasia. Sometimes hyperplasia occurs when there is no apparent underlying endocrinologic disorder. Recent studies have shown that there are two forms of hyperplasia, one (atypical) that is closely linked to adenocarcinoma, being an apparent precursor lesion, and another form (nonatypical) that is largely self-limited with little apparent relationship to carcinoma.[1,3,5,8,10-17]

The subject of epithelial metaplasia is closely linked to the topic of hyperplasia, because so-called metaplasia occurs frequently in hyperplasia.[1,4,18-22] Most of these lesions actually represent alterations of the epithelium that are either a degenerative or regenerative "change" and not truly metaplastic. These cellular changes are not unique to hyperplasia, however, and occur in a variety of other conditions. These alterations often mimic the cellular features of hyperplasia and therefore complicate the interpretation.

Refinements in the classification of endometrial hyperplasia and related cellular changes reflect our increased understanding of endometrial pathology. Introduction of new terminology and classification, however, is always met with resistance, and statements such as "I *used* to understand hyperplasia" express the frustration of some pathologists and gynecologists who are trying to utilize these new terms. The current classification and recognition of superimposed non-hyperplastic cellular changes actually assist in correctly diagnosing hyperplasia. This chapter reviews the current classification and morphologic features of endometrial hyperplasia as well as their differential diagnosis. Related epithelial changes (metaplasia) and artifactual alterations are included, since they are an integral part of the differential diagnosis.

Terminology and Classification of Hyperplasia

The diagnosis and management of endometrial hyperplasia have been unnecessarily complicated by the use of a wide variety of terms and histologic classifications. Terms such as adenomatous hyperplasia, atypical hyperplasia, and carcinoma in situ have been employed by different authors for the same lesions, and, conversely, different investigators have used the same term to describe different lesions.[3,6,10,15–18,23] The distinction of atypical hyperplasia from well-differentiated adenocarcinoma has been further clouded by the term "carcinoma in situ."[15,17,23] The confusion resulting from the use of different classifications has often precluded comparison of data between institutions and has created problems in communication between the gynecologist and the pathologist. Recently, the World Health Organization (WHO) and the International Society of Gynecologic Pathologists (ISGYP) have promoted one classification of endometrial hyperplasia that has gained widespread acceptance (Table 9.1).[1,4,24] The basic feature of this classification is the separation of hyperplasia into non-

atypical and atypical forms. The glandular complexity has secondary importance. Thus, hyperplasia without atypia and atypical hyperplasia are both divided into simple and complex categories. These latter terms give a general assessment of the degree of gland crowding and irregularity.

Although the terminology of "adenomatous hyperplasia" is retained parenthetically for complex patterns with or without cytologic atypia, the term "adenomatous" is best avoided because of its nonstandardized use in earlier publications. Lesions previously classified as carcinoma in situ are now included in the category of atypical hyperplasia, and the former term has been abandoned. Consequently, borderline lesions are classified as either atypical hyperplasia or invasive well-differentiated adenocarcinoma. With the use of a single classification, refined morphologic criteria, and better understanding of the behavior of these lesions, the diagnosis of hyperplasia in a biopsy specimen should allow the gynecologist to individualize patient management.

Pathologic Features of Hyperplasia

All types of hyperplasia share certain morphologic features. They all show an increase in the gland-to-stroma ratio, irregularities in gland shape, and variation in gland size.[1,4,5,25,26] In addition, mitotic activity is evident, although the level is variable and often less than that observed in proliferative endometrium. The uterus is often, but not invariably, enlarged, and tissue obtained at curettage may be considerable, sometimes yielding enough to fill three or more tissue cassettes. On the other hand there may be a limited volume of tissue, especially from office-based biopsies. Accordingly, volume alone does not influence the diagnosis.

Architectural alterations, characterized by glandular complexity and the amount of stroma separating the glands, distinguish simple and complex forms of hyperplasia, regardless of the presence of atypia. Hyperplasia is generally a diffuse abnormality, involving much of the endometrium, but also may display an exuberant, heaped-up growth, resulting in polypoid configurations. At times, hyperplasia, especially atypical hyperplasia, may be focal, possibly due to

TABLE 9.1. World Health Organization classification of endometrial hyperplasia.

Hyperplasia (without atypia)
Simple
Complex (adenomatous)
Atypical hyperplasia
Simple
Complex (adenomatous)

differences in estrogen and progesterone receptor content of the endometrium.

In hyperplasia, ectatic vascular channels (venules) are often present in the superficial stroma beneath the surface epithelium. The pathogenesis of this change is not well understood but appears to be associated with nonphysiologic, noncyclical endometrial growth. Morphologic evidence of active breakdown and bleeding (Chapter 5) also may be present around thrombosed ectatic venules.

Hyperplasia Without Atypia

Simple Hyperplasia

In simple hyperplaia, previously referred to as "cystic" or "mild" hyperplasia, many, but not all, of the proliferating glands are dilated and cystic, with irregular size and shape, yet separated by abundant stroma (Table 9.2). The glandular architectural changes are characterized by

TABLE 9.2. Morphologic features of hyperplasia without atypia.

Cytologic features
Nuclei
Pseudostratified
Cigar-shaped to oval with smooth contours
Uniform chromatin distribution
Small to indistinct nucleoli
Mitotic activity, variable amount
Cytoplasm
Variable, often amphophilic
Glands
Irregular, variable size, some dilated
Branching, infolding and outpouching
Simple hyperplasia
Haphazardly spaced in abundant stroma
Complex hyperplasia
Closely spaced with decreased stroma
Highly irregular outlines
Frequent associated features
Polypoid growth
Ciliated cells
Ectatic venules
Breakdown and bleeding

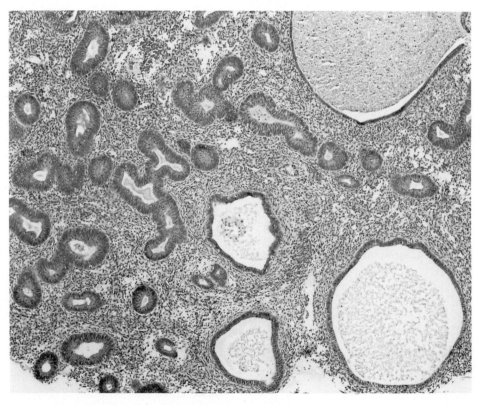

FIGURE 9.1. Simple hyperplasia. Irregular glands showing marked variation in size and shape are separated by abundant stroma. Several cystic glands are present in this field.

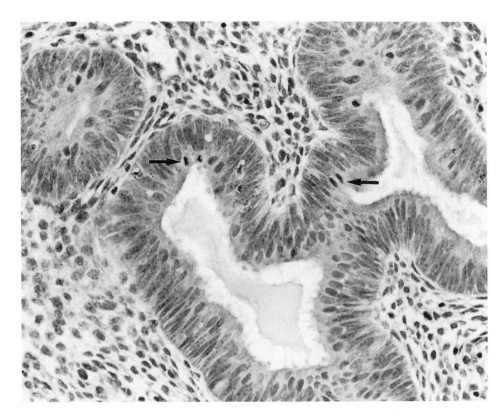

FIGURE 9.2. Simple hyperplasia. The glandular cell nuclei are oval and pseudostratified with uniform outlines, lacking cytologic atypia. Nucleoli are indistinct. Both glandular and stromal cells are cytologically similar to those of proliferative phase endometrium. Note mitotic figures (*arrows*).

varying degrees of irregular branching with infoldings and outpouchings of the glands. (Fig.9.1).

The cells lining the irregular glands cytologically resemble those of the proliferative endometrium (Fig. 9.2). They are columnar with amphophilic cytoplasm and have pseudostratified nuclei that maintain their orientation to the underlying basement membrane. Nuclei are oval with smooth contours, evenly dispersed chromatin, and small, inconspicuous nucleoli. Mitotic activity can be quite variable, but the mitotic rate has no influence on the diagnosis of simple hyperplasia. Cilia (ciliated cell change) often are seen along the luminal border of glands as well as along the surface epithelium. Squamous metaplasia may also be present, although this change is relatively infrequent in hyperplasia without atypia.

By definition, considerable stroma is present in simple hyperplasia. The stroma resembles that seen in the proliferative phase of the normal menstrual cycle, consisting of small, oval cells with scant cytoplasm. Like the glands, the stroma shows mitotic activity. When the hyperplasia is polypoid, the stroma may contain thick-walled arteries similar to those seen in polyps. The superficial stroma in simple hyperplasia typically contains dilated venules, and these can be numerous when the hyperplasia is exuberant and polypoid.

Complex Hyperplasia

In contrast to simple hyperplasia, complex hyperplasia, previously termed "moderate" or "adenomatous" hyperplasia, shows more densely crowded glands. In addition, the glands may demonstrate increased structural complexity with more outpouchings and infoldings (Fig. 9.3). Usually the glands are closely apposed and often show back-to-back crowding, although some small amount of intervening stroma is always

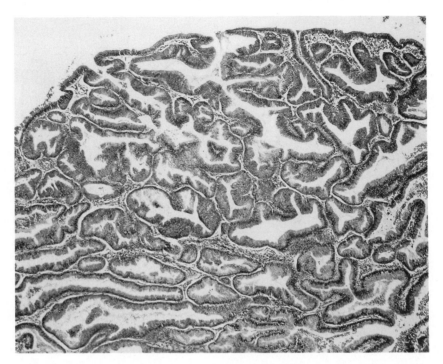

FIGURE 9.3. Complex hyperplasia. The glands are closely packed, lacking the abundant stroma seen in simple hyperplasia.

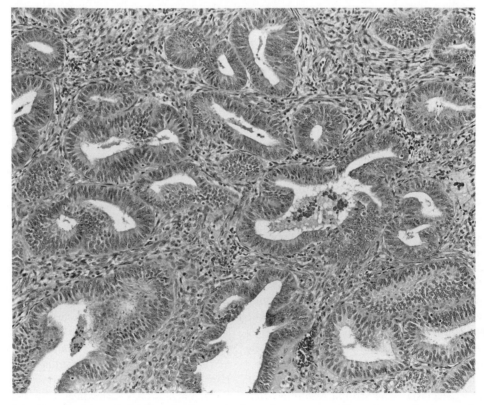

FIGURE 9.4. Complex hyperplasia. The glands vary in size and are separated by only a small amount of stroma.

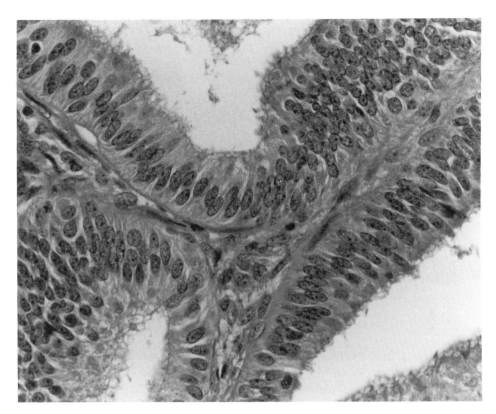

FIGURE 9.5. Complex hyperplasia. Although the glands are separated by scant stroma, the nuclei remain small and pseudostratified with oval contours, resembling cells in the normal proliferative phase.

present (Fig. 9.4). It is the degree of glandular crowding, however, that separates complex from simple hyperplasia. Cystic glands can involve a portion of the endometrium in complex hyperplasia, and mixtures of simple and complex hyperplasia often coexist.

Cytologically the glands in complex hyperplasia are identical to those in simple hyperplasia (Table 9.2). The cells are pseudostratified, with oval nuclei, small and inconspicuous nucleoli, and a variable amount of mitotic activity (Fig. 9.5). Thus, architecture alone separates simple and complex hyperplasia.

Sometimes the glands are somewhat crowded and irregular but not densely packed, and it is not clear whether the process should be termed simple or complex hyperplasia. When the distinction between complex and simple hyperplasia is not clear, we recommend classifying the lesions as simple hyperplasia.

Atypical Hyperplasia

Atypical hyperplasia can have simple or complex architectural patterns.[1,12] In contrast to nonatypical hyperplasia, however, most cases of atypical hyperplasia have a complex pattern with closely packed glands (complex atypical hyperplasia) (Figs. 9.6–9.10). The glands tend to be highly irregular in size and shape (Table 9.3). Papillary infolding or tufts lacking a fibrovascular core may project into the lumen (Figs. 9.7 and 9.8). Although they may be complex and closely packed, the glands in atypical hyperplasia are surrounded by stroma. Even with an apparent back-to-back glandular arrangement, each gland has a basement membrane with a thin rim of stroma separating it from adjacent glands. In some cases, however, the glands are widely dispersed (simple atypical hyperplasia (Fig. 9.11). In these instances glands displaying no cyto-

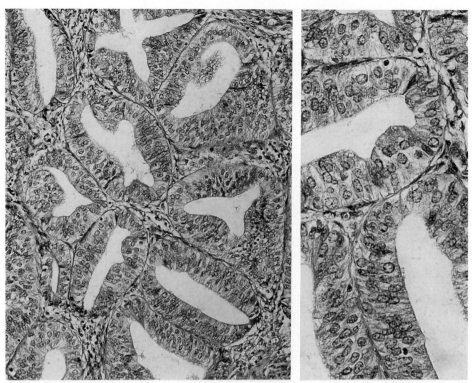

FIGURE 9.6. Complex atypical hyperplasia. *Left*: The glands are closely spaced, with little intervening stroma. *Right*: The lining epithelium shows atypia, characterized by rounded, stratified nuclei with loss of polarity. The cytoplasm is eosinophilic.

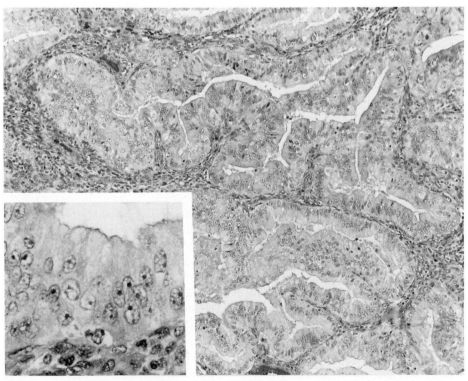

FIGURE 9.7. Complex atypical hyperplasia. The glands are highly irregular, but a small amount of stroma encompasses each gland. The cells show atypia with stratified nuclei that have prominent nucleoli. *Inset*: The nuclei are vesicular with chromatin clumped along the nuclear membrane. The cells also have abundant, eosinophilic cytoplasm.

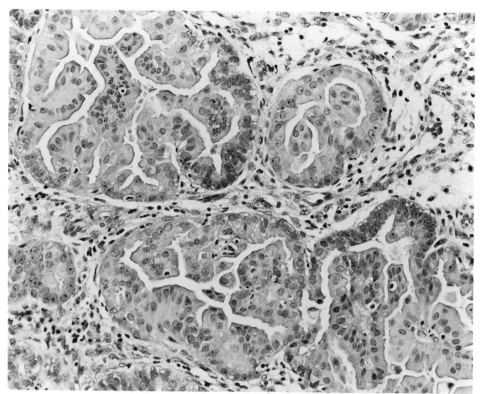

FIGURE 9.8. Complex atypical hyperplasia. The complex glands have multiple papillary tufts of eosinophilic cells that project into the lumen. The glandular cells have rounded nuclei with prominent nucleoli. A small amount of stroma separates the glands.

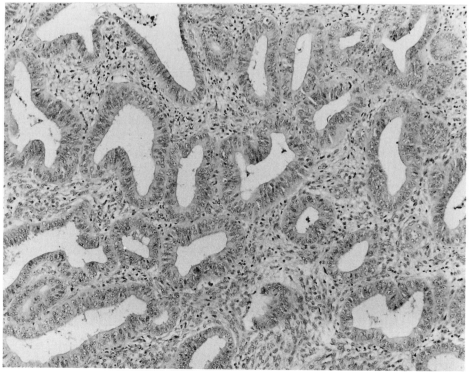

FIGURE 9.9. Complex atypical hyperplasia. The glands are not highly convoluted but are closely spaced and vary in size and shape.

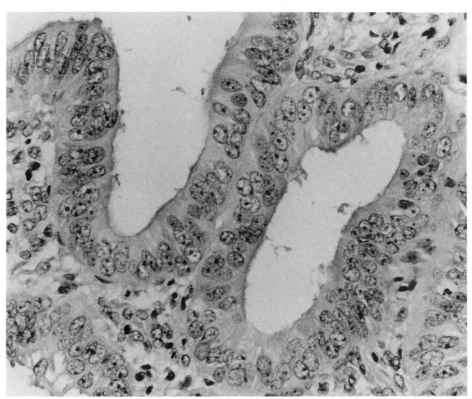

FIGURE 9.10. Complex atypical hyperplasia. High magnification shows glandular nuclei with features of atypia. The nuclei are rounded and vesicular, with prominent nucleoli. They have a haphazard distribution. The cells contain a moderate amount of pale cytoplasm. Same case as Fig. 9.9.

TABLE 9.3. Morphologic features of atypical hyperplasia.

Cytologic features[a]
  Nuclei
    Stratification with loss of polarity
    Enlarged, rounded with irregular shapes
    Coarsening of chromatin creating a vesicular appearance
    Prominent nucleoli
    Mitotic activity, variable amount
  Cytoplasm
    Eosinophilia, diffuse or focal
Glands
  Irregular, variable size, some dilated
  Simple atypical hyperplasia
    Haphazardly spaced in abundant stroma
  Complex atypical hyperplasia
    Closely spaced with decreased stroma
    Highly irregular outlines
Frequent associated features
  Papillary infoldings into glands (no bridging)
  Decreased stroma
  Ciliated cells
  Squamous change

[a] Atypical nuclei should be readily apparent, involving most of the cells lining affected glands.

logic atypia may be admixed with those showing cytologic atypia.

The diagnosis of atypia is based on specific nuclear features (Table 9.3). The nuclei are enlarged and rounded rather than oval and may have irregular nuclear membranes (Figs. 9.7, 9.10, and 9.11). The chromatin is dispersed and forms clumps along the nuclear membrane, resulting in a distinctive vesicular appearance. These vesicular nuclei are highly characteristic of endometrial atypia. Nucleoli may be prominent. The nuclei often show true stratification, with loss of polarity in relation to the basement membrane, that contrasts with the pseudostratification shown by nuclei of nonatypical hyperplasia. The stratification ranges from two to four cells in thickness.

The cytoplasm of the atypical glandular cells often is abundant and eosinophilic. This eosinophilia, a helpful feature when present, is not specific by itself for atypical hyperplasia. Sometimes with atypia the cells are highly stratified, yet the

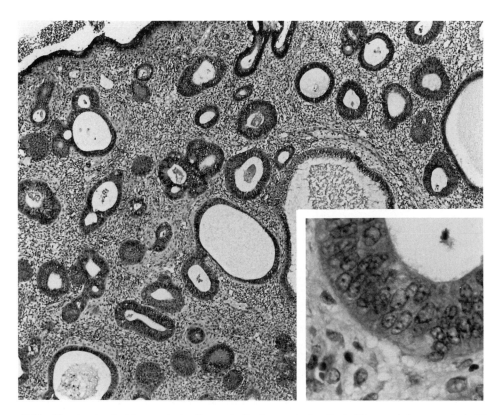

FIGURE 9.11. Simple atypical hyperplasia. Several of the glands are cystic, and there is a moderate amount of intervening stroma. Some of the cystic glands lack nuclear atypia, but the lesion still represents atypical hyperplasia. *Inset*: The nuclei are typical. They are round, vesicular, and stratified. In this case the cells lack abundant eosinophilic cytoplasm.

eosinophilia of the cytoplasm is less pronounced. Epithelial cellular changes often are found in atypical hyperplasia [see below, Epithelial Cytoplasmic Change (Metaplasia)]. Ciliated cells frequently are seen, at least focally, and other epithelial changes, such as secretory or mucinous change, occasionally will be found. Squamous metaplasia can be focal or extensive in atypical hyperplasia. When present, squamous metaplasia sometimes fills and expands the glands, accentuating the crowded appearance and leaving only a partial rim of columnar gland cells (Fig. 9.12). Often the squamous cells partially bridge the lumen, yielding an apparent cribriform pattern. The squamous epithelium by itself has no influence on diagnosis or prognosis of endometrial lesions, however. The cytologic features and architecture of the glands determine the diagnosis. For these reasons, the nuclear rather than the cytoplasmic features of the glandular cells are more important for the diagnosis of hyperplasia.

Atypical hyperplasia also can be focally present in tissue along with nonatypical hyperplasia.[13] The minimal criteria for diagnosis of focal atypia have not been defined. Nonetheless, for focal atypia to be a significant finding, it should be a readily discernible lesion present in a background of clearly hyperplastic glands with irregular sizes and shapes. In equivocal cases where there is a question of focal atypia in a background of simple or complex hyperplasia, there often are atypical nuclei focally distributed in many glands. In other cases the apparent atypia is confined to only a few glands. In either case a diagnosis of atypical hyperplasia is best limited to those cases in which clearly atypical nuclei are readily identified without diligent searching. Furthermore, the cytologic changes of atypia should involve most of the epithelium lining the glands. In equivocal cases, we recommend that atypia not be diagnosed unless clearly atypical nuclei involve most of the epithelium, lining several well-visualized glands in cross

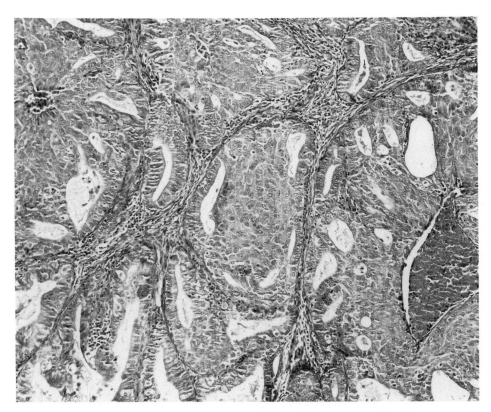

FIGURE 9.12. Complex atypical hyperplasia with squamous change. Many of the glands are partially filled with nonkeratinizing squamous epithelium that bridges the lumen. There is central necrosis of the squamous change in the gland at the right of the field, a finding that has no significance in the diagnosis. Each gland is separated by a thin rim of stroma.

section. Surface epithelium should be avoided for establishing the diagnosis of these borderline cases.

Differential Diagnosis

A number of artifacts, as well as a variety of benign and malignant lesions, can be confused with hyperplasia, especially in endometrial biopsies. Artifactual changes to glands include fragmentation during biopsy or curettage, active bleeding with stromal collapse, and poor orientation. With any of these artifacts, the glands can appear irregular and crowded on casual inspection. Fragmented proliferative or normal late secretory glands may be closely positioned during embedding and sectioning, giving the illusion of crowded, disorganized glands with irregular shapes and sizes. The artifact of "telescoping," resulting in a "gland within a gland" appearance, frequently occurs in association with fragmentation (Chapter 2) This change can be mistaken for hyperplasia, since it often occurs in proliferative endometrium. Glandular and stromal breakdown and bleeding distorts the tissue, causing irregular crowding of glands around areas of collapse that can be mistaken for hyperplasia. Likewise, basalis has irregular glands that focally resemble the glands in hyperplasia. These potential pitfalls of interpretation are avoided by ensuring that the tissue on which the diagnosis is based has intact glands and stroma without areas of breakdown. Surface epithelium is an important anatomic landmark to orient the tissue, thereby avoiding misinterpretations of artifactual changes (Chapter 2).

Disordered proliferative endometrium frequently enters into the differential diagnosis of hyperplasia, especially simple hyperplasia. Some pathologists use the term "disordered proliferative" to avoid assigning the term "hyperplasia" to a case. The disordered proliferative endometrium has mild irregularities in gland patterns that do not fulfull the quantitative criteria for simple hyperplasia. Often this type of case represents estrogen-stimulated endometrium from anovulatory cycles that shows focal glandular irregularities (Chapter 5). We use the term in those cases where only a few glands are dilated or branched, being confined to no more than scattered foci within functionalis. Other areas show tubular to tortuous proliferative glands. With diffuse glandular irregularities, the process is better classified as hyperplasia.

Polyps are another frequent source of confusion in the differential diagnosis of hyperplasia. Many polyps represent focal hyperplasia of the basalis that contains irregular glands (Chapter 8). In addition, they may show ciliated cell or squamous change. Nonetheless, they are separated from diffuse hyperplasia because they are generally not estrogen-related abnormalities. In general, polyps are focal lesions, and the surrounding endometrium is normal. The polypoid shape, dense stroma, and thick-walled vessels are helpful features in recognizing the ordinary polyp. In summary, it is the focal nature of the polyp that separates this lesion from the more diffuse hyperplasia. Sometimes, however, it is difficult to make this distinction with certainty in a small biopsy. Repeat curettage and hysteroscopy may be necessary to establish the correct diagnosis.

In atypical hyperplasia the differential diagnosis is broader than in nonatypical hyperplasia. At one end of the spectrum, the cytologic changes of atypia must be distinguished from benign abnormalities, such as eosinophilic syncytial change. At the other end of the spectrum, the differential diagnosis includes well-differentiated adenocarcinoma, since both lesions are often composed of closely packed glands with cytologic atypia. Typically, the benign cellular changes that mimic atypia are those that result in cytoplasmic eosinophilia, since the cells of atypical hyperplasia also frequently have eosinophilic cytoplasm [see below, Epithelial Cytoplasmic Change (Metaplasia)].

Endometritis may at times result in glandular changes that mimic hyperplasia with atypia (Chapter 7). In cases with marked inflammation, especially those with acute and chronic inflammation, the glands will show reactive changes with an irregular distribution in a reactive, spindle stroma. The reactive process includes cytologic changes with enlarged, stratified nuclei, but these are generally focal. With endometritis the glands are not irregular and crowded unless there is fragmentation artifact. Usually these reactive changes associated with inflammation occur in premenopausal patients.

The *atypical polypoid adenomyoma* (Chapter 8) also enters into the differential diagnosis, because in this lesion the glands are highly irregular and the cytologic changes of the epithelium are similar to those of atypical hyperplasia. In atypical adenomyoma the smooth muscle cells around the glands set this lesion apart from atypical hyperplasia. Instead of endometrial stroma, as is seen in hyperplasia, this lesion contains smooth muscle in short, interlacing fascicles. Immunohistochemical stains for desmin or actin can assist in the diagnosis of this lesion by demonstrating the smooth muscle.

In addition to these specific alterations that may be confused with true atypical hyperplasia, there are occasional situations where normal, nonhyperplastic endometrium can be confused with an atypical proliferation. Often in such cases, the cells lining glands of proliferative endometrium can appear atypical at high magnification; the nuclei seem to be stratified and rounded, and show a coarse chromatin distribution. Artifactual distortion of the tissue also may yield changes that superficially resemble atypical proliferations. For example, there is a peculiar artifact of biopsies in which the glandular cells appear to be stratified, with a hobnail-like pattern (Fig. 9.13). In addition, mitotically active cells protrude into the lumen. This hobnail-like artifact usually involves only a few glands, generally occurring at the edge of tissue fragments while the remainder of the tissue is free of the abnormality. It usually is found in fragmented proliferative endometrium and can be mistaken for atypia unless the overall pattern of normal gland architecture is recognized and fragmented areas are avoided.

When atypia is suspected, it is important to identify areas with glands and surrounding intact stroma. Here, if atypical hyperplasia is present,

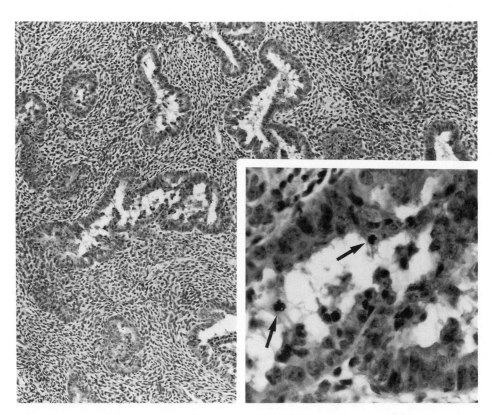

FIGURE 9.13. Hobnail-like artifact of proliferative endometrium. Curettings of proliferative endometrium show a focus where glandular epithelium appears stratified and disorderly. Although appearing worrisome at first glance, this artifact typically occurs as a focal finding at the edge of tissue fragments in curettings. This change does not represent atypia. *Inset*: The glandular cells have a hobnail appearance as they become detached. A few of the cells contain mitotic figures (*arrows*).

the glands should have the architectural as well as the cytologic features of hyperplasia that establish the diagnosis. If the glands in these foci are tubular and lack the irregular outlines and altered gland-to-stroma ratio of hyperplastic glands, the apparent atypia probably has no clinical significance. Also, it is important to determine if the nuclei in areas with intact, architecturally normal proliferative glands appear the same as those in the apparently atypical hyperplasia areas. If the nuclei in the hyperplastic areas resemble those in the normal proliferative endometrium, then the diagnosis of atypical hyperplasia is suspect. Multiple levels through the tissue block can help resolve equivocal cases. If step sections do not resolve the question, then additional sampling such as a dilatation and curettage may be necessary, especially if the first specimen was an office-based biopsy.

Finally, it is important for the pathologist who is attempting to differentiate normal variations and artifacts from true atypia to consider the clinical history. Atypical hyperplasia is unusual in premenopausal women unless they have a history of anovulation associated with obesity or polycystic ovaries.[7–9] Conversely, atypical glandular proliferations become more common in perimenopausal or postmenopausal patients. Consequently, foci of apparent gland cell atypia in premenopausal women should be viewed very conservatively, considering the possibility of artifact. In the postmenopausal patient, critical study also is necessary, but with the consideration that subtle gland cell changes may actually represent atypia.

Once true atypia is identified and benign lesions that mimic hyperplasia are excluded, the

TABLE 9.4. Follow-up comparing cytologic and architectural abnormalities in 170 patients.[a]

Type of hyperplasia	No. of patients	Regressed		Persisted		Progressed to carcinoma	
		No.	(%)	No.	(%)	No.	(%)
Simple	93	74	(80)	18	(19)	1	(1)
Complex	29	23	(80)	5	(17)	1	(3)
Simple atypical	13	9	(69)	3	(23)	1	(8)
Complex atypical	35	20	(57)	5	(14)	10	(29)

[a] Adapted with permission of Kurman et al.[12]

differential diagnosis includes well-differentiated adenocarcioma. A diagnosis of well-differentiated carcinoma is established easily when there is myometrial invasion, but this is a very rare finding in curettings. Thus, a diagnosis of carcinoma is based on identifying invasion of endometrial stroma, but this is a subtle change in well-differentiated neoplasms. There are three criteria, any of which identifies endometrial stromal invasion: 1) an irregular infiltration of glands associated with an altered fibroblastic stroma (desmoplastic response); 2) a confluent glandular pattern in which individual glands, uninterrupted by stroma, merge and create a cribriform pattern; and 3) an extensive papillary pattern.[1,2,27] Increasing degrees of nuclear atypia, mitotic activity, and stratification in curettings also are associated with a higher frequency of carcinoma but are of limited value compared to the main criterion of stromal invasion. These criteria for determining the presence of invasion allow the diagnosis of atypical hyperplasia or carcinoma to be made more objectively. The specific histologic features of these patterns of stromal invasion in well-differentiated adenocarcinoma are discussed further and illustrated in the next chapter.

Behavior of Endometrial Hyperplasia

Hyperplasia without atypia, simple or complex, usually is a self-limited lesion that will regress. Atypical hyperplasia, however, is associated with the development of adenocarcinoma.[5,10–16,28,29] In one study that examined untreated hyperplasia in detail, 80% of both simple and complex hyperplasia cases without atypia regressed (Table 9.4).[12] Furthermore, the risk of progression to carcinoma was slight, 1% in simple hyperplasia and 3% in complex hyperplasia. Approximately 60% of cases of atypical hyperplasia also regressed, but the risk of progression to carcinoma was significantly greater compared to hyperplasia without atypia (Table 9.4). In the same study, 8% of cases of simple atypical hyperplasia and 29% of cases of complex atypical hyperplasia progressed to carcinoma. These differences in progression rates between simple and complex atypical hyperplasia did not achieve statistical significance, but overall there was a 23% rate of progression to carcinoma of atypical hyperplasia compared to 2% in hyperplasia without atypia, and this was a statistically significant difference. Accordingly, the presence of atypia is the most important prognostic feature for endometrial hyperplasia. Other studies also find that 17% to 25% of patients who undergo a hysterectomy soon after the diagnosis of atypical hyperplasia at biopsy have well-differentiated adenocarcinoma in the uterus.[13,27,29] When adenocarcinoma is present following a biopsy diagnosis of atypical hyperplasia, the neoplasm is almost always well differentiated, focal, and either confined to the endometrium or minimally invasive into the myometrium.[13,27,29]

Epithelial Cytoplasmic Change (Metaplasia)

Epithelial cytoplasmic alterations, commonly designated metaplasia, often occur in the endometrium. The term "metaplasia" refers to transformation of cells to a type not normally found in an organ. By this definition, most of the alterations commonly classified as endometrial metaplasia do not qualify as such. Consequently, some of the cytologic transformations of the epithelium previously referred to as endometrial metaplasia are better classified as a "change." The latter term has the advantage of offering a descriptive designation without implying a specific mechanism of development. Since these "changes" are especially common in hyperplasia, it is important that they be recognized and clearly separated from more significant glandular abnormalities. "Changes" vary from squamous differentiation to other benign cytoplasmic transformations, such as secretory-like vacuolization, to degenerative or reparative processes. Eosinophilic syncytial change is an example of this latter group.[30] This change, discussed in greater detail in Chapter 5, appears to be a de-generative/regenerative process related to endometrial breakdown.

There are five general categories of cytoplasmic transformations that occur in the endometrium: squamous, ciliated cell, eosinophilic, mucinous, and secretory (clear cell and hobnail cell) change.[1,20,26] The terminology for these changes continues to evolve as greater experience with them is gained. For example, ciliated cell change has also been termed tubal metaplasia, and the terms eosinophilic and pink cell change are synonymous. The relative frequencies of these cytoplasmic changes are difficult to determine. Ciliated and squamous change are the most widely recognized, but in our experience eosinophilic change is the most common of the nonspecific cellular changes.

Squamous and ciliated cells are generally found in endometria that show signs of estrogenic stimulation, especially hyperplasia.[19-21] They are

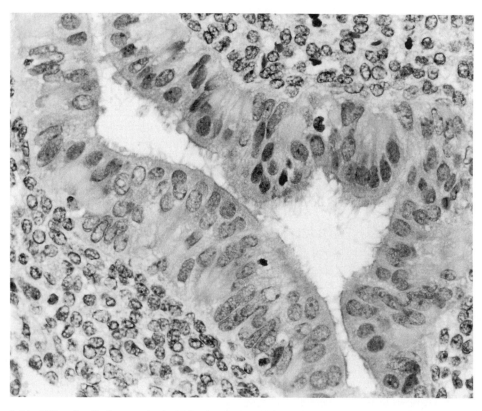

FIGURE 9.14. Ciliated cell change. A gland in simple hyperplasia is lined by ciliated cells. The cytoplasm is eosinophilic and some nuclei are enlarged and rounded. The nuclei lack features of atypia: they have smooth, uniform contours, a delicate chromatin pattern, and tiny nucleoli.

also found in low-grade endometrial carcinoma,[31,32] although squamous differentiation can occur in association with all grades of endometrial carcinoma. The association of cytoplasmic change with hyperplasia and carcinoma suggests that many forms of cytoplasmic differentiation or transformation are induced by chronic estrogen stimulation. Cytoplasmic changes also may be associated with trauma, polyps, or inflammation, however. Occasionally these cellular changes may be found in atrophy with no other known underlying pathology. It is important to recognize the various types of cellular change and determine whether they accompany hyperplasia or not, since these changes by themselves have no neoplastic potential.

Squamous differentiation (squamous metaplasia) often is nonkeratinizing, forming so-called morules because of their three-dimensional resemblance to mulberries.[33] The squamous epithelium is rarely keratinized in hyperplasia, keratinization occurring more frequently in adenocarcinoma with squamous differentiation (Chapter 10). The nonkeratinizing morules have a characteristic appearance, forming solid nests of bland eosinophilic cells that fill gland lumens (Fig. 9.12) (see also Chapter 8, Figs. 8.4, 8.5, and 8.12, and Chapter 10, Fig. 10.6). The cells have uniform, round to oval nuclei with small nucleoli and rare or absent mitoses. The nuclei are centrally placed in dense, eosinophilic cytoplasm. When the squamous change forms morules, the gland is largely filled with a round to oval mass of uniform cells with indistinct cell borders. The intraglandular nests of squamous epithelium may show central necrosis, but this feature has no effect on the diagnosis or prognosis of the lesion. Squamous change predominantly occurs within gland lumens, and in most cases surface epithelium shows minimal involvement. Surface squamous change is occasionally observed secondary to inflammation.

Ciliated cell change (tubal metaplasia) is arguably not a true metaplasia, since ciliated cells are nor-

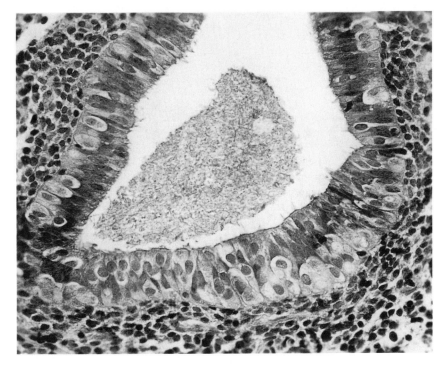

FIGURE 9.15. Ciliated cell change. The epithelial lining of this endometrial gland resembles that of the fallopian tube. The luminal border is sharply demarcated where some of the cells have a dense cytoplasmic cuticle. Some nuclei are slightly enlarged and rounded, but they lack the coarsely clumped chromatin and irregular nuclear contours seen with atypia.

mally present along the surface epithelium, being most numerous in proliferative endometrium.[34] Glands lined by ciliated cells are not normal, however. Ciliated cells usually are prominent in endometrium stimulated by unopposed estrogen. Hyperplasia may or may not be present. These cells often are interspersed in small groups among nonciliated columnar cells, but sometimes they are extensive and line most of the gland. Ciliated cells have pale to eosinophilic cytoplasm (Fig. 9.14). The luminal border of these cells may show a cuticle of dense cytoplasm formed by the ciliary basal bodies (Fig. 9.15). Often the nuclei are mildly stratified, yet they remain cytologically bland with round to oval shapes, an even chromatin distribution, and small nucleoli. The rounding and slight nuclear enlargement that characteristically occur should not be considered as evidence of atypia. Mitoses generally do not occur in ciliated cells.

Eosinophilic (pink) cell change also is common. This change actually represents several types of cytoplasmic transformation. Eosinophilic cells may be a variant of ciliated cells, squamous cells, or oncocytes as well as eosinophilic syncytial change.[1,4] All of these cytoplasmic transformations are without clinical consequence, per se. Eosinophilic cytoplasm also is a frequent feature of glands in atypical hyperplasia and low-grade adenocarcinoma, however, so it is important to determine if there is a coexisting neoplastic process.

Eosinophilic cell change that resembles ciliated cell change is common. In this situation the cells are columnar or slightly rounded and have a moderate amount of pale pink cytoplasm, resembling the cytoplasm of ciliated cells but lacking luminal cilia (Fig. 9.16). Eosinophilic cell change also merges with squamous change in some cases; here the cells become more rounded to polygonal and pavement-like, resembling cells seen in squa-

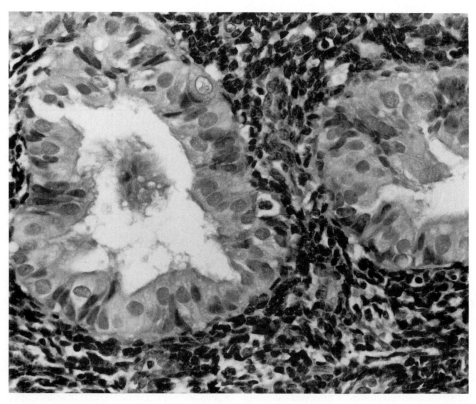

FIGURE 9.16. Eosinophilic cell change. The cells have abundant eosinophilic cytoplasm and small, round to oval nuclei. This pattern resembles ciliated cell change, but the cells lack visible cilia. In this case the finding was seen focally in an abnormal secretory phase pattern with breakdown. No hyperplasia was present.

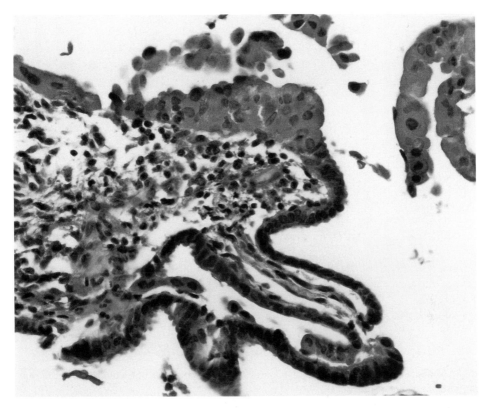

FIGURE 9.17. Eosinophilic cell change. Endometrium in a postmenopausal patient shows partial replacement of atrophic epithelium by cells with abundant granular eosinophilic cytoplasm, resembling oncocytes. The nuclei lack atypical features, and mitotic figures are absent. This alteration, by itself, has no significance.

mous differentiation but lacking the solid, morule-like growth pattern. Other cases show eosinophilic cells with abundant, granular cytoplasm that resemble oncocytes or Hurthle cells seen in other organs (Fig. 9.17). In all these forms of eosinophilic cell change, the nuclei are often round rather than oval and somewhat stratified. Luminal cell borders are sharply demarcated. The nuclei are smaller and more uniform and lack the irregular nuclear membrane, chromatin condensation along the membrane, and prominent nucleoli that characterize cells with true cytologic atypia. As in other forms of cytoplasmic change, mitoses are extremely rare. Occasionally, eosinophilic cell change occurs in nonestrogenic patterns such as atrophy.

As noted above, eosinophilic syncytial change is not a metaplastic transformation, yet it has been commonly described as such. In several studies this cellular alteration has been termed "papil-lary syncytial metaplasia," "surface syncytial change," or an "early" form of squamous metaplasia.[4,26,30,25] The classification of these eosinophilic cells as a metaplastic phenomenon is due to the fact that the syncytial aggregation of eosinophilic cells in this change superficially resembles the cytologic features of the cells in squamous metaplasia. Eosinophilic syncytial change should not be mistaken for squamous metaplasia or interpreted as an "early" form of squamous differentiation, however. The constant association of eosinophilic syncytial change with breakdown and bleeding indicates that this change is degenerative and regenerative rather than metaplastic.[30] Syncytial change is recognized by its prominent localization along surface epithelium, although it may also occur in glands (see Chapter 5, Figs. 5.5–5.7). Eosinophilic syncytial change usually is accompanied by karyorrhectic-debris, neutrophils, and adjacent glandular and

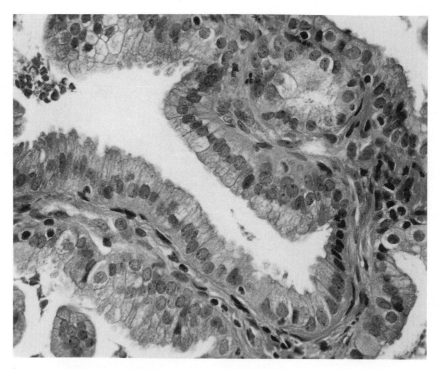

FIGURE 9.18. Mucinous change. The glandular epithelial cells contain vacuoles of mucin in the supranuclear cytoplasm, resembling endocervical cells.

stromal breakdown with stromal collapse. Futhermore, in this change, nuclei have a haphazard distribution, whereas with the other cytoplasmic changes, nuclei generally have a uniform distribution.

Mucinous change is characterized by the presence of abundant mucinous cytoplasm, resembling normal endocervical glandular cells (Fig. 9.18). Often with this change the epithelium is also thrown into small papillary projections. This pattern is not as common as the other cytoplasmic changes and is seen most often in association with atypical hyperplasia or carcinoma. These cells are columnar, with basal nuclei and abundant pale supranuclear cytoplasm that contains mucin. Histochemical stains, such as mucicarmine or periodic–acid Schiff with diastase digestion, demonstrate the abundant cytoplasmic mucin. As in ciliated cell change and eosinophilic change, the nuclei remain small and uniform, although they may contain small nucleoli. Mitotic figures are infrequent. Very rarely mucinous change can include transformation into goblet cells, and the change has been designated "intestinal metaplasia."

Secretory and clear cell change is very infrequent once progestin-related effects are excluded. This is almost invariably a focal alteration, limited to scattered glands. As the names imply, the cells contain clear, glycogen-rich cytoplasm and resemble those found in secretory or gestational endometrium (Fig. 9.19). Rarely the cells develop a hobnail pattern with nuclei that protrude into the gland lumen, and this pattern resembles the Arias-Stella reaction (Fig. 9.20). The secretory/clear cell change usually occurs in endometrium that shows estrogenic effects that can range from a proliferative pattern to carcinoma. Sometimes secretory endometrium shows extensive cytoplasmic clear cell change that exceeds the amount of vacuolization seen during normal luteal phase development, and this, too, can be considered a form of clear cell change.

Diffuse secretory changes sometimes occur in hyperplasia, and this has been called "secretory hyperplasia" (Fig. 9.21). This process can be seen

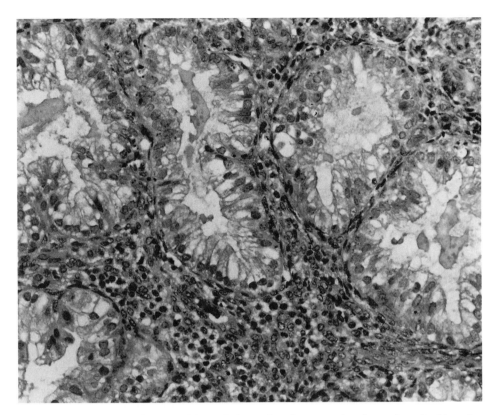

FIGURE 9.19. Secretory change. The glandular cells have abundant vacuolated cytoplasm in this endometrium with glandular and stromal breakdown. The patient was not pregnant. In contrast to mucinous change, cytoplasmic vacuoles are irregular and the cells have ragged luminal borders.

in the premenopausal or perimenopausal patient with hyperplasia who has sporadic ovulation or who has been treated with progestins; however, some examples are found with no evidence of either ovulation or exogenous progestin use. Regardless of the cause, in secretory hyperplasia the glands maintain the disordered architecture of hyperplasia, but they also show secretory changes with variably vacuolated cytoplasm and luminal secretions. Atypia is difficult to recognize in these cases, because the secretory changes result in differentiation of the gland cells. In such cases, rebiopsy may be necessary to assess the endometrium after the secretory change has resolved.

Rarely, the endometrium may show papillary proliferations composed of papillary processes with fibrovascular cores and a lining of cuboidal to low columnar epithelium with no atypia.[4] This change, termed "papillary proliferation,"[4] is ex-

tremely unusual and has not received clinicopathologic study with long-term follow-up. Nonetheless, it appears to be a benign alteration.

Differential Diagnosis

Squamous, ciliated cell, and the various types of eosinophilic cell change all may superficially resemble the epithelium in atypical hyperplasia, or even well-differentiated adenocarcinoma, because they have pale, often pink cytoplasm and nuclei that appear to be stratified.[18,31,32] To complicate matters further, these changes often occur in hyperplastic endometrium. When these cellular changes occur in hyperplasia, their recognition and separation from true glandular atypia requires attention to the nuclear features. With atypia, the nuclei are enlarged, rounded, and vesicular, with irregular nuclear membranes. Often the nuclei are stratified. These cytologic

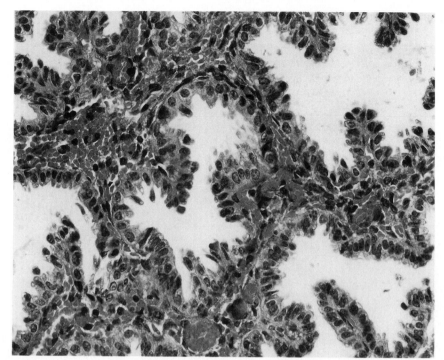

FIGURE 9.20. Hobnail secretory change. The cells show a hobnail pattern that resembles the pattern of secretory exhaustion or Arias-Stella reaction in which secretory vacuoles are absent and the irregular nuclei bulge into the glandular lumen.

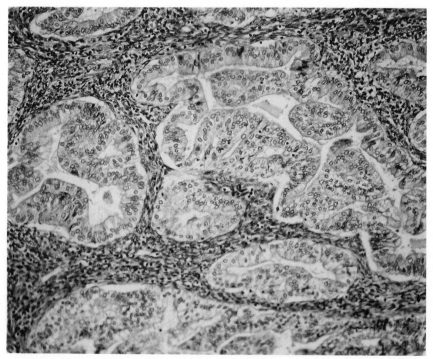

FIGURE 9.21. Secretory change in hyperplasia. Hyperplastic glands show vacuolated cytoplasm indicating secretory change. This pattern often is due to progestin therapy prior to biopsy but may occur in the absence of this history.

findings contrast with the relatively bland nuclear features of the various cellular cytoplasmic changes. Mitoses are very infrequent in the latter, another helpful feature in the differential diagnosis.

Cytoplasmic change may occur in benign, nonhyperplastic endometrium. It may occur in proliferative or secretory endometrium or in other conditions such as endometritis or polyps. In these situations, the lack of hyperplastic glandular architecture is helpful in recognizing these alterations as incidental processes with no biologic significance. Therefore, it is important to assess the overall configuration of the glands and to be certain that intact endometrium without glandular and stromal breakdown is studied in order to determine whether or not variations in cytoplasmic features represent nonspecific "change" or a more significant lesion.

Sometimes in biopsy specimens, small, detached fragments of tissue, foci of squamous or mucinous change may be found that are suggestive of a more significant abnormality, even in the absence of glands with identifiable atypia. Such foci are especially worrisome when they occur in postmenopausal patients, since their endometrium should be atrophic. Detached fragments of squamous or mucinous epithelium may reflect the presence of more significant glandular abnormalities, including atypical hyperplasia or even adenocarcinoma, that have not been adequately sampled. Further sampling, usually by dilatation and curettage, may be necessary to determine the significance of the focal alteration.

Secretory changes in hyperplasia must be distinguished from normal secretory phase patterns that appear abnormal because of fragmentation, haphazard orientation, or crowding (artifactual or real), possibilities that are much more likely than this rare form of hyperplasia. Orientation of the tissue in the sections with regard to surface epithelium, surrounding stroma, and basalis is necessary to avoid this pitfall (Chapter 2).

Clinical Queries and Reporting

Patients with hyperplasia typically present with abnormal uterine bleeding, and the diagnosis establishes a cause for the bleeding. The diagnosis of hyperplasia should be qualified as to whether or not atypia is present using the WHO classification. Although the WHO terminology has achieved widespread use, some pathologists prefer using terminology to which they have become accustomed. Likewise, gynecologists who are not familiar with the current classification may need clarification of the terminology and correlation with the terms for hyperplasia that they have used previously. We recommend using the WHO terminology primarily and appending other terminology parenthetically.

If atypia is present, the gynecologist will be concerned about the possibility of adenocarcinoma, since atypical hyperplasia is a recognized risk factor for adenocarcinoma. Even focal atypia carries a greater risk for the presence or subsequent development of adenocarcinoma. Conversely, hyperplasia without atypia has little neoplastic potential. Hyperplasia, especially without atypia, can be managed conservatively, since these lesions are self-limited. Atypical hyperplasia does not necessarily require hysterectomy either. This lesion can be managed medically with suppressive progestin therapy in young women who wish to retain their fertility and in older women in whom surgery is contraindicated. Close follow-up with endometrial biopsies is necessary to monitor the response to therapy in patients managed medically, however.

Separating cases of hyperplasia according to whether they are simple or complex is of lesser importance than determining the presence or absence of atypia. Often areas of simple hyperplasia and complex hyperplasia are admixed, and these lesions should be classified as mixed simple and complex hyperplasia. In contrast, almost all atypical hyperplasias are complex. They may coexist with nonatypical hyperplasia, but the diagnosis should be based on the worst lesion.

Cellular cytoplasmic changes should be clearly separated from hyperplasia, since they have no effect on prognosis. Changes such as ciliated cells and eosinophilic cells usually do not need to be reported as long as the other underlying conditions are evident. Eosinophilic syncytial change also does not need to be reported, since it is simply a marker of breakdown and bleeding. The importance of these changes lies in their recognition as benign cytoplasmic transformations that should not be classified as atypical lesions. When these changes are specified in the report, it is important to add a comment to explain that the alteration has no clinical significance.

Finally, there are situations in which the biopsy sample may not be sufficient to completely determine the full extent of the underlying abnormality. For example, architectural features may be suggestive, but not conclusive, of hyperplasia, especially when the specimen is small or shows extensive fragmentation. Likewise, nuclear changes may be present that suggest atypia but are inconclusive. In such cases it is best to describe the abnormality as thoroughly as possible, indicating that artifact or limited sampling precludes a definitive diagnosis. A descriptive diagnosis that indicates the uncertainty of the findings is appropriate in these cases.

At other times the distinction between atypical hyperplasia and well-differentiated adenocarcinoma may be difficult because of small amounts of tissue. When the differential is between these two lesions, it is best to issue a diagnosis of atypical hyperplasia and indicate that the findings strongly suggest that a well-differentiated adenocarcinoma is present but that a definitive diagnosis could not be made based on the submitted sample. Follow-up and rebiopsy may be needed to clarify the true nature of the lesion.

References

1. Kurman RJ, Norris HJ: Endometrial hyperplasia and related cellular changes. In: Blaustein's Pathology of the Female Genital Tract. 4th ed. Kurman RJ, ed. New York: Springer-Verlag, 1994; 411–437.
2. Norris HJ, Tavassoli FA, Kurman RJ: Endometrial hyperplasia and carcinoma. Diagnostic considerations. Am J Surg Pathol 1983;7:839–847.
3. Silverberg SG: Hyperplasia and carcinoma of the endometrium. Semin Diagn Pathol 1988;5:135–153.
4. Silverberg SG, Kurman RJ: Tumors of the uterine corpus and gestational trophoblastic disease. Atlas of Tumor Pathology, 3rd series, Fascicle 3. Washington, DC: Armed Forces Institute of Pathology, 1992.
5. Kraus FT: High-risk and premalignant lesions of the endometrium. Am J Surg Pathol 1985; 9(Suppl): 31–40.
6. Welch WR, Scully RE: Precancerous lesions of the endometrium. Hum Pathol 1977;8:503–512.
7. Chamlian DL, Taylor HB: Endometrial hyperplasia in young women. Obstet Gynecol 1970;36: 659–660.
8. Lee KR, Scully RE: Complex endometrial hyperplasia and carcinoma in adolescents and young women 15 to 20 years of age: A report of 10 cases. Int J Gynecol Pathol 1989;8:201–213.
9. McBride JM: Pre-menopausal cystic hyperplasia and endometrial carcinoma. J Obstet Gynaecol Br Emp 1959;66:288–296.
10. Gusberg SB, Kaplan AL: Precursors of corpus cancer. IV. Adenomatous hyperplasia as stage 0 carcinoma of the endometrium. Am J Obstet Gynecol 1963;87:662–677.
11. Hertig AT, Sommers SC: Genesis of endometrial carcinoma. I. Study of prior biopsies. Cancer 1949;2:946–956.
12. Kurman RJ, Kaminski PF, Norris HJ: The behavior of endometrial hyperplasia. A long-term study of "untreated" hyperplasia in 170 patients. Cancer 1985;56:403–412.
13. Tavassoli F, Kraus FT: Endometrial lesion in uteri resected for atypical endometrial hyperplasia. Am J Clin Pathol 1978;70:772–777.
14. Deligdisch L, Cohen CJ: Histologic correlates and virulence implications of endometrial carcinoma associated with adenomatous hyperplasia. Cancer 1985;56:1452.
15. Buehl IA, Vellios KF, Carter JE, Huber CP: Carcinoma in situ of the endometrium. Am J Clin Pathol 1964;42:594–601.
16. Campbell PE, Barter RA: The significance of atypical hyperplasia. J Obstet Gynaecol Br Commonw 1961;68:668–672.
17. Hertig AT, Sommers SC, Bengaloff H: Genesis of endometrial carcinoma. III. Carcinoma in situ. Cancer 1949;2:964–971.
18. Winkler B, Alvarez S, Richart RM, Crum CP: Pitfalls in the diagnosis of endometrial neoplasia. Obstet Gynecol 1984;64:185–194.
19. Crum CP, Richart RM, Fenoglio CM: Adenoacanthosis of the endometrium. A clinicopathologic study in premenopausal women. Am J Surg Pathol 1981;5:15.
20. Hendrickson MR, Kempson RL: Endometrial epithelial metaplasias: Proliferations frequently misdiagnosed as adenocarcinoma. Report of 89 cases and proposed classification. Am J Surg Pathol 1980;4:525–542.

21. Blaustein A: Morular metaplasia misdiagnosed as adenoacanthoma in young women with polycystic ovarian disease. Am J Surg Pathol 1982; 6:223.

22. Clement PB: Pathology of the uterine corpus. Hum Pathol 1991;22:776–791.

23. Vellios F: Endometrial hyperplasia and carcinoma in situ. Gynecol Oncol 1974;2:152–161.

24. Scully RE, Bonfiglio TA, Kurman RJ, Silverberg SG, Wilkinson EJ: International Histological Classification and Typing of Female Genital Tract Tumours. Berlin: Springer-Verlag, 1994.

25. Hendrickson MR, Kempson RL: Surgical pathology of the uterine corpus (Major Problems in Pathology series). Volume 12. Philadelphia: W.B. Saunders, 1980.

26. Buckley CH, Fox H: Biopsy Pathology of the Endometrium. New York: Raven Press, 1989.

27. Kurman RJ, Norris HJ: Evaluation of criteria for distinguishing atypical endometrial hyperplasia from well-differentiated carcinoma. Cancer 1982; 49:2547–2557.

28. Gray LA, Robertson RW Jr, Christopherson WM: Atypical endometrial changes associated with carcinoma. Gynecol Oncol 1974;2:93–100.

29. King A, Seraj IM, Wagner RJ: Stromal invasion in endometrial carcinoma. Am J Obstet Gynecol 1984;149:10–14.

30. Zaman SS, Mazur MT: Endometrial papillary syncytial change. A nonspecific alteration associated with active breakdown. Am J Clin Pathol 1993; 99:741–745.

31. Andersen WA, Taylor PT, Fechner RE, Pinkerton JAV: Endometrial metaplasia associated with endometrial carcinoma. Am J Obstet Gynecol 1987;157:597–604.

32. Kaku T, Tsukamoto N, Tsuruchi N, Sugihara K, Kamura T, et al: Endometrial metaplasia associated with endometrial carcinoma. Obstet Gynecol 1992;80:812–816.

33. Dutra F: Intraglandular morules of the endometrium. Am J Clin Pathol 1959;31:60–65.

34. Masterson R, Armstrong EM, More IAR: The cyclical variation in the percentage of ciliated cells in the normal human endometrium. J Reprod Fertil 1975;42:537–540.

35. Rorat E, Wallach RC: Papillary metaplasia of the endometrium: Clinical and histopathologic considerations. Obstet Gynecol 1984;64:90S–92S.

10
Endometrial Carcinoma

Endometrial adenocarcinoma is the most common malignant tumor of the female genital tract in the United States. This neoplasm represents a biologically and morphologically diverse group of tumors, with differing pathogenesis.[1–3] The typical endometrial adenocarcinoma is well to moderately differentiated, with or without squamous differentiation, and accounts for 80% to 85% of all endometrial carcinomas. The typical patient is perimenopausal or postmenopausal, obese, hypertensive, and diabetic. The low-grade tumors are frequently associated with hyperplasia, especially atypical hyperplasia, conditions that result from unopposed estrogenic stimulation. Unopposed estrogenic stimulation due to anovulatory cycles normally occurs at the time of menopause or in younger women with the Stein–Leventhal syndrome. Unopposed exogenous estrogen use as hormone replacement therapy in older women also predisposes to endometrial carcinoma that tends to be low grade. In hysterectomy specimens these tumors tend to show minimal myometrial invasion, although deep invasion can occur in some cases. The prognosis is generally good, with a 5-year survival of 80% or better.[3]

Another, very different, type of endometrial carcinoma is a high-grade neoplasm that appears to be less related to sustained estrogen stimulation.[1,2] These tumors account for 10% to 15% of all endometrial carcinomas and include histologic subtypes such as serous and clear cell carcinomas along with other carcinomas that show high-grade nuclear features. The tumors tend to occur in older postmenopausal women. They usually invade the myometrium deeply, permeate lymphatic and vascular channels, and may show extrauterine spread at the time of hysterectomy.

Clinicopathologic studies over the past several years have shown the importance of recognizing specific histologic subtypes and accurately grading carcinomas to help predict prognosis and direct treatment.[4–23] Most endometrial tumors diagnosed at biopsy are subsequently treated by extrafascial total abdominal hysterectomy and bilateral salpingo-oophorectomy that allows precise surgical-pathologic staging.[24] Nonetheless, identification of more aggressive tumors is important at the time of biopsy, since these neoplasms have greater potential for metastatic spread, including involvement of the peritoneal surfaces. Therefore, they merit more thorough surgical staging. The clinical relevance of the histologic classification and grading of endometrial carcinoma is reflected in the revised World Health Organization (WHO) histologic classification[25] and the International Federation of Gynecology and Obstetrics (FIGO) staging system.[26]

The morphologic diversity of endometrial carcinoma can lead to problems in the diagnosis of carcinoma in biopsies and curettings. For low-grade carcinoma, distinction from atypical hyperplasia and other benign lesions that mimic carcinoma is an important issue. Identifying and properly classifying aggressive, clinically significant histologic subtypes of endometrial carcinoma is a second important area of biopsy interpretation. Another problem in biopsy interpretation is ascertaining whether the tumor originates in the endometrium or the endocervix. This chapter addresses the general classification, staging, and grading of endometrial carcinoma, the differential diagnosis of benign lesions versus low-grade carcinoma, and the classification of different types of carcinoma once the diagnosis of carcinoma has been established.

TABLE 10.1. World Health Organization (WHO) classification of endometrial adenocarcinoma.

Endometrioid adenocarcinoma, NOS
   Variants
      Ciliated cell
      Secretory
Adenocarcinoma, NOS, with squamous differentiation
Mucinous adenocarcinoma
Serous adenocarcinoma
Clear cell adenocarcinoma
Squamous carcinoma
Undifferentiated carcinoma
Mixed carcinoma[a]
Metastatic carcinoma

NOS, Not otherwise specified.
[a] Tumor with greater than 10% of a second cell type.

Classification, Staging, and Grading

Classification

The current WHO histologic classification recognizes several distinct morphologic forms of carcinoma that are important to identify in biopsies (Table 10.1).[25] Many examples of endometrial adenocarcinoma have the "typical," "usual," or "not otherwise specified (NOS)" pattern referred to as "endometrioid" carcinoma. More than one-half of all endometrial carcinomas have this typical (endometrioid) pattern.[3,7,8] The term "endometrioid" provides a specific designation for this neoplastic pattern, clearly separating it from the other histologic types of endometrial carcinoma. Since endometrioid carcinoma is more widely applied to primary ovarian cancer, however, this terminology for primary uterine neoplasia is potentially confusing to clinicians. Practically, ordinary adenocarcinoma with this pattern is frequently classified as endometrial carcinoma and graded in the microscopic diagnosis.

From 20% to 30% of endometrial carcinomas show an "endometrioid" pattern with squamous differentiation.[15] Previously, these tumors with squamous differentiation were separated into two categories: adenoacanthoma denoted tumors that had cytologically benign-appearing squamous epithelium (squamous metaplasia), and adenosquamous carcinoma denoted tumors that had a cytologically malignant appearing squamous component. More recently, studies have shown that endometrioid carcinomas with or without squamous epithelium behave in the same fashion when stratified according to the grade of the glandular component.[15,16,27] Accordingly, these tumors are best classified as adenocarcinomas with squamous differentiation and graded. The terms "adenoacanthoma" and "adenosquamous carcinoma" are no longer used for endometrial carcinoma.

The other histologic types of endometrial carcinoma are relatively infrequent. Serous and mucinous tumors both account for 5% to 10% of endometrial primaries in most series, and clear cell adenocarcinoma occurs in no more than 5% of all cases.[3]

TABLE 10.2. International Federation of Gynecology and Obstetrics (FIGO) staging of corpus cancer.

Stage	Description
Ia G123	Tumor limited to endometrium
Ib G123	Invasion of less than half of the myometrium
Ic G123	Invasion of more than half of the myometrium
IIa G123	Endocervical glandular involvement only
IIb G123	Cervical stromal invasion
IIIa G123	Tumor invades serosa and/or adenexae and/or positive peritoneal cytology
IIIb G123	Vaginal metastases
IIIc G123	Metastases to pelvic and/or paraaortic lymph nodes
IVa G123	Tumor invasion of bladder and/or bowel mucosa
IVb	Distant metastases including intraabdominal and/or inguinal lymph nodes

Abbreviation: G = Grade.

Staging

In 1988 FIGO revised its staging system from one that was strictly based on clinical evaluation to one based on combined surgical and histopathologic findings.[26] Staging of endometrial carcinoma (corpus cancer) now employs a variety of histologic risk factors, including grade, depth of myometrial invasion, involvement of the cervix. and peritoneal cytology (Table 10.2).[24]

Endometrial carcinoma confined to the corpus is stage I. Based on the presence and amount of myometrial invasion, carcinomas are subdivided into Ia when tumor is limited to the endometrium, Ib when tumor invades less than one-half the myometrium, and Ic when tumor invades more than one-half the myometrium. With cervical invasion the tumor becomes stage II. Stage II is subdivided into IIa when there is endocervical glandular involvement only, and IIb when there is cervical stromal invasion by endometrial carcinoma. Since this assessment is based on the micro-

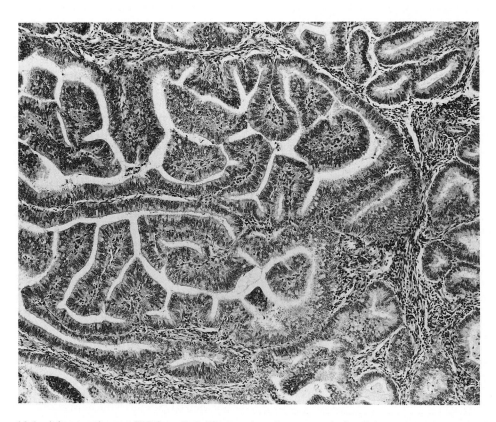

FIGURE 10.1. Adenocarcinoma, FIGO grade 1. The neoplasm is composed of well-formed glands with a confluent pattern. The stroma is desmoplastic. The nuclei are grade 1 with minimal pleomorphism, small nucleoli, and a low mitotic rate.

scopic findings in the hysterectomy specimen, fractional dilatation and curettage (D&C), with curettings of the endometrium and endocervix submitted separately to differentiate stage I and stage II, is no longer necessary.

About three-quarters of all primary endometrial carcinomas are stage I. Although staging is based on surgical–pathologic analysis of the hysterectomy specimen, accurate histologic evaluation of curettings is important, since parameters such as grade and histologic type can influence the planning for surgery, including the extent of surgical staging and lymph node sampling. Furthermore, with a high-grade neoplasm, a gynecologist without extensive experience in operative techniques may wish to have a gynecologic oncologist assist in order that appropriate staging and therapy are performed.

Grading

In addition to identifying specific histologic subtypes in biopsies, the histologic grade provides useful information for predicting prognosis and

planning treatment. Tumors of low histologic grade usually are confined to the corpus at the time of diagnosis, and the overall survival is very good. High-grade tumors, in contrast, are more aggressive. This latter group is more likely to spread beyond the corpus, involve the endocervix or extrauterine structures at the time of diagnosis, and have a poor prognosis.

The traditional grading of endometrial adenocarcinoma standardized by FIGO uses a three-grade system. Until recently, this grading was based solely on architectural features, and architecture still remains the primary feature for grading. Tumors are grade 1 when most (95%) of the tumor forms glands (Fig. 10.1), grade 2 when 6%–50% of the tumor exhibits solid growth (Fig. 10.2), and grade 3 when more than 50% of the tumor has a solid growth pattern (Fig. 10.3). It is important to avoid areas of squamous or "morular" change and evaluate only the glandular components.

The system of architectural grading has been useful, but recent studies suggest that prediction of prognosis can be improved by nuclear grad-

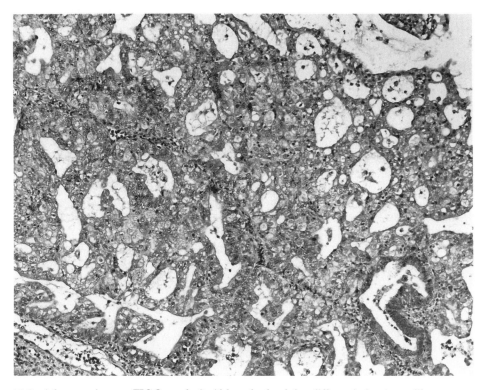

FIGURE 10.2. Adenocarcinoma, FIGO grade 2. Although glandular differentiation is readily apparent, a substantial amount (approximately 20%) of the tumor has a solid growth pattern.

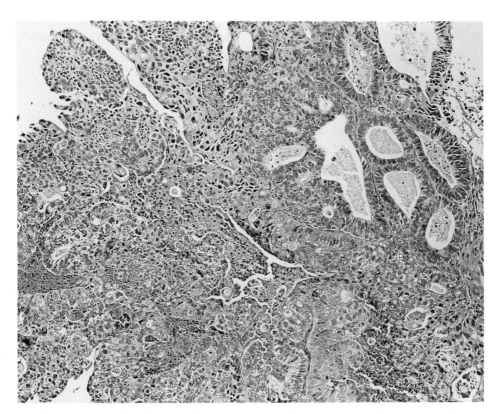

FIGURE 10.3. Adenocarcinoma, FIGO grade 3. A few residual glands are present, but more than 50% of the tumor shows a solid growth pattern with sheets and nests of malignant epithelial cells.

ing. Consequently, FIGO modified the standard architectural grading system to include these considerations.[24,26] Like architectural grading, nuclear grading is somewhat subjective. The grading system is not complex (Table 10.3). Nuclei with small, relatively uniform nuclei and low mitotic activity are grade 1 (Fig. 10.4). Nuclei with features between grade 1 and grade 3 are grade 2 (Fig. 10.5). Highly pleomorphic nuclei with irregular outlines, macronucleoli, and numerous, often abnormal mitotic figures are grade 3 (Fig. 10.6).[6,28]

FIGO recommends that notable nuclear atyp-

ia, inappropriate for the architectural grade, raises an architectural grade 1 or grade 2 tumor by 1 (i.e., grade 1 becomes grade 2, and grade 2 becomes grade 3). Notable nuclear atypia was not defined, but in a recent study it was found that for clinical significance, nuclear atypia should be grade 3. For example, a tumor with grade 2 nuclei but grade 1 architecture would be given a final FIGO grade of 1, whereas an architectural grade 1 tumor with grade 3 nuclei should be given a final FIGO grade of 2.[29]

Other histologic parameters that influence the grade according to the FIGO system are:

1. Nuclear grading takes precedence in serous, clear cell, and squamous carcinoma.
2. Adenocarcinomas with squamous differentiation are graded according to the nuclear grade of the glandular component.

Although these guidelines provide a reasonable baseline for assessing endometrial carcinoma,

TABLE 10.3. Nuclear grading.

Grade 1	Oval/elongated nuclei, fine chromatin, small nucleoli, few mitoses
Grade 2	Features between grades 1 and 3
Grade 3	Enlarged/pleomorphic nuclei, coarse chromatin, prominent nucleoli, many mitoses

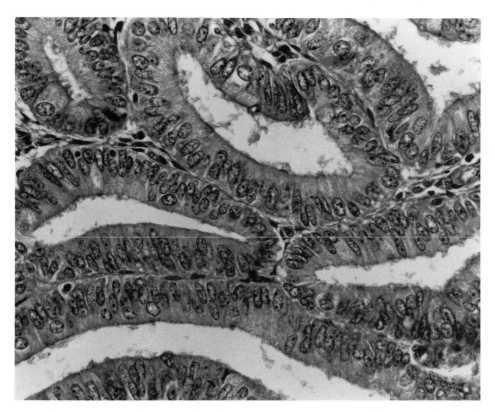

FIGURE 10.4. Adenocarcinoma, nuclear grade 1. Nuclei are round to oval with small nucleoli. The mitotic rate is low.

they require further evaluation. For example, serous carcinoma, by definition, has a high nuclear grade, so the concept of "precedence" of nuclear grading for serous carcinoma has no relevance, in our opinion.

The grade of the tumor from the biopsy specimen agrees with the grade in the hysterectomy in less than 60% of cases, with both apparent undergrading and overgrading of biopsies, as compared to the hysterectomy specimens.[30–32] Overgrading may be due to heterogeneity of the tumor, with the surface component removed at biopsy showing the higher grade. Undergrading in biopsy specimens is most often due to limited sample size. Thus, the biopsy gives a general assessment of the degree of differentiation of a tumor. Treatment decisions are generally based on the grade of the tumor in the hysterectomy specimen. Nonetheless, grading of the biopsy gives the clinician a reasonable expectation of the degree of malignancy to be expected in the hysterectomy specimen. Furthermore, in occasional cases, all or most

of the carcinoma will be removed by biopsy or curettage, so there is insufficient tumor in the hysterectomy for further evaluation.

The utility of nuclear grade in the assessment of endometrial carcinoma has been examined in several reports.[6,8,13,33,34] In general, a correlation between nuclear and architectural grade has been found.[6,7,13,28,33] Nuclear grading in hysterectomy specimens can identify a small subset of nuclear grade 3 tumors that have a poorer prognosis but do not show grade 3 architectural patterns.[29] Some studies suggest that nuclear grading is not an independent index of prognostic utility compared to the FIGO architectural grade.[34] The method of nuclear grading has not been uniform throughout the studies, however, and often has failed to incorporate all cytologic features in determining the final nuclear grade. For example, one study considered a tumor to have high-grade nuclei if it showed "large nucleoli" and "coarsely clumped chromatin," but not necessarily nuclear pleomorphism.[34] In our opinion, however, nu-

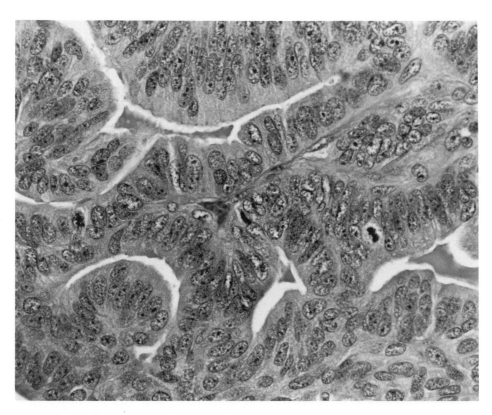

FIGURE 10.5. Adenocarcinoma, nuclear grade 2. In contrast to grade 1, these nuclei are more pleomorphic and have coarser chromatin and larger nucleoli, but they are not as abnormal as grade 3 nuclei. Mitoses are readily identified.

clear grading should consider all features, including pleomorphism. Mitotic activity is an independent histological variable but it is generally increased with nuclear grade, as are abnormal mitotic figures (Table 10.3). Careful nuclear grading provides a useful adjunct to architectural grading in the evaluation of endometrial carcinoma in biopsies and curettings, and appears to have utility for decreasing the amount of upgrading in subsequent hysterectomy specimens. Further study will be needed to determine the ultimate role of nuclear grading in the assessment of endometrial carcinoma.

Important Issues in Interpretation of Biopsies

There are two major concerns in the evaluation of endometrial curettings from the standpoint of a diagnosis of carcinoma. First, is the lesion in the curettings benign or malignant? Second, if the curetting contains a malignant tumor, what are the characteristics of the tumor? The latter consideration includes identification of histologic subtypes of endometrial carcinoma as well as identifying other unsuspected primary carcinomas, especially endocervical carcinoma.

Borderline Lesions and Benign Disorders That Mimic Carcinoma

Since a diagnosis of carcinoma will have an important impact on clinical management, it is necessary for the pathologist to be familiar with the minimal histologic criteria for that diagnosis. One of the most problematic areas is the distinction of atypical hyperplasia (Chapter 8) from well-differentiated adenocarcinoma.[35–38] Separation of these entities is based on identification of specific morphologic criteria that establish the diagnosis of low-grade carcinoma. Hyperplasia without atypia generally is not a problem in the differential diagnosis, since these forms of hyper-

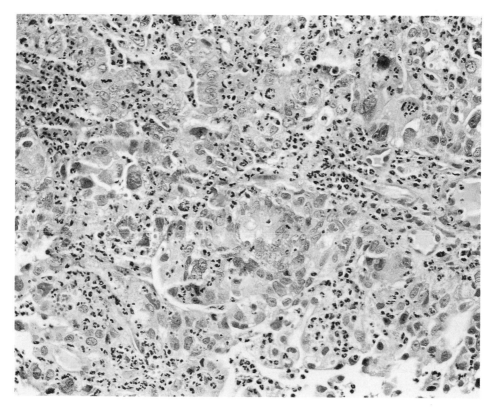

FIGURE 10.6. Adenocarcinoma, nuclear grade 3. Nuclei are markedly enlarged and highly pleomorphic.

plasia do not have nuclear glandular atypia. It is imperative, however, to accurately separate carcinoma from other, benign changes that may mimic neoplasia, including tissue artifacts and pregnancy-related changes.

Criteria for the Diagnosis of Well-Differentiated Adenocarcinoma

Diagnosis of low-grade adenocarcinoma can be difficult at times, because these tumors do not always show clear-cut destructive stromal invasion. Furthermore, invasion into myometrium is rarely demonstrated in biopsies. Nonetheless, invasion is a logical criterion for separating frank adenocarcinoma from atypical hyperplasia or other lesions that mimic adenocarcinoma.

For practical application, specific patterns of stromal and epithelial alterations have been described that reflect "endometrial stromal invasion" and identify carcinoma.[36,39] There are three separate features, any of which indicates stromal invasion in low-grade glandular proliferations:

1. a confluent glandular pattern in which individual glands, uninterrupted by stroma, merge and create a cribriform arrangement;
2. an irregular infiltration of glands associated with an altered fibroblastic stroma (desmolastic response); and
3. an extensive papillary pattern.

Although quantitative features have limited usefulness in endometrial biopsy diagnosis, these specific and objective criteria for invasion also should be quantitatively significant. Therefore, the glandular proliferation that fulfills criteria for well-differentiated adenocarcinoma should be sufficiently extensive to involve at least one-half of a low-power (4×) field, a distance of 2.0 mm. This guideline helps mainly to avoid the problem of tangential sectioning or other arti-

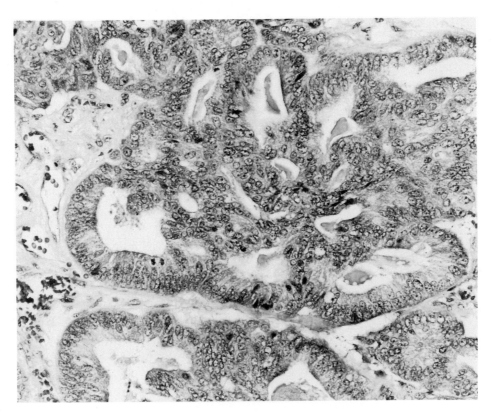

FIGURE 10.7. Well-differentiated adenocarcinoma. Confluent glandular pattern. Confluent glands with a cribriform bridging arrangement. There is no stromal support to the epithelium that bridges the glandular lumens.

facts in establishing the diagnosis of carcinoma. This general rule should not be too rigidly applied, particularly in scant specimens. If the features of "stromal invasion" are clearly evident, a diagnosis of carcinoma should be made even if the diagnostic area does not occupy one-half of a low-power field.

Confluent Glandular Pattern

This pattern reflects invasion by showing a complete absence of stroma between glands. At times a cribriform bridging pattern with true "gland in gland" formation is present. With cribriform growth, trabeculae of columnar cells bridge the lumen, subdividing the lumen into smaller glandular spaces (Fig. 10.7). No stroma supports the bridging cells. A confluent glandular pattern also is represented by large, irregular glands that interconnect continuously throughout the field, exceeding the outline of any acceptable non-neo-plastic gland (Fig. 10.8). Confluent glandular patterns should be identified in areas free of squamous differentiation, since squamous morules may bridge gland lumens, but these do not reflect stromal invasion.

Altered Fibrous or Desmoplastic Stroma

With this change, atypical glands are dispersed in a reactive fibroblastic mesenchyme rather than in endometrial stromal cells (Fig. 10.9). These fibrous stromal cells are different from the usual endometrial stromal cells, being more spindle-shaped and having elongate nuclei. The stroma also contains collagen that compresses the stromal cells and gives an eosinophilic appearance to the stroma (Fig. 10.10). The fibrous change also leads to retraction and distortion of the normal architecture, resulting in a haphazard glandular pattern. Dense stroma in polyps, alteration of the stroma associated with marked inflammation,

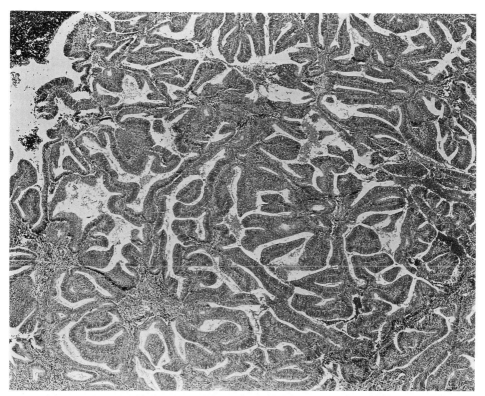

FIGURE 10.8. Well-differentiated adenocarcinoma. Confluent glandular pattern. Large irregular and branching glands interconnect continuously throughout the field.

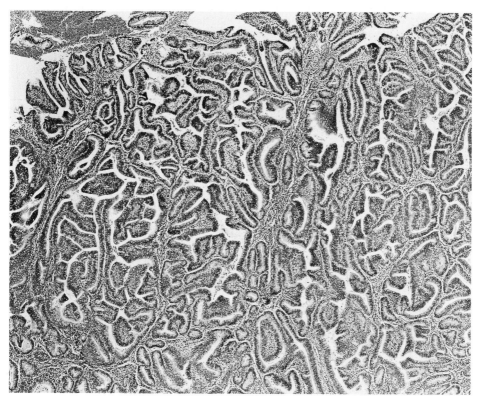

FIGURE 10.9. Well-differentiated adenocarcinoma. Desmoplastic stroma. A fibroblastic mesenchyme encompasses the neoplastic glands.

193

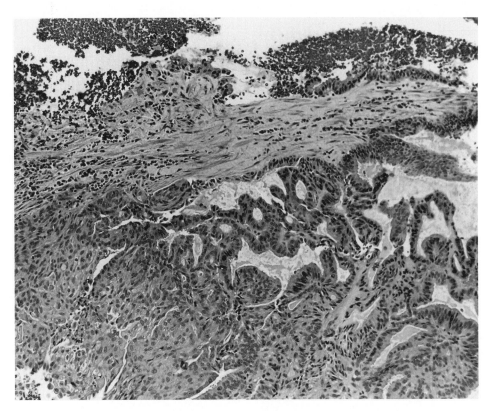

FIGURE 10.10. Well-differentiated adenocarcinoma. Desmoplastic stroma. The stroma supporting the malignant glands is composed of elongated fibroblasts and collagen. Squamous change is present in the lower portion of the field.

the stroma of the atypical polypoid adenomyoma, and stroma of the lower uterine segment all may mimic the desmoplastic response of carcinoma. In these types of cases, where desmoplasia is difficult to evaluate, other features of carcinoma, such as a confluent glandular pattern, should be used in establishing an unequivocal diagnosis of malignancy.

Extensive Papillary Pattern

The extensive papillary growth pattern is characterized by delicate, elongate, branching papillary fronds (Fig. 10.11). The fronds have thin, fibrous cores. These papillary structures are much more elaborate and branching than the small papillary tufts that may occur in the glands of atypical hyperplasia. Papillary tufts also lack fibrovascular cores. The diffuse papillary pattern distinguishes this form of adenocarcinoma from focal alterations, such as papillary arrangements in eosino-

philic syncytial change (Chapter 5). Serous papillary adenocarcinoma is readily separated from this well-differentiated neoplasm by its high-grade nuclear features and extensive papillary tufting (see below).

Originally, another pattern, squamous masses, in which sheets of bland squamous cells form irregular coalescent nests throughout the stroma, was proposed as a criterion for invasion.[36] This pattern is rare by itself, however, and not useful for recognizing carcinoma in most cases. When this pattern is present, other areas usually show confluent glandular patterns or an altered (desmoplastic) stroma.

Applying these criteria for invasion to establish the diagnosis of well-differentiated adenocarcinoma yields a clinically significant diagnosis of carcinoma, when present. One study found that in curettings with well-differentiated adenocarcinoma, defined by at least one of these features of

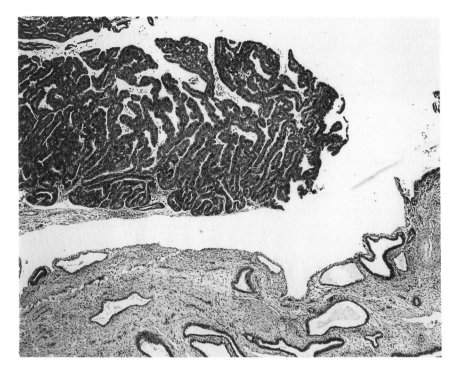

FIGURE 10.11. Well-differentiated adenocarcinoma. Extensive papillary pattern. This low-grade adenocarcinoma with a villoglandular pattern forms multiple delicate papillae.

invasion, subsequent hysterectomy specimens showed residual adenocarcinoma in one-half of the cases.[36] Usually the residual carcinoma was well differentiated, but in about one-third of cases the tumor was grade 2 or 3, and in one-quarter of the cases with tumor, the myometrium was deeply invaded. In another study that used the same criteria to assess "stromal invasion," 16% of patients without stromal invasion in endometrial samples had myometrial invasion in the hysterectomy specimens, whereas 62.5% of patients with invasion in the biopsy had myometrial invasion.[40] These studies show the utility of these criteria for determining the presence of well-differentiated adenocarcinoma.

Epithelial Cytoplasmic Change

Benign cytoplasmic changes and metaplasia also may yield changes that can be confused with endometrial carcinoma.[39,41–45] This differential diagnosis is most likely to occur in the presence of prominent squamous or eosinophilic cell change, especially in specimens with considerable tissue

fragmentation. These cytoplasmic changes can occur in a variety of conditions, including polyps, hyperplasia, inflammation, and nonspecific glandular and stromal breakdown, as well as in carcinoma.[39,43–50] Consequently, carcinoma should only be diagnosed when there is a glandular proliferation that fulfills, at a minimum, the histologic criteria for well-differentiated carcinoma described previously or if the lesion shows unequivocal features of malignancy with cytologic features of grade 2 or 3 carcinoma. Detached epithelial fragments, especially when they lack significant nuclear atypia, should not be diagnosed as carcinoma. These epithelial changes may occur in carcinoma, however, and equivocal cases require processing of additional tissue. Cytoplasmic change is discussed in greater detail in Chapter 9.

Atypical Polypoid Adenomyoma

The atypical polypoid adenomyoma can be confused with carcinoma of the endometrium because the lesion shows atypical glands, usually with squamous morules, in smooth muscle that can be confused with carcinoma invading the myometrium (Chapter 8).[51–53] Myometrial invasion is rarely seen in curettings, however. Furthermore, the orderly pattern of the smooth muscle of the atypical polypoid adenomyoma contrasts with the desmoplasia typically associated with neoplasia. In those rare cases where the differential includes the atypical polypoid adenomyoma and adenocarcinoma, it is important to note that a confluent or cribriform pattern does not occur in the atypical polypoid adenomyoma. Immunohistochemical stains for actin or desmin can help to demonstrate the smooth muscle in the atypical adenomyoma and distinguish it from the fibroblastic desmoplasia of carcinoma.

Pregnancy and the Arias-Stella Reaction

In pregnancy, crowded secretory glands, especially those that display the Arias-Stella reaction, may yield a pattern that resembles carcinoma, especially clear cell carcinoma. This potential pitfall is best avoided by considering the patient's age. For any premenopausal patient, the possibility of non-neoplastic lesions, such as the Arias-Stella reaction, is much more likely than carcinoma. The clinical history often clarifies the diagnosis in questionable cases.

Several microscopic features also help in the recognition of the Arias-Stella reaction (Chapter 3). This lesion tends to be multifocal, admixed with secretory glands, and does not form a discrete lesion. Usually decidua is present, too. In addition, this change lacks the features of invasion, such as confluent glands, an extensively papillary pattern, or altered stroma. The nuclei in the Arias-Stella reaction generally appear to be degenerated, with smudged chromatin, and mitotic figures are infrequent. Other pregnancy-related cytologic changes, such as vacuolated cytoplasm and optically clear nuclei, also may be found in the epithelial cells when the Arias-Stella reaction is present.

Tissue Artifacts, Contaminants, and Necrosis

Tissue artifacts can yield worrisome patterns that may mimic carcinoma. For example, the artifactual crowding and distortion of glands that occur during biopsy can result in glands becoming closely apposed (Chapter 2). Likewise, breakdown and bleeding distorts the normal architecture and presents a variety of cytologic alterations, including eosinophilic syncytial change (see above). Cervical contaminants, especially endocervical squamous metaplasia, prominent detached fragments of endocervical epithelium, or microglandular hyperplasia, may become mixed with endometrial tissue in curettings and yield a complex pattern that can mimic carcinoma at first glance. These tissue artifacts usually are not a major problem in the differential diagnosis, however, since they are generally focal and admixed with normal endometrium. In menstrual endometrium, where there is more diffuse and extensive breakdown, the possibility of mistaking the pattern for adenocarcinoma is greater. In such cases it is important to attempt to identify secretory glandular changes and intact endometrium that is not showing breakdown. Furthermore, the clinical history, including the patient's age and menstrual status, can be very helpful in recognizing a menstrual pattern that may not be obvious at first inspection.

Fragmentation and artifacts also occur in curettings containing adenocarcinoma. When this occurs, the diagnosis of carcinoma still can be made if the epithelial cells demonstrate high nuclear grade. Those areas where glands are attached to surrounding mesenchymal tissue and are free of the changes of breakdown and bleeding demonstrate the true relationship of the glands to each other. To reliably identify malignancy in equivocal cases, however, it is best to evaluate the features that establish the diagnosis of well-differentiated adenocarcinoma in clearly intact areas.

Actual tumor necrosis rarely, if ever, occurs in well-differentiated tumors. This form of necrosis is often seen in high-grade tumors, but in these cases the histologic and nuclear features readily identify the lesion as carcinoma. Conversely, much of the necrosis that is commonly encountered in biopsy material is unique to the endometrium and actually reflects breakdown rather than necrotic tumor. The necrosis associated with bleeding and breakdown is apparent in low-grade carcinoma but often occurs in benign conditions, too, regardless of cause. Because tissue breakdown and necrosis are so ubiquitous in endometrial tissue, the finding of this pattern of necrosis is not helpful in establishing the diagnosis of neoplasia. Another pattern of necrosis can be seen in the center of nests of squamous change (morules). Central necrosis in areas of squamous change can occur in benign lesions, including any form of hyperplasia, polyps, and the atypical polypoid adenomyoma. Consequently, the necrosis associated with squamous change has no significance and does not indicate malignancy. In contrast to low-grade carcinoma, high-grade carcinomas and mixed mesodermal tumors can show extensive tumor-associated necrosis, but in these cases the tumor cells show marked cytologic atypia that assists in the diagnosis.

Malignant Neoplasms—Classification of the Tumor

Once the diagnosis of carcinoma is established, it is important that the tumor be properly classified in order to identify aggressive forms of carcinoma. Also, since the biopsy or curettage is generally a blind procedure with no direct visualization of the neoplasm, it is important to ascertain whether or not the carcinoma is primary in the endometrium or if it arises in the cervix. Finally, especially if the tumor displays an unusual pattern, the possibility of a metastasis from another site should be considered.

Clinically Important Histologic Subtypes

Typical (Endometrioid) Carcinoma

With this pattern the glands are similar to those seen in atypical hyperplasia. These tumors have a moderate amount of eosinophilic to amphophilic cytoplasm (Fig. 10.12).[3,41] The luminal border of the glands often is ill-defined. Glands may contain a small amount of mucin or necrotic debris (Fig. 10.13). This type of adenocarcinoma often shows a glandular pattern with prominent cribriform

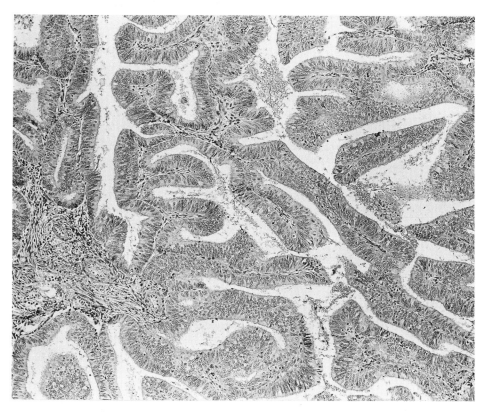

Figure 10.12. Adenocarcinoma. Typical (endometrioid) pattern. Classic "endometrioid" pattern with the glands lined by cells with pale cytoplasm and stratified nuclei. This well-differentiated tumor also shows villoglandular papillary features.

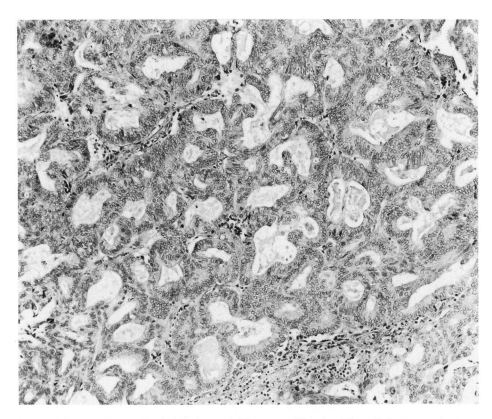

FIGURE 10.13. Adenocarcinoma. Typical (endometrioid) pattern. The glandular cells have a moderate amount of eosinophilic cytoplasm. The mucoid contents within the glandular lumens do not affect the classification of the carcinoma.

bridging, but not infrequently it may display a papillary pattern that has been referred to as "villoglandular" (Figs. 10.11 and 10.12).[3,54,55] In these papillary tumors, the cells are columnar and perpendicular to the fibrovascular core. Nuclei are cigar-shaped and relatively bland (see below, Serous Carcinoma for further discussion of papillary patterns).

Variants of endometrioid carcinoma include ciliated carcinoma and secretory carcinoma.[3,41] Ciliated carcinoma is a very rare neoplasm in which the invasive glands are lined by cells with cilia along the luminal border.[3,56,57] Its significance lies in the recognition that cilia do not always indicate a benign lesion.

In the secretory variant of endometrial adenocarcinoma, the neoplastic glands are lined by cells with vacuolated cytoplasm (Fig. 10.14).[3,5,9,58] Cytoplasmic vacuolization is a feature also seen in many clear cell carcinomas (see below, Clear Cell

Carcinoma), but it is important to separate the low-grade secretory carcinoma from clear cell carcinoma, which is generally a high-grade neoplasm. In secretory carcinoma, clear vacuoles fill the subnuclear or supranuclear cytoplasm, and the cells resemble those seen in normal early secretory phase. The nuclei usually show minimal atypia, although the glands fulfill the criteria for invasion. These rare tumors have an excellent prognosis. Secretory carcinoma can occur in premenopausal or postmenopausal patients.

Foam cells often are present in the stroma of endometrioid carcinoma or its variants, especially when they are low grade.[41,59] The presence of foam cells by themselves does not influence the diagnosis or the classification of endometrial carcinoma, since foam cells can occur in a variety of benign conditions in which there is abnormal glandular and stromal breakdown (Chapter 5). Some endometrial carcinomas show a marked

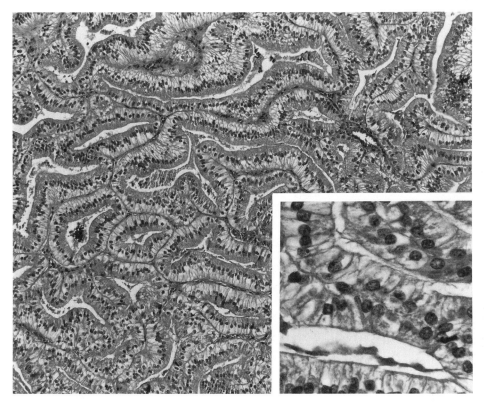

FIGURE 10.14. Secretory carcinoma. This variant shows neoplastic glandular cells with extensive subnuclear vacuoles, superficially resembling early secretory phase endometrium. *Inset*: The secretory changes are accompanied by low-grade nuclei.

neutrophilic infiltrate. Polymorphonuclear leukocytes can be intimately admixed with the tumor, and the tumor cells can show apparent phagocytosis of neutrophils. The neutrophilic response has no known effect on prognosis.

Adenocarcinoma with Squamous Differentiation

Squamous differentiation commonly occurs in tumors with a typical (endometrioid) glandular pattern.[3] It is rarely, if ever, associated with serous or clear cell carcinoma. At least 10% of the tumor should have squamous features for it to qualify as adenocarcinoma with squamous differentiation. Typically the squamous epithelium is intimately admixed with glands (Fig. 10.15).

The squamous epithelium can have low-grade nuclear features resembling the squamous change seen in benign lesions and in atypical hyperplasia. Carcinomas with this pattern have been termed "adenoacanthoma" in the past. Conversely, the squamous component can show cytologic features of malignancy. This latter group, with cytologically malignant squamous epithelium, has been termed "adenosquamous carcinoma."

In the low-grade (adenoacanthoma) neoplasms, the squamous changes often include so-called morules, rounded masses of bland squamous cells largely filling the lumens of the malignant glands (Fig. 10.16). These squamous cells are incompletely differentiated and have eosinophilic cytoplasm and indistinct cell borders. The nuclei are uniform, bland, and lack prominent nucleoli; they do not palisade. Mitotic figures are infrequent. The squamous cells can show intercellular bridges, but this finding is infrequent. Often these squamous nests are nonkeratinizing, but keratinization may be present.

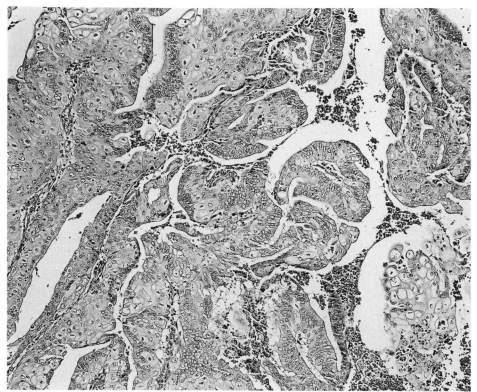

FIGURE 10.15. Adenocarcinoma with squamous differentiation. Multiple foci of squamous change are interspersed in this well-differentiated (FIGO grade 1) adenocarcinoma.

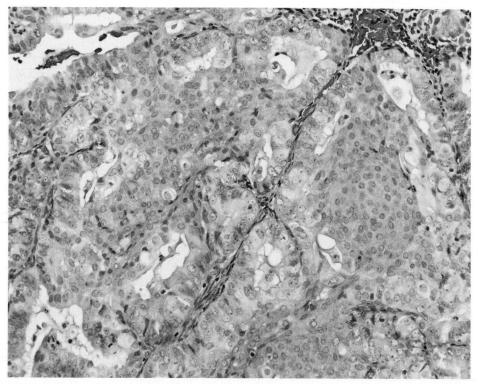

FIGURE 10.16. Adenocarcinoma with squamous differentiation. Central nests of squamous epithelium form morules in well-differentiated adenocarcinoma. The nuclear grade of the glandular and the squamous element is the same (grade 1).

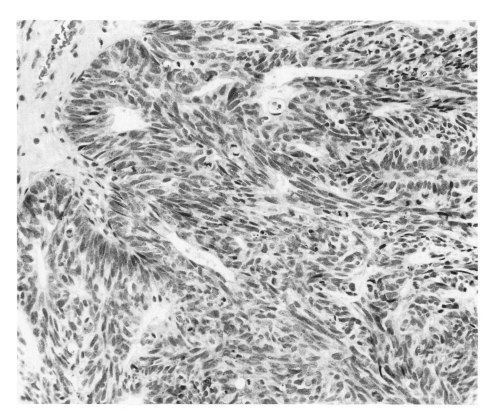

FIGURE 10.17. Adenocarcinoma with squamous differentiation. Gland lumens are partially obliterated by spindle-shaped squamous cells. The squamous component is cytologically malignant, with multiple mitoses and no keratinization. The spindle pattern should not be mistaken for a sarcomatous component.

When the squamous component appears malignant, the change usually is associated with a neoplasm that is grade 2 or 3. Portions of the tumor may show squamous carcinoma without glandular differentiation. Tumors with a cytologically malignant squamous component often are composed of nests of spindle-shaped cells that obliterate gland lumens (Fig. 10.17). Keratinization and squamous pearl formation are frequently apparent. Abundant keratin formation may even incite a foreign body response. Mitotic activity often is brisk in the squamous component. Not surprisingly, studies in the past have demonstrated that adenoacanthoma has an excellent prognosis and adenosquamous carcinoma a poor prognosis.

Despite the apparent dichotomy between the growth patterns of adenoacanthoma and adenosquamous carcinoma, a clear distinction between the cytologically benign and malignant squamous epithelium is not always possible. The squamous component often shows mild degrees of atypia and scattered mitotic figures (Fig. 10.18). In these cases the cytologic features exceed the "benign" appearance required for a diagnosis of adenoacanthoma but do not have all the characteristics of malignancy required for a diagnosis of adenosquamous carcinoma. Furthermore, this squamous change, since it occurs in adenocarcinoma, is malignant, regardless of its histology. Studies have shown that when these tumors are stratified by grade and depth of myometrial invasion, the presence of squamous epithelium does not alter the prognosis when compared to endometrioid carcinoma lacking squamous epithelium.[15,16,27] Accordingly, it is the grade of the glandular component that has prognostic significance. For these reasons, the term "adenocarcinoma with squamous differentiation" is preferred. These tumors should be graded 1, 2, or 3

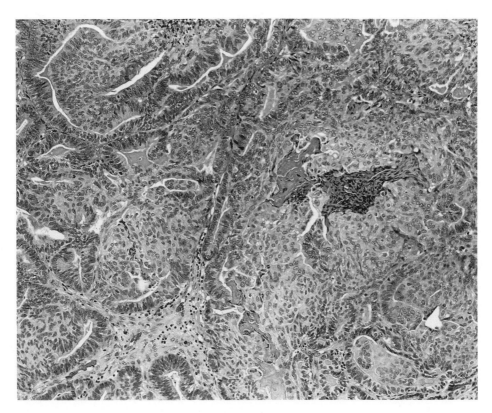

FIGURE 10.18. Adenocarcinoma with squamous differentiation. In this tumor the squamous cell nuclei are intermediate between grade 1 and grade 3 (compare to Figs. 10.16 and 10.17). The glandular component showed features of moderately differentiated (FIGO grade 2) adenocarcinoma.

based on the architectural and nuclear features of the glandular component.

Mucinous Carcinoma

Mucinous carcinoma of the endometrium has a glandular architecture resembling endometrioid carcinoma but is composed of cells containing abundant intracytoplasmic mucin (Fig. 10.19).[3,10,11,41,60] Mucinous carcinomas tend to be well to moderately differentiated, and they frequently have a papillary or villous architecture. Portions of these carcinomas often appear extremely well differentiated, because the mucinous cytoplasm results in basal alignment of the nuclei with minimal nuclear stratification, but usually the sections show transitions to areas with a more typical endometrioid pattern. Foam cells are also often associated with these tumors.

The presence of extracellular and luminal mu-

cin is not used in establishing the diagnosis of endometrial mucinous carcinoma. Furthermore. the presence of cytoplasmic mucin should be extensive, involving greater than 50% of the cells for a tumor to be classified as mucinous carcinoma, since some mucin production is present in most endometrial carcinomas.[11,61] Special stains for epithelial mucin, such as mucicarmine or the periodic acid-Schiff (PAS) with diastase digestion, can be helpful to demonstrate the mucin. Up to 9% of all stage 1 endometrial carcinomas are of the mucinous type according to these criteria.[11]

The morphologic features of low-grade mucinous carcinoma overlap with the patterns of so-called secretory carcinoma, because both types of tumors have abundant pale cytoplasm and basal nuclei with minimal stratification. In mucinous carcinoma the cells contain cytoplasmic mucin, whereas in secretory carcinoma the cytoplasmic vacuoles contain glycogen. The distinction is

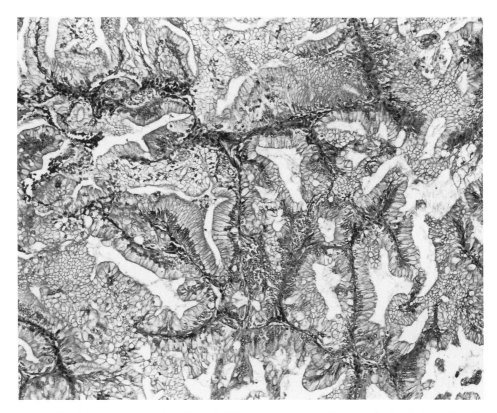

FIGURE 10.19. Mucinous carcinoma. In this well-differentiated tumor, the glandular cells have abundant cytoplasmic mucin. Nuclei are oriented along the basal portion of the cells, resulting in a resemblance to endocervical epithelium.

largely academic, however, since tumor grade rather than cytoplasmic differentiation determines prognosis. These neoplasms show no difference in behavior from endometrioid tumors of similar grade.[11]

Since the cell population of mucinous carcinoma resembles endocervical epithelium, with basal nuclei and abundant supranuclear cytoplasm that contains mucin, the differential diagnosis often includes endocervical adenocarcinoma. This differential is discussed in greater detail below.

Endocervical-Like Endometrial Carcinoma

Occasional well-differentiated mucinous endometrial carcinomas have patterns that mimic cervical microglandular hyperplasia.[62] These tumors are composed of numerous small mucinous glands (Fig. 10.20). Some examples also contain

acute inflammatory cells in the lumens and the intervening stroma. These tumors have minimal cytologic atypia and mitotic activity, thus closely resembling endocervical microglandular hyperplasia. The endometrial neoplasms typically show a transition to ordinary endometrial adenocarcinoma, which facilitates the diagnosis. In addition, the criteria outlined below for distinguishing endometrial and endocervical primaries also help in the recognition of these carcinomas.

Endometrial Versus Endocervical Carcinoma

At times it is difficult to determine whether carcinoma in an endometrial biopsy involves the endometrium, the endocervix, or both sites. Assigning a primary site is important, because endometrial carcinoma confined to the corpus is managed differently from endocervical carcinoma. The usual therapy for endometrial carcinoma is extra-fascial total abdominal hysterectomy and bilateral salpingo-oophorectomy. In contrast, surgical management of invasive endocervical carcinoma is a radical hysterectomy and pelvic lymph node dissection, an operation with potential for greater morbidity.

If the tumor in the endometrial biopsy has the typical endometrioid pattern and the clinical information, such as older age and uterine enlargement, is consistent with an endometrial cancer, there is little question regarding the primary site. In contrast, if the tumor has a pattern that also may be found in the cervix, such as mucinous, clear cell, or extensive squamous differentiation, then determination of the primary site is more difficult.

Squamous differentiation can be prominent in primary endometrial carcinoma and adenosquamous carcinoma is a well-recognized variant of endocervical carcinoma. Consequently, when curettings show a mixture of glandular and squamous components, the differential diagnosis often includes endometrial and endocervical primary sites. Adenocarcinoma with a squamous component at each site has different histologic features. In endometrial carcinoma, the squamous element often is intimately associated with glands, appearing to arise in and differentiate from the glands. The glandular element typically predominates in endometrial carcinomas. In contrast, in endocervical adenosquamous carcinoma, the squamous element usually predominates and glandular differentiation is more subtle. Furthermore, the cervical neoplasms do not show the prominent nests of morular growth ("adenoacanthoma pattern") with squamous differentiation confined to gland lumens that are very frequent in endometrial adenocarcinoma.

Added evidence in favor of an endometrial primary carcinoma is the presence of associated hyperplasia. Conversely, the presence of cervical intraepithelial neoplasia or endocervical adenocarcinoma in situ, as well as transitions to normal endocervical epithelium, supports the diagnosis of cervical carcinoma. In addition, in a fractional curettage, if more tumor is present in the endometrial fraction, it is more likely that the neoplasm arises in the endometrium. Conversely, the endocervical fraction contains the bulk of

the tumor when the primary tumor is in the endocervix.

Some immunohistochemical stains can help to distinguish endometrial from endocervical primary tumors. Carcinoembryonic antigen (CEA) often is present in endocervical carcinomas but is less common in endometrial primary tumors.[63-65] The majority of endocervical carcinomas show abundant, diffuse intracellular CEA reactivity, whereas only about half of endometrial carcinomas contain CEA, and this reactivity is usually focal and at the luminal surface. The opposite reactivity is found with vimentin.[66] Endometrial tumors selectively express this intermediate filament to a far greater extent than endocervical carcinoma. Histochemical stains for mucin have little value in determining the primary site, however, since endometrial adenocarcinoma often shows at least focal cytoplasmic mucin and some endocervical adenocarcinomas show little cytoplasmic mucin.

If the morphologic features do not clearly establish the primary site, clinical information often resolves the problem. The presence or absence of gross tumor involving the cervix is important information. If tumor clinically involves the cervix, then the issue of primary site is largely irrelevant. The tumor can be managed as a cervical neoplasm.[24] If the tumor is occult, other information, such as age and menopausal status, can be helpful. Endometrial carcinoma usually occurs in older patients with an average age of 55 to 60 years. Endometrial carcinoma is unusual before the menopause unless the patient has a predisposing condition, such as the Stein–Leventhal syndrome. Endocervical adenocarcinoma, in contrast, has a much wider age range, with many tumors occurring in premenopausal women. The average age is between 45 and 55 years.

Serous Carcinoma

Serous carcinoma is recognized by its marked nuclear atypia and its resemblance to ovarian serous carcinoma.[17,20,54,67-70] Like their ovarian counterparts, these tumors often have a highly papillary growth pattern (Fig. 10.21). The fibrotic papillary fronds are lined by a stratified layer of cells with a high nuclear/cytoplasmic

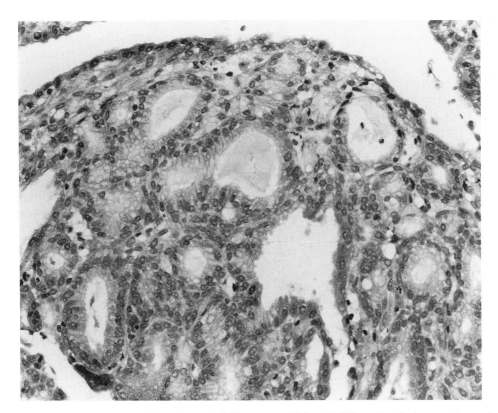

FIGURE 10.20. Adenocarcinoma with endocervical-like pattern. This well-differentiated adenocarcinoma is composed of anastomosing small glands that have a superficial resemblance to microglandular hyperplasia of the cervix. Transitions to ordinary endometrial adenocarcinoma in other fields help to establish the correct diagnosis.

TABLE 10.4. Histologic features of serous carcinoma.

Complex, coarse, or fine papillae
Irregular, gaping glands
Papillary tufting
High nuclear/cytoplasmic ratio
Marked nuclear pleomorphism
Numerous and abnormal mitoses
Macronucleoli
Clear cell component[a]
Psammoma bodies[a]

[a] Nonspecific features found in approximately a third of serous carcinoma.

ratio and high-grade nuclei (Table 10.4). The malignant cells also form complex papillary tufts that may be present as free-floating clusters of cells. The papillae have a coarse appearance, with thick fibrotic cores lined with highly epithelial atypical cells (Fig. 10.22). These papillary tufts often lack stroma and are composed of dense papillary aggregates of tumor cells. Psammoma bodies are present in up to one-third of cases.[54] Because of the papillary growth, serous carcinoma can appear deceptively well differentiated in the endometrium, although these are high-grade, aggressive neoplasms. Serous carcinoma was originally considered a predominantly papillary neoplasm, but further studies have shown that it is morphologically diverse.[68] In some cases the papillae are long and slender instead of short and coarse. The tumor may even be primarily composed of glands, and the lumens have an irregular, gaping appearance (Fig. 10.23).

It is the combination of a papillary or gaping glandular pattern and the marked nuclear atypia that identifies serous carcinoma. The nuclei are hyperchromatic and pleomorphic with macronucleoli and many mitoses (Fig. 10.24). Abnormal mitotic figures are frequent. Some nuclei are highly lobulated, with deep nuclear clefts. In

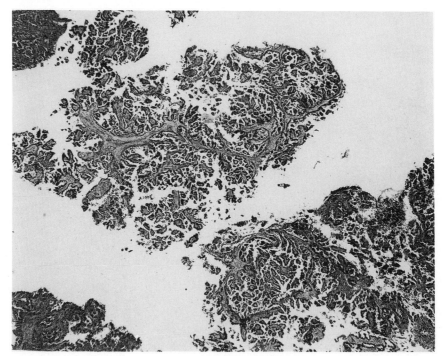

FIGURE 10.21. Serous carcinoma. Arborizing papillae with multiple papillary tufts are a frequent characteristic of this tumor. Many of the papillae appear as free-floating clusters of cells.

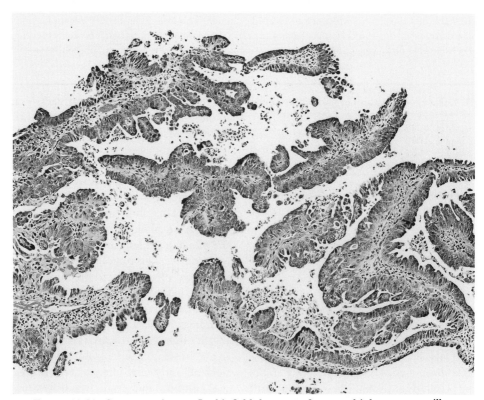

FIGURE 10.22. Serous carcinoma. In this field the tumor forms multiple coarse papillae.

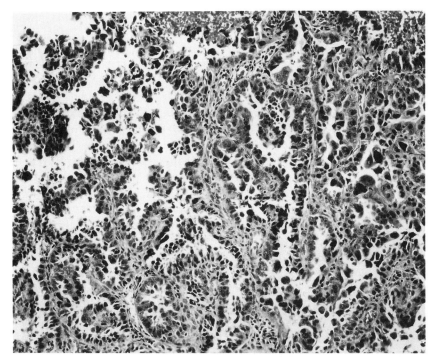

FIGURE 10.23. Serous carcinoma. This tumor is composed of gaping glands and papillae with papillary tufts. There is marked nuclear pleomorphism and high nuclear grade. These are constant features of serous carcinoma.

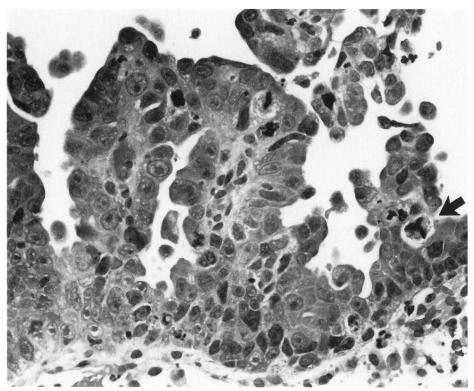

FIGURE 10.24. Serous carcinoma. The nuclei are grade 3. There is a high nuclear/cytoplasmic ratio, and numerous mitoses with abnormal forms. A tripolar mitosis is present (*arrow*).

some cases the chromatin appears smudged at low magnification. The cells of serous carcinoma tend to be rounded, and they often have abundant granular, eosinophilic cytoplasm. Areas displaying the features of serous carcinoma but containing clear cells, i.e., clear cell carcinoma, are seen in up to one-third of cases (see below, Clear Cell Carcinoma).

Since these tumors are almost always composed of high-grade nuclei, nuclear grading as recommended by FIGO is probably not relevant. The diagnosis of serous carcinoma itself establishes the presence of highly malignant carcinoma.

Several other histologic subtypes of endometrial carcinoma, including low-grade endometrioid tumors, also may show papillary growth, yielding the so-called villoglandular pattern.[3,12,28,41,54,71] The papillary endometrioid tumors have low- to moderate-grade nuclei (see above, Grading) and often grow in long, slender branching papillary fronds (Figs. 10.11, 10.12, 10.25, and 10.26). The lining cells are columnar and do not form papillary tufts. In contrast, the papillae in serous carcinoma tend to be small and coarse, although it is the high nuclear grade that is most useful for identifying this neoplasm. To avoid confusion between these papillary tumors with different cytologic features and prognosis, we recommend not using the term "papillary" as a diagnostic term for any type of endometrial carcinoma.

Serous carcinoma is a highly malignant form of endometrial carcinoma that usually occurs in older women, with a median age in the seventh decade.[12,54,70–73] These tumors often invade the myometrium deeply and permeate lymphatic or vascular spaces. Not uncommonly, this neoplasm can be superficial and minimally invasive, however, and even may be confined to an endometrial polyp.[74] Even with no or minimal myometrial

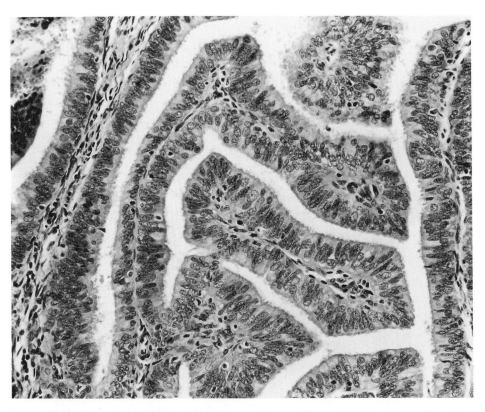

FIGURE 10.25. Well-differentiated villoglandular adenocarcinoma. The nuclei lining the papillae have grade 1 features, in contrast to the high nuclear grade seen in serous carcinoma. Nuclei are round to oval and exhibit minimal pleomorphism.

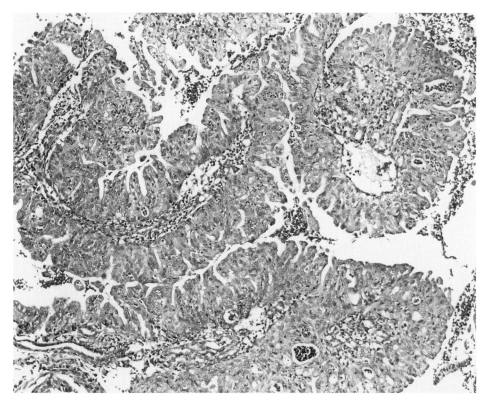

FIGURE 10.26. Moderately differentiated adenocarcinoma with papillary features. Typical ("endometrioid") adenocarcinoma with a papillary pattern. The nuclei lack the high nuclear grade that is characteristic of serous carcinoma.

invasion, serous carcinoma can disseminate widely.[8,12,54,67,68,71]

Patients with serous carcinoma often either have peritoneal spread at the time of laparotomy or relapse with peritoneal carcinomatosis, so in this regard they behave like their ovarian counterparts. Occasional cases also appear to be multifocal, with associated ovarian serous carcinoma at the time of diagnosis. Because of their aggressive growth, even when superficial or confined to polyps, tumors showing both endometrioid and serous patterns with at least 25% of the tumor containing a serous component should be classified as serous carcinoma.

Clear Cell Carcinoma

In clear cell carcinoma, the majority of the cells have clear, vacuolated cytoplasm due to the presence of glycogen.[3,5,9,18,19,22,41] This tumor can have a variety of growth patterns, including tubular, cystic, papillary, and solid (Figs. 10.27–10.29). In some cases the clear cytoplasm is inconspicuous and the nuclei bulge into the lumens of the malignant glands, forming so-called hobnail cells (Fig. 10.28). Clear cell carcinoma also occurs in the ovary, cervix, and vagina. In the ovary or cervix, clear cell tumors in older women have similar patterns to those found in the endometrium, but in the vagina and cervix of women exposed to in utero diethylstibestrol (DES), the tubulocystic pattern predominates.

Many examples of clear cell carcinoma appear to be closely related to serous carcinoma, and, as mentioned above, this tumor pattern may be admixed with serous carcinoma.[54] The similarity with serous carcinoma is reflected in the high nuclear grade of many clear cell tumors. Especially in the papillary and solid patterns, the nuclei generally are pleomorphic with marked atyp-

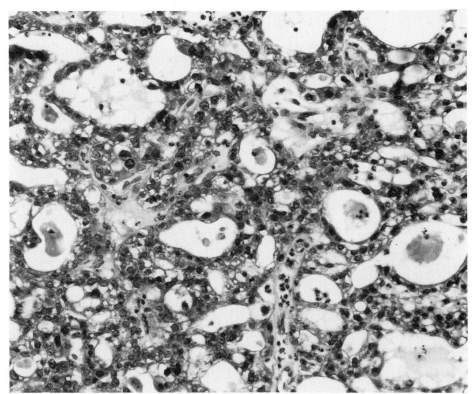

FIGURE 10.27. Clear cell carcinoma. Tubular pattern in which most of the cells contain clear cytoplasm. There is nuclear enlargement and pleomorphism, a frequent finding in clear cell carcinoma.

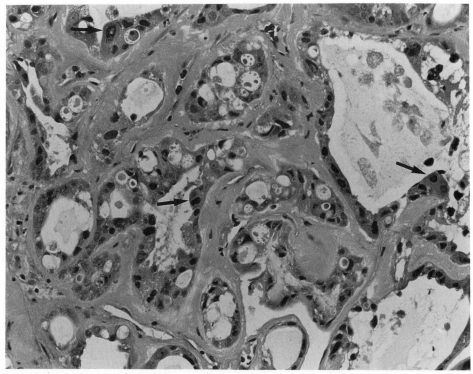

FIGURE 10.28. Clear cell carcinoma. The clear cytoplasm is less conspicuous, and the nuclei bulge, hobnail fashion, into the glandular lumens (*arrows*). The hyalinized stroma is an occasional feature of clear cell carcinoma.

210

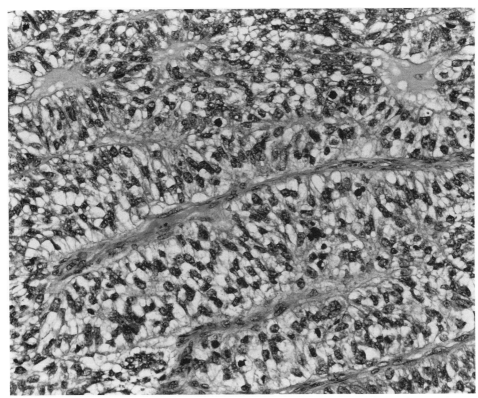

FIGURE 10.29. Clear cell carcinoma. Solid pattern with highly vacuolated cytoplasm. The nuclei are not as pleomorphic as those shown in Fig. 10.27. This case also could be classified as poorly differentiated endometrioid carcinoma with secretory change and illustrates the overlap between clear cell and secretory patterns.

ia. Macronucleoli and abnormal mitotic figures usually are present. In these cases, the close relationship of serous and clear cell carcinoma indicates that these two cell types may be different morphologic expressions of a carcinoma with the same biologic behavior. Occasionally, these tumors, like serous carcinoma, contain psammoma bodies. This form of clear cell adenocarcinoma is another aggressive variant of endometrial cancer.[5,9] It, like serous carcinoma, tends to occur in older patients and has a high relapse rate.

Some examples of clear cell carcinoma do not show high nuclear grade, however, and appear to represent a variant of endometrioid carcinoma with clear cell change (Fig. 10.29). These latter tumors often show tubulocystic growth. The cells lining the tubules and cysts may be hobnail-shaped, cuboidal, or flattened and generally have bland nuclei. This pattern of clear cell differentiation should be separated from the aggressive,

serous-like clear cell carcinoma. This distinction is based on the papillary pattern and high-grade nuclei in the serous-related clear cell carcinoma. The variation in the morphologic forms of clear cell carcinoma illustrates the utility of nuclear grading (Table 10.3) when evaluating this type of endometrial carcinoma.

Occasional cases of high-grade clear cell carcinoma show focal areas that appear well differentiated and resemble secretory carcinoma, and it is important to thoroughly sample apparent low-grade secretory or clear cell tumors to determine if they have foci with grade 3 nuclei that indicate a more aggressive neoplasm.

Mixed Mesodermal Tumor

The distinction between a malignant mixed mesodermal tumor (MMMT) and high-grade carcinoma may at times be difficult. In MMMTs the epithelial element usually has features of high-grade endometrial adenocarcinoma, often serous or clear cell carcinoma, although endometrioid patterns, including carcinoma with squamous differentiation, may be found. It is important to identify a sarcomatous component, however, since the MMMTs are even more aggressive than high-grade carcinomas. In such cases, as-certaining the presence of a malignant stromal component, a feature discussed in Chapter 11, becomes important. Often, the sarcomatous com-ponent is readily identified, especially when het-erologous elements, such as cartilage or rhabdo-myoblasts, are present. In many cases, however, the malignant stroma is composed only of spindle cells, identified as malignant by their cellularity, nuclear atypia, and high mitotic activity, that may be intimately associated with, yet distinct from, the carcinomatous component. In these cases, use of a keratin immunohistochemical stain can be helpful for distinguishing the carcinomatous from the sarcomatous component, since the sar-comatous elements are generally negative or only focally positive for keratin.

Rare Carcinomas

Primary squamous carcinoma of the endome-trium does occur, but is rare.[75,76] To diagnose this entity, it is necessary to exclude a primary cervical carcinoma (see below, Endometrial Ver-sus Endocervical Carcinoma). Primary verrucous squamous cell carcinoma also has been reported to arise in the endometrium.[77]

Undifferentiated carcinomas show no evidence of glandular or squamous differentiation.[78] They account for less than 2% of endometrial pri-maries. Some undifferentiated carcinomas have features resembling small cell carcinoma of the lung, whereas others are composed of large cells that range from polygonal to spindle in shape. Undifferentiated carcinoma often has a diffuse growth pattern with extensive necrosis. With the small cell pattern, the neoplastic cells have scant cytoplasm and hyperchromatic nuclei with indis-tinct nucleoli.[79] These neoplasms may show neu-roendocrine differentiation.[80–84] Some tumors with a small cell component show an admixture with typical adenocarcinoma.[79] The large cell variant is composed of sheets of large epithelial cells that have a moderate amount of cytoplasm and large vesicular nuclei and prominent nucle-oli. Rarely, carcinomas show unusual patterns of differentiation, such as osteoclastic-type giant cells or trophoblast.[55,83] Other rare histologic types include glassy cell and giant cell carci-noma.[83–85] These high-grade malignancies most often occur in older patients.

On occasion an endometrial neoplasm is dif-ficult to classify. Small tissue samples or extensive necrosis may limit the histologic evaluation. Im-munohistochemistry has little utility for subclas-sification of endometrial carcinomas, although keratin reactivity can help determine whether or not a malignant tumor represents a carcinoma.

Metastatic Carcinoma

The most common extrauterine carcinomas that metastasize to or extend into the endometrium arise in the ovary, breast, or gastrointestinal tract, especially the colon.[86–88] Metastases from other primary sites are rare, but on occasion a tumor from the stomach, pancreas, or other vis-ceral site metastasizes to the endometrium. It is very unusual for tumors from these sites to present with abnormal vaginal bleeding and to be diag-nosed first on an endometrial biopsy.

Separating metastatic ovarian carcinoma from an endometrial primary tumor can be especially difficult, since virtually all patterns of primary endometrial carcinoma can occur in primary ovarian epithelial carcinoma.[89,90] In particular, serous and endometrioid carcinomas are com-mon in the ovary, and these tumors are histolog-ically identical to their endometrial counterparts. Despite these difficulties, the question of ovarian metastasis versus an endometrial primary site in a biopsy or curetting is infrequent. This differential is most likely to occur when the biopsy shows a serous carcinoma, usually with psammoma bod-ies. In such cases it may be impossible to exclude an ovarian primary site, but metastatic tumor presenting in biopsies is extremely infrequent compared to a primary endometrial serous carci-noma. Furthermore, cases with involvement of the endometrium and ovary often appear to rep-resent synchronous primary tumors rather than metastases. Metastatic lesions should be consid-ered, however, when the amount of tumor is rel-

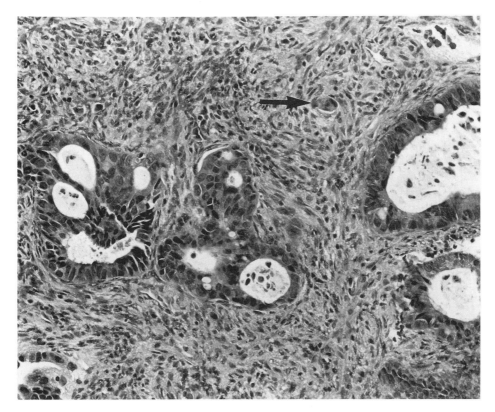

FIGURE 10.30. Metastatic colon carcinoma. Irregular glands with sharply delimited luminal borders are haphazardly distributed in a reactive, fibroblastic stroma. This pattern can closely mimic an endometrial primary, but the haphazard distribution of the glands in markedly desmoplastic stroma suggests a metastasis from a gastrointestinal primary. Also, the small nests of malignant cells (*arrow*) are not typical of endometrial carcinoma.

atively scant and is admixed with more abundant fragments of benign, nonhyperplastic endometrium. Also, clinical history of an adnexal mass should alert the pathologist to the possibility of primary ovarian neoplasia.

Metastatic carcinoma from other sites, while rare, can be problematic. Occasionally, colon carcinoma may involve the endometrium and closely simulate a uterine primary tumor, having an "endometrioid" pattern (Fig. 10.30). In such cases a history of a known extrauterine primary tumor or a mass lesion in the bowel can be essential for establishing the correct diagnosis. Colon adenocarcinoma may have a so-called garland-like arrangement of glands surrounding areas of "dirty" necrosis composed of cellular debris that helps in recognizing the tumor. The glands of metastatic colon carcinoma have a sharp luminal border. Endometrial carcinoma, on the other hand, typically does not show much necrosis in glandular lumens, and the cells have an ill-defined, fuzzy luminal border in routine sections. Mucin stains have little utility in determining the primary site, since endometrial carcinoma can have abundant cytoplasmic mucin. Immunohistochemical stains for CEA may be helpful in helping to establish whether the tumor is metastatic from the gastrointestinal tract or is primary in the endometrium. In general, colon primaries are diffusely positive for CEA while endometrial carcinomas are not.

Metastatic breast carcinoma, while rare, can be especially difficult to diagnose. These tumors typically infiltrate in solid sheets or small groups in a linear, Indian file pattern, often sparing glands and diffusely invading the stroma (Fig. 10.31). The neoplastic cells may resemble stromal cells or inflammatory cells, lacking the organoid ar-

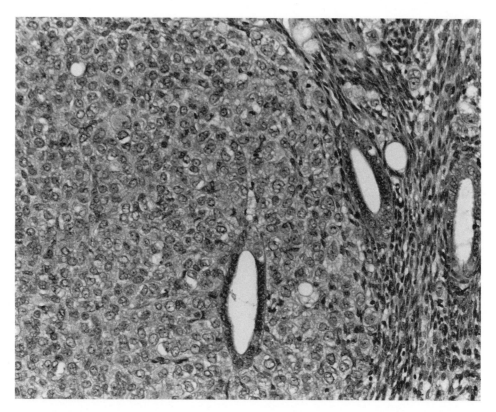

FIGURE 10.31. Metastatic breast carcinoma. A solid sheet of cells representing metastatic breast carcinoma infiltrates the endometrium. The pattern could be mistaken for an aggregate of stromal or inflammatory cells, and special stains for mucin and keratin may be needed to establish the diagnosis. The residual glands show progestin effect with glandular atrophy secondary to therapy for breast carcinoma.

rangements seen in most carcinomas. In such cases, immunohistochemical stains for keratin and histochemical stains for mucin are useful for demonstrating the epithelial origin of the cells.

Clinical Queries and Reporting

It is important to clearly establish the diagnosis of atypical hyperplasia versus well-differentiated adenocarcinoma whenever possible. A biopsy diagnosis of atypical hyperplasia may be managed medically with progestin therapy and periodic resampling of the endometrium. This conservative management is possible, since many lesions are reversible. A biopsy diagnosis of well-differentiated adenocarcinoma, in contrast, clearly establishes the presence of malignancy. Although the criteria for distinguishing atypical hyper-

plasia from well-differentiated adenocarcinoma have general quantitative guidelines, the diagnosis should also be placed in the appropriate clinical context. In younger, premenopausal patients, a conservative approach is appropriate when the biopsy shows an atypical lesion that may represent well-differentiated adenocarcinoma. Several studies have shown that these lesions, even if they fulfill criteria for adenocarcinoma, are indolent and possibly reversible with progestin therapy. Thus, in the premenopausal patient under 40 years of age, it is especially important to be certain that a lesion at least fulfills the minimal criteria for well-differentiated adenocarcinoma before establishing a diagnosis of malignancy. If the glands are atypical but do not clearly show features of "stromal invasion" as defined earlier, then the lesion is best classified as atypical hyperplasia. These patients can be managed conservatively and rebiopsied, and often the lesions will regress. In older postmenopausal women, atypical glands should be viewed even more suspiciously for the possibility of underlying carcinoma, and criteria for the histologic diagnosis of carcinoma can be applied more liberally. Most of these patients are best treated by a total abdominal hysterectomy and bilateral salpingo-oophorectomy if they are candidates for surgery.

Once the diagnosis of endometrial adenocarcinoma is made, the gynecologist often needs information on several other aspects of the tumor. Whenever possible, the FIGO grade of endometrial carcinoma in biopsies should be given. For example, low-grade adenocarcinoma usually is confined to the endometrium and myometrium, and extrauterine spread is unlikely. Conversely, high-grade carcinoma, including aggressive histologic subtypes of serous and clear cell carcinoma, has greater potential for showing extrauterine spread at the time of hysterectomy. If grading is not possible due to limited sampling, necrosis or other distortion of the tissue, this should be noted.

Classifying the tumor according to histologic subtype is important. When the tumor has the typical "endometrioid" or mucinous pattern, the type of tumor has little clinical significance by itself. These distinctions have more relevance to the pathologist than to the clinician. Squamous differentiation, too, has little clinical significance once the tumor is graded but may be relevant to note for histologic correlation with any subsequent metastases or recurrences. On the other hand, serous and high-grade clear cell carcinomas are aggressive tumors that are important to identify. The diagnosis of these tumors should indicate to the clinician that there is an increased risk for deep myometrial invasion and metastases.

Mixed carcinomas have at least 10% of a second cell type. An example would be a mixture of endometrioid and serous patterns. If 25% or more of such tumor is composed of serous carcinoma, then it should be classified as such, since these mixed neoplasms behave the same as pure serous carcinoma. Otherwise it can be termed a "mixed carcinoma," with a note describing the different types of carcinoma present.

The amount of tumor in the specimen and associated lesions such as hyperplasia or polyps are potentially useful data. For example, a small amount of tumor may alert the clinician to difficulties in accurate grading. The presence of associated hyperplasia suggests estrogenic effects that may influence the method of therapy. Accordingly, the presence of hyperplasia should be included in the report. Should the tumor suggest a metastatic process, the report should clearly indicate this and suggest the primary sites, if possible.

References

1. Smith M, McCartney AJ: Occult, high-risk endometrial cancer. Gynecol Oncol 1985;22:154–161.
2. Bokhman JV: Two pathogenetic types of endometrial carcinoma. Gynecol Oncol 1983;15:10.
3. Kurman RJ, Zaino RJ, Norris HJ: Endometrial carcinoma. In: Blaustein's Pathology of the Female Genital Tract. 4th ed. Kurman RJ, ed. New York: Springer-Verlag, 1994;439–486.
4. Alberhasky RC, Connelly PJ, Christopherson WM: Carcinoma of the endometrium. IV. Mixed adenosquamous carcinoma. Am J Clin Pathol 1982;77:655–664.
5. Christopherson WM, Alberhasky RC, Connelly PJ: Carcinoma of the endometrium. I. A clinicopathologic study of clear cell carcinoma and secretory carcinoma. Cancer 1982;49:1511–1523.
6. Christopherson WM, Connelly PJ, Alberhasky RC: Carcinoma of the endometrium. V. An analysis of prognosticators in patients with favorable subtypes and stage I disease. Cancer 1983;51:1705–1709.
7. Connelly PJ, Alberhasky RC, Christopherson WM: Carcinoma of the endometrium. III. Analysis of 865 cases of adenocarcinoma and adenoacanthoma. Obstet Gynecol 1982;59:569–575.
8. Hendrickson M, Ross J, Eifel PJ, Cox RJ, Martinez A, et al: Adenocarcinoma of the endometrium: An analysis of 256 cases with carcinoma limited to the uterine corpus. I. Pathology review and analysis of prognostic variables. Gynecol Oncol 1982;13:373–392.
9. Kurman RJ, Scully RE: Clear cell carcinoma of the endometrium. An analysis of 21 cases. Cancer 1976;37:872–882.
10. Melhem MF, Tobon H: Mucinous adenocarcinoma of the endometrium: A clinico-pathological review of 18 cases. Int J Gynecol Pathol 1987;6:347–355.
11. Ross JC, Eifel PJ, Cox RS, Kempson RL, Hen-

drickson MR: Primary mucinous adenocarcinoma of the endometrium. A clinicopathologic and histochemical study. Am J Surg Pathol 1983;7:715–729.

12. Chen JL, Trost DC, Wilkinson EJ: Endometrial papillary adenocarcinomas: Two clinicopathological types. Int J Gynecol Pathol 1985;4:279.

13. Mittal KR, Schwartz PE, Barwick KW: Architectural (FIGO) grading, nuclear grading, and other prognostic indicators in Stage I endometrial adenocarcinoma with identification of high-risk and low-risk groups. Cancer 1988;61:538–545.

14. Wilson TO, Podratz KC, Gaffey TA, Malkasian GD, O'Brien PC, et al: Evaluation of unfavorable histologic subtypes in endometrial adenocarcinoma. Am J Obstet Gynecol 1990;162: 418–426.

15. Zaino RJ, Kurman R, Herbold D, Gliedman J, Bundy BN, et al: The significance of squamous differentiation in endometrial carcinoma—Data from a Gynecologic Oncology Group study. Cancer 1991;68:2293–2302.

16. Abeler VM, Kjorstad KE: Endometrial adenocarcinoma with squamous cell differentiation. Cancer 1992;69:488–495.

17. Abeler VM, Kjorstad KE: Serous papillary carcinoma of the endometrium: A histopathological study of 22 cases. Gynecol Oncol 1990;39:266–271.

18. Abeler VM, Kjorstad KE: Clear cell carcinoma of the endometrium: A histopathological and clinical study of 97 cases. Gynecol Oncol 1991; 40:207–217.

19. Webb GA, Lagios MD: Clear cell carcinoma of the endometrium. Am J Obstet Gynecol 1987;156: 1486–1491.

20. Dunton CJ, Balsara G, McFarland M, Hernandez E: Uterine papillary serous carcinoma. A review. Obstet Gynecol Survey 1991;46:97–102.

21. Fanning J, Evans MC, Peters AJ, Samuel M, Harmon ER, et al: Endometrial adenocarcinoma histologic subtypes: Clinical and pathologic profile. Gynecol Oncol 1989;32:288–291.

22. Kanbour-Shakir A, Tobon H: Primary clear cell carcinoma of the endometrium. A clinicopathologic study of 20 cases. Int J Gynecol Pathol 1991;10:67–78.

23. Kadar N, Malfetano JH, Homesley HD: Determinants of survival of surgically staged patients with endometrial carcinoma histologically confined to the uterus: Implications for therapy. Obstet Gynecol 1992;80:655–659.

24. DiSaia PJ, Creasman WT: Clinical Gynecologic Oncology. 4th ed. St. Louis: Mosby-Year Book, 1993.

25. Scully RE, Bonfiglio TA, Kurman RJ, Silverberg SG, Wilkinson EJ: International Histological Classification and Typing of Female Genital Tract Tumours. Berlin: Springer-Verlag, 1994.

26. Creasman WT: New gynecologic cancer staging. Obstet Gynecol 1990;75:287–288.

27. Demopoulos RI, Dubin N, Noumoff J, et al: Prognostic significance of squamous differentiation in stage I endometrial adenocarcinoma. Obstet Gynecol 1986;68:245–250.

28. Christopherson WM, Alberhasky RC, Connelly PJ: Carcinoma of the endometrium: II. Papillary adenocarcinoma: A clinical pathologic study of 46 cases. Am J Clin Pathol 1982; 77:534–540.

29. Zaino RJ, Kurman RJ, Diana KL, Morrow P: The utility of the revised International Federation of Gynecology and Obstetrics histologic grading of endometrial carcinoma using a defined nuclear grading system: A Gynecologic Oncology Group study. Cancer 1994; In press:

30. Daniel AG, Peters WA, III: Accuracy of office and operating room curettage in the grading of endometrial carcinoma. Obstet Gynecol 1988; 71:612–614.

31. Cowles TA, Magrina JF, Masterson BJ, Capen CV: Comparison of clinical and surgical staging in patients with endometrial carcinoma. Obstet Gynecol 1985;66:413–416.

32. Piver MS, Lele SB, Barlow JJ, Blumenson L: Paraaortic lymph node evaluation in stage I endometrial cancer. Obstet Gynecol 1982;59:97–100.

33. Nielsen AL, Thomsen HK, Nyholm HCJ: Evaluation of the reproducibility of the revised 1988 International Federation of Gynecology and Obstetrics grading system of endometrial cancers with special emphasis on nuclear grading. Cancer 1991; 68:2303–2309.

34. Zaino RJ, Silverberg SG, Norris HJ, Bundy BN, Morrow CP, et al: The prognostic value of nuclear versus architectural grading in endometrial adenocarcinoma. A Gynecologic Oncology Group study. Int J Gynecol Pathol 1994;13:29–36.

35. Hendrickson MR, Ross JC, Kempson RL: Toward the development of morphologic criteria for well-differentiated adenocarcinoma of the endometrium. Am J Surg Pathol 1983;7:819–838.

36. Kurman RJ, Norris HJ: Evaluation of criteria for distinguishing atypical endometrial hyperplasia from well-differentiated carcinoma. Cancer 1982; 49:2547–2557.

37. Norris HJ, Tavassoli FA, Kurman RJ: Endometrial hyperplasia and carcinoma. Diagnostic considerations. Am J Surg Pathol 1983;7:839–847.

38. Kraus FT: High-risk and premalignant lesions

of the endometrium. Am J Surg Pathol 1985;9 (Suppl):31–40.

39. Kurman RJ, Norris HJ: Endometrial hyperplasia and related cellular changes. In: Blaustein's Pathology of the Female Genital Tract. 4th ed. Kurman RJ, ed. New York: Springer-Verlag, 1994; 411–437.

40. King A, Seraj IM, Wagner RJ: Stromal invasion in endometrial carcinoma. Am J Obstet Gynecol 1984;149:10–14.

41. Silverberg SG, Kurman RJ: Tumors of the uterine corpus and gestational trophoblastic disease. Atlas of Tumor Pathology, 3rd series, Fascicle 3. Washington, DC: Armed Forces Institute of Pathology, 1992.

42. Winkler B, Alvarez S, Richart RM, Crum CP: Pitfalls in the diagnosis of endometrial neoplasia. Obstet Gynecol 1984;64:185–194.

43. Crum CP, Richart RM, Fenoglio CM: Adenoacanthosis of the endometrium. A clinicopathologic study in premenopausal women. Am J Surg Pathol 1981;5:15.

44. Hendrickson MR, Kempson RL: Endometrial epithelial metaplasias: Proliferations frequently misdiagnosed as adenocarcinoma. Report of 89 cases and proposed classification. Am J Surg Pathol 1980;4:525–542.

45. Blaustein A: Morular metaplasia misdiagnosed as adenoacanthoma in young women with polycystic ovarian disease. Am J Surg Pathol 1982; 6:223.

46. Andersen WA, Taylor PT, Fechner RE, Pinkerton JAV: Endometrial metaplasia associated with endometrial carcinoma. Am J Obstet Gynecol 1987;157:597–604.

47. Clement PB: Pathology of the uterine corpus. Hum Pathol 1991;22:776–791.

48. Zaman SS, Mazur MT: Endometrial papillary syncytial change. A nonspecific alteration associated with active breakdown. Am J Clin Pathol 1993; 99:741–745.

49. Kaku T, Tsukamoto N, Tsuruchi N, Sugihara K, Kamura T, et al: Endometrial metaplasia associated with endometrial carcinoma. Obstet Gynecol 1992;80:812–816.

50. Rorat E, Wallach RC: Papillary metaplasia of the endometrium: Clinical and histopathologic considerations. Obstet Gynecol 1984;64:90s–92s.

51. Kurman RJ, Mazur MT: Benign diseases of the endometrium. In: Blaustein's Pathology of the Female Genital Tract. 4th ed. Kurman RJ, ed. New York: Springer-Verlag, 1994;367–409.

52. Mazur MT: Atypical polypoid adenomyomas of the endometrium. Am J Surg Pathol 1981;5: 473–482.

53. Young RH, Treger T, Scully RE: Atypical polypoid adenomyoma of the uterus. A report of 27 cases. Am J Clin Pathol 1986;86:139–145.

54. Hendrickson M, Ross J, Eifel P, Martinez A, Kempson R: Uterine papillary serous carcinoma. A highly malignant form of endometrial adenocarcinoma. Am J Surg Pathol 1982;6:93–108.

55. Clement PB, Scully ER: Endometrial hyperplasia and carcinoma. In: Tumors and Tumorlike Lesions of the Uterine Corpus and Cervix. Clement PB, Young RH, eds. New York: Churchill Livingstone, 1993;181–264.

56. Hendrickson MR, Kempson RL: Ciliated carcinoma—A variant of endometrial adenocarcinoma. A report of 10 cases. Int J Gynecol Pathol 1983;2:1–12.

57. Gould PR, Li L, Henderson DW, Barter RA, Papadimitriou JM: Cilia and ciliogenesis in endometrial adenocarcinomas. Arch Pathol Lab Med 1986;110:326–330.

58. Tobon H, Watkins GJ: Secretory adenocarcinoma of the endometrium. Int J Gynecol Pathol 1985; 4:328–335.

59. Dawagne MP, Silverberg SG: Foam cells in endometrial carcinoma. Gynecol Oncol 1982;13:67–75.

60. Tiltman AJ: Mucinous carcinoma of the endometrium. Obstet Gynecol 1980;55:244–247.

61. Czernobilsky B, Katz Z, Lancet M, Gaton E: Endocervical type epithelium in endometrial carcinoma: A report of 10 cases with emphasis on histochemical methods for differential diagnosis. Am J Surg Pathol 1980;4:481–489.

62. Young RH, Scully RE: Uterine carcinomas simulating microglandular hyperplasia. A report of six cases. Am J Surg Pathol 1992;16:1092–1097.

63. Cohen C, Shulman G, Budgeon LR: Endocervical and endometrial adenocarcinoma: An immunoperoxidase and histochemical study. Am J Surg Pathol 1982;6:151-157.

64. Tamimi HK, Gown AM, Kimdeobald J, Figge DC, Greer BE, et al: The utility of immunocytochemistry in invasive adenocarcinoma of the cervix. Am J Obstet Gynecol 1992;166:1655–1662.

65. Maes G, Fleuren GJ, Bara J, Nap M: The distribution of mucins, carcinoembryonic antigen, and mucus-associated antigens in endocervical and endometrial adenocarcinomas. Int J Gynecol Pathol 1988;7:112–122.

66. Dabbs DJ, Geisinger KR, Norris HT: Intermediate filaments in endometrial and endocervical carcinomas. The diagnostic utility of vimentin patterns. Am J Surg Pathol 1986;10:568–576.

67. Lee KR, Belinson JL: Recurrence in noninvasive endometrial carcinoma. Relationship to uterine papillary serous carcinoma. Am J Surg Pathol 1991;15:965–973.

68. Sherman ME, Bitterman P, Rosenshein NB, Delgado G, Kurman RJ: Uterine serous carcinoma—A morphologically diverse neoplasm with unifying clinicopathologic features. Am J Surg Pathol 1992;16:600–610.

69. Lee KR, Belinson JL: Papillary serous adenocarcinoma of the endometrium: A clinicopathologic study of 19 cases. Gynecol Oncol 1992;46:51–54.

70. Carcangiu ML, Chambers JY: Uterine papillary serous carcinoma—A study of 108 cases with emphasis on the prognostic significance of associated endometrioid carcinoma, absence of invasion, and concomitant ovarian carcinoma. Gynecol Oncol 1992;47:298–305.

71. Sutton GP, Brill L, Michael H, et al: Malignant papillary lesions of the endometrium. Gynecol Oncol 1987;27:294–304.

72. Chambers JT, Merino M, Kohorn EI, et al: Uterine papillary serous carcinoma. Obstet Gynecol 1987;69:109.

73. Jeffrey JF, Krepart GV, Lotocki RJ: Papillary serous adenocarcinoma of the endometrium. Obstet Gynecol 1986;67:670.

74. Silva EG, Jenkins R: Serous carcinoma in endometrial polyps. Mod Pathol 1990;3:120–128.

75. Simon A, Kopolovic J, Beyth Y: Primary squamous cell carcinoma of the endometrium. Gynecol Oncol 1988;31:454–461.

76. Melin JR, Wanner L, Schulz DM, Cassell EE: Primary squamous cell carcinoma of the endometrium. Obstet Gynecol 1979;53:115–119.

77. Ryder DE: Verrucous carcinoma of the endometrium—A unique neoplasm with long survival. Obstet Gynecol 1982;59:78S–80S.

78. Abeler VM, Kjorstad KE, Nesland JM: Undifferentiated carcinoma of the endometrium. A histopathologic and clinical study of 31 cases. Cancer 1991;68:98–105.

79. Huntsman DG, Clement PB, Gilks CB, Scully RE: Small-cell carcinoma of the endometrium: A clinicopathologic study of sixteen cases. Am J Surg Pathol 1994;18:364–375.

80. Olson N, Twiggs L, Sibley R: Small-cell carcinoma of the endometrium: Light microscopic and ultrastructural study of a case. Cancer 1982;50:760–765.

81. Paz RA, Frigerio B, Sundblad AS, Eusebi V: Small-cell (oat cell) carcinoma of the endometrium. Arch Pathol Lab Med 1985;109:270–272.

82. Manivel C, Wick MR, Sibley TK: Neuroendocrine differentiation in mullerian neoplasms. An immunohistochemical study of a "pure" endometrial small-cell carcinoma and mixed mullerian tumor containing small-cell carcinoma. Am J Clin Pathol 1986;86:438–443.

83. Pesce C, Merino MJ, Chambers JT, Nogales F: Endometrial carcinoma with trophoblastic differentiation. An aggressive form of uterine cancer. Cancer 1991;68:1799–1802.

84. Jones MA, Young RH, Scully RE: Endometrial adenocarcinoma with a component of giant cell carcinoma. Int J Gynecol Pathol 1991;10:260–270.

85. Arends J, Willebrand D, Gans HJD, Swaen GJV, Bosman FT: Adenocarcinoma of the endometrium with glassy cell features—Immunohistochemical observations. Histopathology 1984;8:873–879.

86. Kumar A, Schneider V: Metastases to the uterus from extrapelvic primary tumors. Int J Gynecol Pathol 1983;2:134–140.

87. Kumar NB, Hart WR: Metastases to the uterine corpus from extagenital cancers. A clinicopathologic study of 63 cases. Cancer 1982;50:2163–2169.

88. Mazur MT, Hsueh S, Gersell DJ: Metastases to the female genital tract. Analysis of 325 cases. Cancer 1984;53:1978–1984.

89. Ulbright TM, Roth LM: Metastatic and independent cancers of the endometrium and ovary: A clinicopathologic study of 34 cases. Hum Pathol 1985;16:28–34.

90. Eifel P, Hendrickson M, Ross J, Ballon S, Martinez A, et al: Simultaneous presentation of carcinoma involving the ovary and uterine corpus. Cancer 1982;50:163–170.

11
Other Tumors

Uterine tumors other than benign polyps or carcinoma are rarely encountered in endometrial biopsies and curettings. The classification in Table 11.1 lists most of these other neoplasms. Among this group of tumors, malignant mixed mesodermal tumors (MMMTs) are the most common malignancy, yet they account for only 1% to 2% of all uterine neoplasms.[1-4] The MMMT typically arises in the endometrium and is often first diagnosed by biopsy or curettage. The remaining tumors are extremely infrequent in endometrial curettings. Even submucosal leiomyomas are only rarely sampled by an endometrial biopsy or curettage. It has been reported that prior to a hysterectomy the diagnosis of endometrial stromal sarcoma is missed in 20% of cases,[5] and, similarly for leiomyosarcoma, inaccurate or inconclusive diagnosis on curettings ranges from 20% to 80%.[5-7] Although these tumors have morphologic features that readily assist in their recognition, it is often impossible to classify them accurately from biopsy material alone.

Malignant Mixed Mesodermal Tumor (Carcinosarcoma)

The MMMT is a highly malignant, biphasic tumor consisting of both epithelial and mesenchymal components. It is predominantly a neoplasm of the postmenopausal patient. The median age at diagnosis is about 65 years.[1,3] As with endometrial carcinoma, the patient with MMMT typically presents with postmenopausal bleeding. The uterus is almost always enlarged, and the tumor may present as a polypoid mass that prolapses through the cervical os.

Clinically these tumors have been treated as sarcomas.[4] Current data using immunohistochemical, tissue culture, and genetic analysis indicate that these neoplasms have many similari-

TABLE 11.1. Uterine tumors other than carcinoma that may be found in biopsies and curettings.

Mixed epithelial–stromal tumors
  Malignant mixed mesodermal tumor (MMMT)
    (carcinosarcoma)
  Adenofibroma
  Adenosarcoma
Stromal tumors
  Stromal nodule
  Low-grade stromal sarcoma
  High-grade stromal sarcoma
Smooth muscle tumors
  Leiomyoma
  Variants of leiomyoma
  Tumorlets
  Leiomyosarcoma
Other neoplasms
  Lymphoma/leukemia
  Rare tumors

---

carcinomatous and sarcomatous elements are reactive for keratin and epithelial membrane antigen (EMA), although immunostaining is less diffuse in the sarcomatous foci.[8,10–12,14,15] Vimentin immunoreactivity also is found in both the carcinoma and sarcoma elements, even though it is more extensive in the spindle cell areas. In addition, the tumors spread like carcinomas rather than sarcomas, and the metastases are almost always carcinoma, even if the bulk of the primary tumor is sarcomatous.[9,10] Thus the behavior of MMMTs is dictated by the epithelial component. Nonetheless, these neoplasms are very aggressive and should be specifically classified as MMMTs whenever possible.

Pathologic Features

MMMTs are biphasic tumors characterized by a combination of carcinoma and sarcoma.[1,3,7a,9,10,16–21] Usually the components are intimately admixed, with nests and masses of car-

ties to carcinomas and may therefore represent metaplastic or sarcomatoid carcinomas.[1,3,8–3] Immunohistochemical studies show that both the

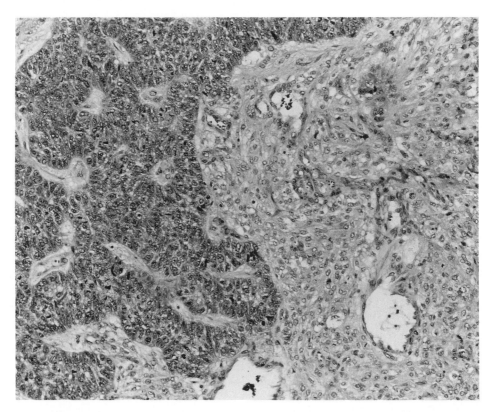

FIGURE 11.1. Malignant mixed mesodermal tumor. This typical pattern shows a mixture of poorly differentiated adenocarcinoma, endometrioid-type (*left*), and a sarcomatous stroma (*right*).

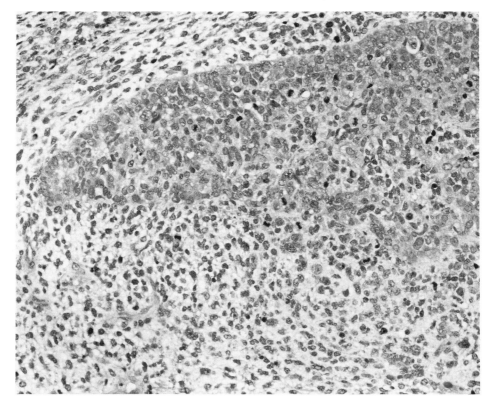

FIGURE 11.2. Malignant mixed mesodermal tumor. A solid nest of poorly differentiated adenocarcinoma, endometrioid-type, merges into a sarcomatous stroma in the lower portion of this field.

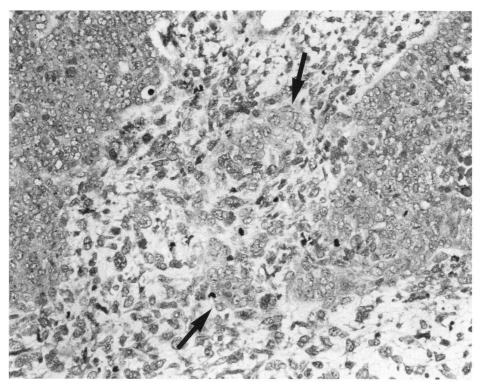

FIGURE 11.3. Malignant mixed mesodermal tumor. Sheets of poorly differentiated carcinoma blend into the sarcoma. Several ill-defined clusters of cells (*arrows*) are difficult to classify as carcinoma or sarcoma.

cinoma separated by a malignant spindle cell stroma (Fig. 11.1). The carcinoma often appears to blend into the sarcoma, with the cells at the interface lacking clear features of either carcinoma or sarcoma (Figs. 11.2 and 11.3). Occasionally, however, the two cell types are seen as separate foci of carcinoma and sarcoma in tissue samples.

The carcinomatous component of MMMT typically is a high-grade adenocarcinoma that often has serous or clear cell features (Fig. 11.4). Some tumors, however, have a typical "endometrioid" pattern and may show squamous change. The epithelial component rarely may have a pattern of pure squamous carcinoma.

The sarcomatous component can display a variety of patterns that have been referred to as either homologous or heterologous.[1,16,18,19] The sarcoma is considered homologous when it shows differentiation toward mesenchymal

cells normally present in the uterus. Often the homologous sarcoma resembles fibrosarcoma or malignant fibrous histiocytoma composed of interlacing primitive spindle cells (Fig. 11.4), but at times it may have features of endometrial stromal sarcoma or leiomyosarcoma. The sarcoma is considered heterologous when it is differentiated into cell types not normally found in the uterus (Fig. 11.5). The usual heterologous components are rhabdomyosarcoma, chondrosarcoma, or osteosarcoma. Other heterologous components, including liposarcoma or even glia, may rarely be found.[22,23]

Some MMMTs have sarcomatous component that contains large cells with abundant, eosinophilic cytoplasm. These large cells superficially resemble rhabdomyoblasts, but they lack sarcomeric filaments and are not immunoreactive for desmin or myoglobin. Other MMMTs may have dense eosinophilic hyaline material be-

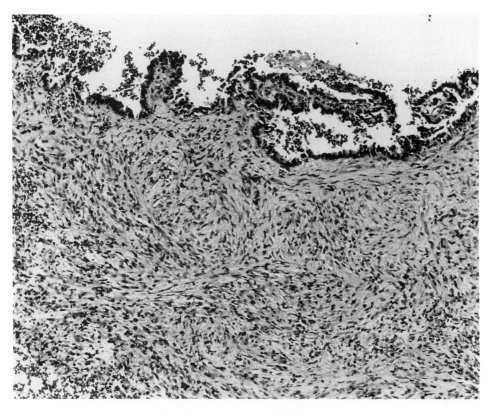

FIGURE 11.4. Malignant mixed mesodermal tumor. The carcinomatous component is serous type with coarse papillae, and the mesenchyme shows undifferentiated sarcoma composed of irregular and haphazard spindle-shaped cells. The primitive spindle cells of the sarcomatous component resemble malignant fibrous histiocytoma.

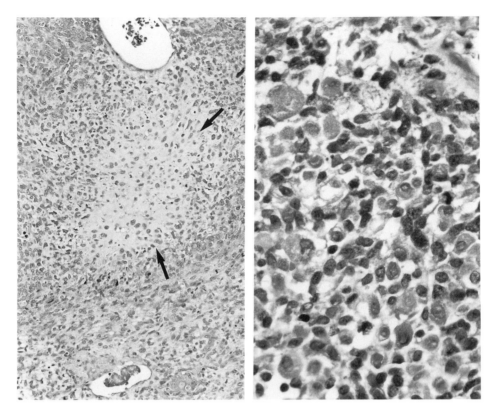

FIGURE 11.5. Heterologous elements in malignant mixed mesodermal tumors. *Left*: A nodule of cartilaginous differentiation (*arrows*) is seen in an area of otherwise undifferentiated sarcoma. *Right*: A focus of rhabdomyosarcoma is present showing multiple rhabdomyoblasts with abundant eosinophilic cytoplasm. Although cross striations are not seen in this field, immunohistochemical stains for desmin and myoglobin demonstrated cytoplasmic muscle filaments.

tween the spindle cells that is suggestive, but not diagnostic, of osteosarcoma, lacking unequivocal osteoid with osteoblastic-like stromal cells. Neither large, eosinophilic cells nor hyaline stroma should be construed as evidence of heterologous differentiation unless the pattern shows clearly diagnostic features. The distinction, however, is largely academic, as discussed below.

Rarely an MMMT may show well-differentiated carcinoma, a relatively low-grade sarcoma, or a combination of both instead of the high-grade patterns usually seen in the carcinoma and sarcoma of MMMTs (Figs. 11.6 and 11.7). These tumors nonetheless show features of malignancy in both the glands and the stroma. The glands show, at a minimum, the features of well-differentiated adenocarcinoma as outlined earlier (see Chapter 9). Low-grade sarcoma lacks high cellularity and nuclear pleomorphism but shows a cellular population of enlarged mesenchymal cells and a high mitotic rate of four or more mitoses per 10 high-power fields (HPFs).

Differential Diagnosis

For most cases of MMMT, the differential diagnosis centers mainly on carcinoma. The mesenchymal component may be indistinct or difficult to differentiate from undifferentiated carcinoma, carcinoma with a spindle cell component, or high-grade adenocarcinoma with squamous differentiation (adenosquamous carcinoma). In the latter case of adenocarcinoma with squamous change, the squamous component may have a spindle appearance with swirling aggregates of elongate, nonkeratinizing squamous cells. The squamous

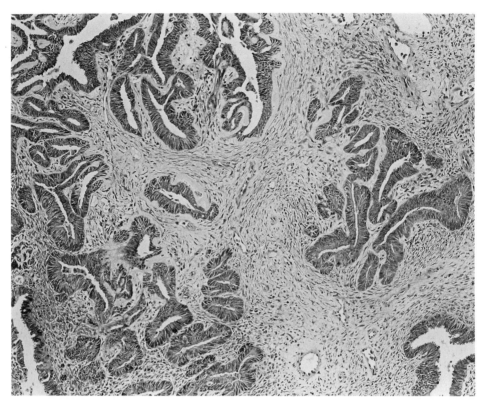

FIGURE 11.6. Malignant mixed mesodermal tumor. In this case the malignant glands appear well differentiated, and the stroma lacks the marked cellularity often seen in these neoplasms.

component is within the center of the glands, in contrast to the sarcoma of the MMMT, which surrounds the glands (see Chapter 10, Fig. 10.17). At times the squamous element may be extensive and efface glandular structures, thereby simulating a sarcoma. Immunohistochemical stains for keratin should help resolve the diagnosis, as discussed below.

In some cases the sarcoma is only focal in the curettings and is eclipsed by a dominant carcinomatous element. Careful study of all the material may be necessary to correctly diagnose an MMMT with a subtle sarcomatous component. In other cases the MMMT is difficult to recognize, because the sarcoma blends imperceptibly into the carcinomatous component, and the sarcoma is difficult to distinguish from poorly differentiated carcinoma. In these cases, the malignant spindle cells have an indistinct interface with the epithelial component, and there is a zone of cells that are indeterminate in their differentiation into

epithelium or mesenchyme (Figs. 11.2 and 11.3). We have found that this feature, the merging of spindle cells into the clearly carcinomatous component, is especially useful for recognizing MMMTs in cases where the sarcoma is largely eclipsed by the carcinoma.

It is important to scrutinize the stroma between glands or nests of carcinomatous epithelium to determine whether the mesenchyme has malignant features, such as increased cellularity, pleomorphic nuclei, and a high mitotic rate. Non-neoplastic mesenchyme in adenocarcinoma either resembles normal endometrial stromal or shows desmoplasia, with cells developing fibroblast-like characteristics. Benign mesenchymal cells have a low mitotic rate; stromal cellularity may be mildly increased, but the nuclei remain oval and uniform with indistinct chromatin. Sarcomatous tissue, in contrast, shows increased cellularity, the nuclei are irregular and closely packed, and mitotic figures are numerous, usu-

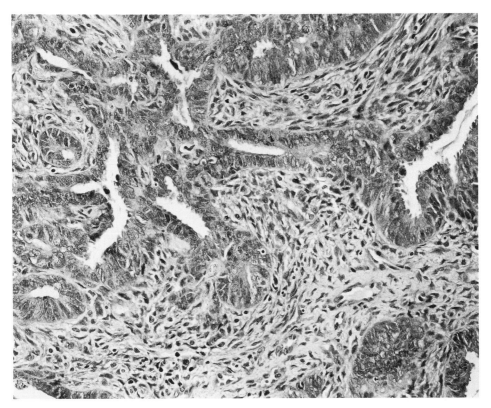

FIGURE 11.7. Malignant mixed mesodermal tumor. Well-formed but malignant glands blend into a sarcomatous stroma. Although both the carcinoma and the sarcoma lack high-grade features, both components are malignant, establishing the diagnosis of mixed mesodermal tumor (same case as Fig. 11.5).

ally in the range of four or more per 10 HPFs. Atypical mitoses often are present.

In questionable cases where the distinction between MMMT and poorly differentiated adenocarcinoma is not clear by routine histology, immunohistochemical stains for keratin, EMA, and vimentin can be useful for demonstrating the biphasic pattern of the MMMT.[8,10–12,14,15,24] The epithelial component shows intense and generalized reactivity for keratin and EMA, as noted earlier, and although the epithelial markers are also present in the sarcomatous component, this staining is less intense. Keratin and EMA immunostains are especially useful, since they highlight the mixed population of carcinoma and sarcoma in the MMMT. Mesenchymal markers also can help to identify an MMMT by highlighting the sarcomatous areas. Vimentin often is present in both the carcinoma and the sarcoma areas, but it is more diffuse in the latter, and this antibody, like

keratin and EMA, accentuates the biphasic growth of the MMMT. Actin, muscle-specific actin, and desmin immunostains are useful for demonstrating muscle differentiation in the spindle cell population. Desmin and myoglobin also assist in demonstrating rhabdomyoblasts.[24,25]

Clinical Queries and Reporting

MMMT is an important diagnosis, because the tumor is highly aggressive. Correct diagnosis prior to hysterectomy alerts the gynecologist to the high likelihood of extrauterine spread at the time of laparotomy. In addition, the gynecologist may wish to stage the patient with an MMMT more thoroughly. The question of heterologous versus homologous sarcoma in an MMMT is of less importance than the recognition of the MMMT. Heterologous elements have no influence on the prognosis.

In some cases biopsy or curettage may show a tumor with features that suggest an MMMT but are not conclusive. This problem is most often seen when the sections show adenocarcinoma with foci of cellular spindle cells around the glands. The spindle cell component may show increased mitotic activity but is not conclusive for a sarcomatous element. In such cases it is best to clearly describe the changes and to indicate the possibility that the tumor may be an MMMT. The knowledge that the tumor may be an MMMT often is sufficient for clinical management in specimens with equivocal features, since a hysterectomy will be performed. The entire uterus can then be studied in greater detail to determine whether a sarcomatous component is present.

An occasional case demonstrates only high-grade sarcoma with no definite epithelial elements, despite immunohistochemical analysis. In these cases the differential diagnosis includes a pure sarcoma or an MMMT with predomi-nance of the sarcomatous component. Practically, this distinction is not important for directing further therapy. Both types of tumor are high-grade malignancies with a similar poor prognosis. Consequently when the tumor type is not clear-cut, diagnosis of "malignant tumor" with a comment indicating the differential should be made. The diagnosis usually is clarified by the study of additional tissue. If the patient is a candidate for surgery, hysterectomy usually is attempted to stage the tumor, and the neoplasm can be fully assessed by examining the entire uterus.

Mullerian Adenofibroma and Adenosarcoma

Adenofibroma and adenosarcoma are related tumors.[1,3,16,26–31] Both are biphasic tumors with benign glands regularly distributed in a cellular mesenchyme. The adenofibroma is benign

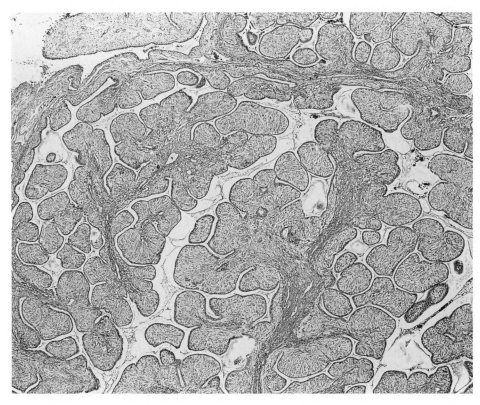

FIGURE 11.8. Adenofibroma. The tumor is characterized by branching bulbous papillary fronds with a thin epithelial lining and sparsely cellular stroma.

whereas the adenosarcoma has low-grade malignant features. These are rare neoplasms that usually arise in the corpus, but about 10% of the tumors originate in the endocervix. They generally occur in postmenopausal patients, although approximately 30% of these tumors are found in patients under the age of 50. Rare cases have occurred in teenagers. A few cases of adenosarcoma have been associated with estrogen use, the Stein–Leventhal syndrome, or prior pelvic irradiation.[26] One reported case of adenosarcoma was associated with tamoxifen use.[32] On clinical examination, adenosarcoma typically is a large, polypoid tumor that expands the endometrial cavity and often prolapses through the cervical os.[26,28,33]

Adenofibroma may recur within the uterus but does not metastasize or extend beyond the uterus. Adenosarcoma, however, recurs in the vagina or pelvis in as many as 25% of cases and sometimes disseminates widely as a high-grade sarcoma. Although the terminology suggests that there is a clear histologic difference between the benign adenofibroma and the malignant adenosarcoma, many of these tumors have borderline features that make separation of the two tumor types difficult. Of the two, adenosarcoma is much more common, accounting for more than 90% of all tumors in this group of adenofibroma and adenosarcoma.[3] Hysterectomy is the treatment of choice for adenosarcoma, but adenofibroma may be managed more conservatively with repeat curettage and hysteroscopy.

Pathologic Features

Adenofibroma is characterized by benign cytologic features of the epithelium and stroma.[28,30,31] The

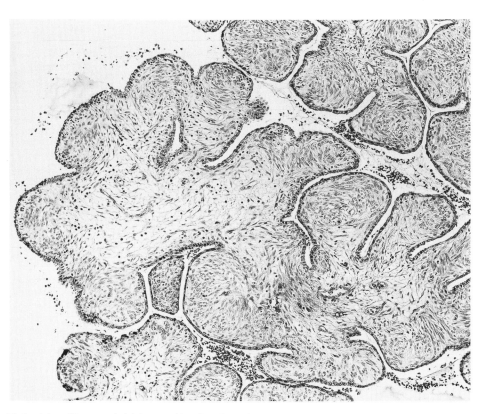

FIGURE 11.9. Adenofibroma. At high magnification the tumor shows bland fibrous stroma covered by cuboidal epithelium. Both glandular and stromal elements lack malignant features. It is important that the entire tumor have these features and that there be no areas of increased cellularity or stromal atypia in order to establish the diagnosis of adenofibroma.

tumor shows a characteristic pattern of broad-based papillary fronds covered with bland epithelium and supported by widely distributed spindle cells (Fig. 11.8). Low columnar epithelium lines large polypoid fronds of sparsely cellular mesenchyme and also forms small glandular infoldings into the stroma. The epithelium lacks atypia or mitotic activity. The mesenchyme is composed of widely spaced spindle cells that also lack mitotic activity (Fig. 11.9).

Adenosarcoma has a similar low-power growth pattern to adenofibroma characterized by leaf-like fronds of mesenchyme covered by cuboidal to columnar epithelium (Fig. 11.10). In adenosarcoma, however, the stroma is more cellular, a feature indicating low-grade malignant growth (Fig. 11.11).[1,3,16,26,28,29] This tumor has irregular, often large glands that form gaping cystic spaces. Besides the surface papillary growth, the glands often have broad-based papillary infoldings into the lumen. In adenosarcoma, glands and surface

epithelium lack cytologic features of malignancy, although they usually appear hyperplastic, with mitotic activity and slight nuclear atypia. Usually the glands have an endometrioid appearance, but they may show eosinophilic, mucinous, squamous, or clear cell change.

In adenosarcoma, the sarcomatous component usually resembles endometrial stromal sarcoma with plump spindle cells in a rich vascular background, but the mesenchyme may have features of fibrosarcoma or leiomyosarcoma and may show heterologous elements. The cellularity of the stroma often is accentuated around the glands, forming hypercellular cuffs with less cellular mesenchyme farther away from the glands. The mitotic rate in the stroma is variable, and the reported cases have ranged between one and 40 mitoses per 10 HPFs. Most cases show four or more mitoses per 10 HPFs, but any convincing mitotic activity of as little as two or more mitoses per 10 HPFs is sufficient to establish a diagnosis of

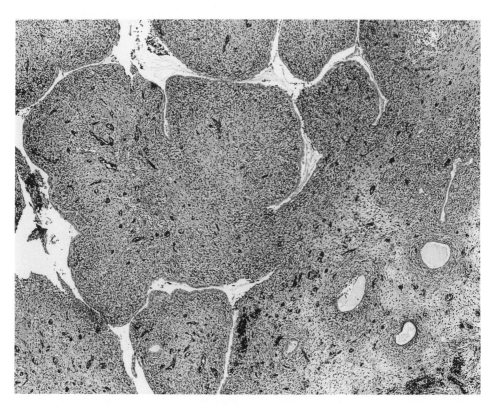

FIGURE 11.10. Adenosarcoma. The tumor is composed of large papillary fronds and glands in a highly cellular stroma. In this case the stroma resembles endometrial stroma.

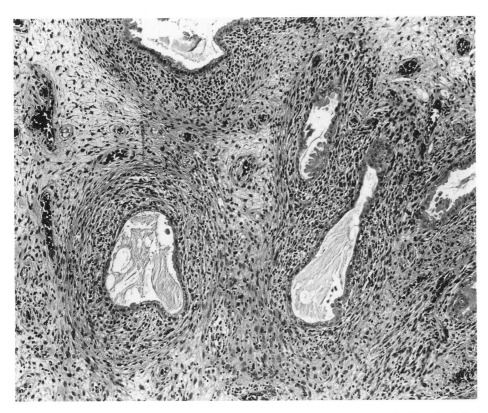

FIGURE 11.11. Adenosarcoma. The stroma forms hypercellular cuffs around the glands. The glands lack malignant cytologic features.

adenosarcoma in a case that shows an otherwise typical growth pattern.[26]

Up to 20% of adenosarcomas have a heterologous element, such as cartilage, fat, osteoid, or rhabdomyoblasts, that appears to have no influence on the overall prognosis of the tumor.[26] In occasional cases adenosarcoma shows overgrowth of sarcoma, either stromal sarcoma or, less commonly, leiomyosarcoma or rhabdomyosarcoma.[29,34] Adenosarcoma with stromal overgrowth is important to recognize, since this tumor has a higher frequency of myometrial invasion, recurrence, and metastases than the typical adenosarcoma.[34]

Adenosarcoma may also show sex cord-like elements characterized by ribbons or nests of cells, sometimes with tubule formation, resembling ovarian sex cord tumors.[35] These patterns also may include cells with abundant clear to foamy cytoplasm.

Differential Diagnosis

The distinction of adenofibroma from adenosarcoma may be difficult, because the mitotic rate is relatively low in some cases of adenosarcoma. As mentioned above, in biopsy material virtually any convincing mitotic activity in an otherwise characteristic tumor indicates a diagnosis of adenosarcoma. In our experience, adenofibroma is an extraordinarily rare diagnosis in biopsy and curettage specimens and should only be made when no mitoses are found in the stroma. In occasional cases, however, the distinction between the two lesions may be extremely difficult, even with repeated evaluations, and hysterectomy is necessary to allow thorough sampling and ensure complete removal of the lesion.

Either adenofibroma or adenosarcoma may resemble an endometrial polyp. In contrast to polyps, these lesions characteristically have a leaflike configuration, and the biopsy consists of large fragments of tissue. The increased cellularity of the stroma and periglandular cuffing in adenosarcoma are helpful features in the differential diagnosis. If a patient has a history of recurrence of apparent endometrial polyps, especially large polyps, the differential diagnosis should include adenosarcoma, since recurrency of ordinary polyps is unusual.

The atypical polypoid adenomyoma may resemble adenosarcoma because of its mixture of atypical glands in a cellular mesenchyme (Chapter 8). Unlike adenosarcoma, the mesenchyme of the atypical polypoid adenomyoma is composed of short, interlacing fascicles of smooth muscle cells. The atypical polypoid adenomyoma is, in general, a smaller lesion, lacking the leaflike papillary fronds of adenosarcoma. In addition, many of the glands in the atypical polypoid adenomyoma show nests of nonkeratinizing squamous (morular) change.

Clinical Queries and Reporting

Because adenofibroma and adenosarcoma are unusual neoplasms, a comment regarding the nature of the tumor is warranted. The comment can include a brief description with a statement regarding the mitotic rate of the stroma. Other salient features of adenosarcoma, such as heterologous elements or sarcomatous overgrowth, should be noted in a comment. Sarcomatous overgrowth is an especially important feature, since it is associated with a higher rate of recurrence. A telephone call can help to clarify the diagnosis for a gynecologist who is not familiar with the entity.

In small samples it may be difficult to establish the diagnosis of either adenofibroma or adenosarcoma, since these neoplasms often have relatively bland cytologic features. If the morphologic features suggest either of these entities but are not clearly diagnostic, the gynecologist should be informed of the differential in order to allow further evaluation as clinically indicated. Often with this information the clinician may elect to proceed with a hysterectomy in the perimenopausal or postmenopausal patient. Hysteroscopy, magnetic resonance imaging (MRI), and repeat cu-

rettage can be performed in young women in whom conservative management is desirable.

Stromal Tumors

Tumors in this category include the benign stromal nodule, low-grade stromal sarcoma, and high-grade stromal sarcoma.[1,16,36–43] These neoplasms often involve the endometrium, so they may be sampled by endometrial biopsy or curettage. Low-grade stromal sarcoma recurs in up to one-half of cases, often in the pelvis or abdomen following hysterectomy.[37–39,42,44–46] Relapses may occur many years after hysterectomy. This lesion also has been termed "endolymphatic stromal myosis" or "stromatosis."[38,44,47,48] High-grade stromal sarcomas are aggressive neoplasms that spread widely.[1,37,39,40,43] Most patients with high-grade stromal sarcoma succumb within 3 years.

Stromal tumors occur over a wide age range, with a mean age in the fifth decade in most studies. The majority of low-grade stromal sarcomas occur in women under the age of 50 years,[44] whereas high-grade stromal sarcoma generally occurs in older women.[37,43] These tumors frequently present with abnormal bleeding, although they may present with pelvic pain, with other, nonspecific complaints, or even with distant metastases to the lung or other sites.[38–40,42] As noted previously, many cases are not detected by curettage and are only diagnosed in hysterectomy specimens.[37]

Stromal Nodule and Low-Grade Stromal Sarcoma

The stromal nodule and low-grade stromal sarcoma are composed of cells that resemble endometrial stroma of the normal proliferative phase.[1,36,37,39,41] Cytologically these lesions are identical and are distinguished by their growth patterns (see below). The cells are oval and uniform and are supported by a prominent network of small vascular spaces (Figs. 11.12 and 11.13). The mitotic rate is variable, but most tumors show no more than three mitotic figures per 10 HPFs. Some tumors can show high mitotic counts, however, and mitotic counts are not a criterion to distinguish stromal nodules, low-grade, or high-

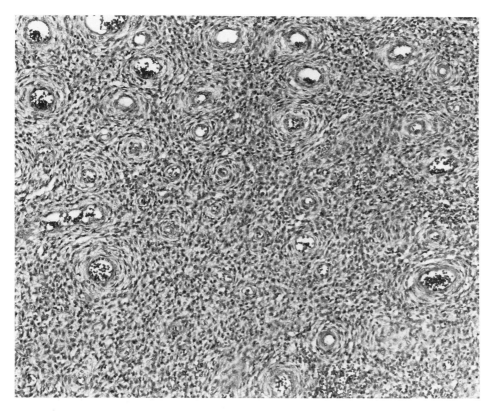

FIGURE 11.12. Low-grade stromal sarcoma. The tumor is composed of a uniform population of oval mesenchymal cells that resemble the stromal cells of proliferative phase endometrium in a background of multiple small vessels. The circumferential orientation of the stromal cells around the blood vessels is a characteristic feature.

grade stromal sarcoma.[36] Stromal nodules and low-grade stromal sarcoma do not show necrosis or cellular pleomorphism (Fig. 11.12). Small amounts of smooth muscle may be interspersed between areas with typical stromal differentiation, but this finding does not alter the diagnosis. In fact, immunohistochemical stains show reactivity of many of the cells for actin and desmin, demonstrating muscle-like properties, even where this is not apparent by light microscopy.[49,50]

The stromal nodule is distinguished from the low-grade stromal sarcoma by the growth pattern, a feature that usually cannot be appreciated in curettings.[1,36,39,41] The stromal nodule is a circumscribed tumor with a rounded, pushing interface with the myometrium or endometrium. Low-grade stromal sarcoma, in contrast, has an infiltrative pattern of growth, showing irregular invasion of the myometrium, often accompanied by endovascular growth.

Low-grade stromal tumors may show sex cord-like patterns with nests and trabeculae of condensed cells forming distinctive epithelial-like patterns that resemble ovarian sex cord tumors (Fig. 11.14).[39,41,50–52] These epithelioid nests often form anastomosing trabeculae that yield a plexiform pattern. The nests and cords may be solid or they may form tubules with a central lumen. Immunohistochemical stains for actin and desmin show reactivity in the sex cordlike areas that resembles that found in the spindle cell component.[49,50,52] Sex cordlike areas also may be immunoreactive for keratin.[50]

Stromal tumors may also show scattered foci of benign endometrial glands and may even show extensive endometrial glandular differentiation, but the presence of glands does not alter the diagnosis.[53] Tumors with this finding should not be classified as carcinosarcomas, since the glands are benign. Stromal tumors with glandular differ-

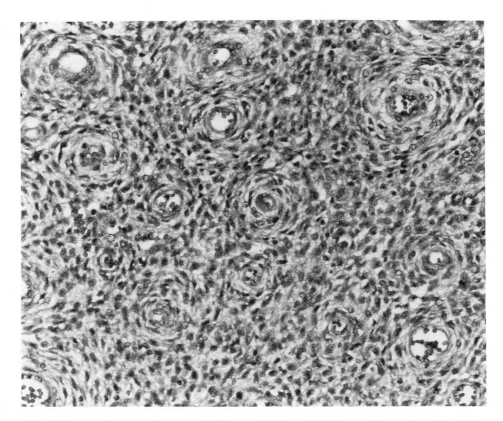

FIGURE 11.13. Low-grade stromal sarcoma. Higher magnification of the tumor shows a monotonous population of cells with small nuclei and scant cytoplasm. In this case mitotic figures are infrequent, but the cytologic features rather than the mitotic rate establish the diagnosis of a low-grade stromal tumor. The pattern in this field could represent either a stromal nodule or a low-grade stromal sarcoma. To firmly establish the diagnosis of low-grade stromal sarcoma, it is necessary to identify infiltrating margins or endovascular growth, features that usually cannot be assessed in curettings.

entiation are distinguished from adenosarcomas by their growth pattern, their lack of leaflike polypoid fronds, and the presence of a prominent vascular framework in the tumor. They resemble low-grade endometrial stromal sarcoma except for the glandular differentiation.

High-Grade Stromal Sarcoma

High-grade stromal sarcoma is a tumor with obvious malignant characteristics, including increased cellularity, pleomorphism, nuclear atypia, and a high mitotic rate.[1,37,40,43] Atypical mitotic figures and foci of necrosis usually are present. An occasional tumor shows some resemblance to low-grade stromal sarcoma, with a population of more uniform ovoid cells but with a high mitotic rate and necrosis. Many of these tumors, however, demonstrate nuclear pleomorphism and marked atypia, features that result in little resemblance to normal endometrial stroma. The term "high-grade undifferentiated sarcoma" has been proposed for these tumors, since their histogenetic relationship to endometrial stroma is less certain.[43] Regardless of terminology, this is an aggressive, high-grade sarcoma with a grave prognosis and is therefore important to recognize.

Differential Diagnosis

Stromal nodules and low-grade stromal sarcomas have very characteristic histologic features that limit the differential diagnosis to only a few other lesions. It is most important, however, to attempt

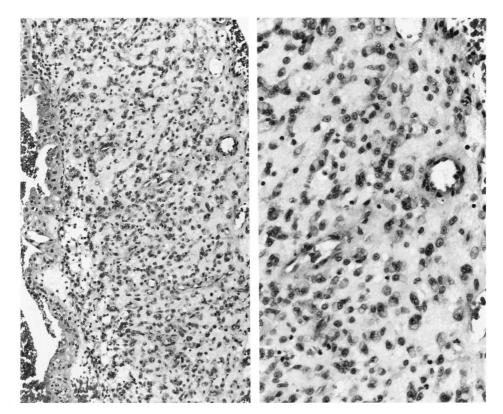

FIGURE 11.14. Low-grade stromal sarcoma. *Left*: Portion of low-grade stromal sarcoma has an epithelioid pattern in which the cells show a vague plexiform arrangement with interlacing linear arrays. A small amount of endometrial surface epithelium is present to the left of the field. *Right*: At high magnification the cells have epithelioid qualities with discernible cell borders. The cells remain monotonous, however, and are distributed around a network of many small vascular spaces.

to distinguish these tumors from each other. The growth pattern determines whether a tumor is a stromal nodule or a low-grade stromal sarcoma. Usually this feature is not discernible in biopsy material, since the interface with normal tissues is, at best, fragmented. Endovascular growth and infiltrative growth cannot be evaluated in biopsies. For these reasons it may not be possible to distinguish between these lesions in biopsy material (see below, Clinical Queries and Reporting).

Most high-grade stromal sarcomas are less differentiated and lack a monotonous cell population. In these cases it may be difficult to determine whether the tumor is a high-grade stromal sarcoma or another type of sarcoma, such as leiomyosarcoma. Practically, this distinction usually makes little difference, since the clinical management rests upon the recognition of high-grade

sarcoma rather than the histologic subtype. If the differential includes poorly differentiated or undifferentiated carcinoma with a sheetlike proliferation of small, monotonous cells, immunostains for keratin, EMA, actin, and desmin should resolve the question. Stromal tumors show reactivity for actin and desmin while carcinoma does not. Keratin may be focally positive in stromal tumors, so focal reactivity for this antigen does not necessarily indicate carcinoma. EMA, however, in our experience, is more specific as a marker for carcinoma and is not found in smooth muscle or stromal cells.

At times stromal tumors show foci of smooth muscle, and sometimes there is a prominent mixture of stromal and smooth muscle spindle cells. For practical purposes these tumors should be classified as stromal tumors, since their behavior will be similar to that of a pure stromal neoplasm. Immunohistochemical stains have limited utility in the diagnosis, since stromal tumors without obvious smooth muscle differentiation show immunoreactivity for actin and desmin.[49,50,54] If immunohistochemical stains are employed to help make the distinction, then the diagnosis of a smooth muscle tumor should be reserved for those cases that show extensive cytoplasmic staining for actin and desmin.

Cellular leiomyomas (see below) can be difficult to distinguish from low-grade stromal tumors, since both lesions show closely spaced, small, spindle-shaped cells. In curettings cellular leiomyomas are very unusual, however, and stromal tumors are more likely to be biopsied. Low-grade stromal tumors also show the characteristic pattern of uniform cells in a network of small vascular channels, which is distinctive for stromal tumors but not for smooth muscle neoplasms. Conversely, smooth muscle tumors have a fascicular pattern with interlacing bundles of elongate cells.

Occasionally, aggregates of histiocytes from the uterine cavity may present as a sheet of monotonous cells in an endometrial biopsy that can superficially mimic a proliferation of stromal cells. Despite the resemblance at low magnification, masses of histiocytes lack the vascular framework that uniformly accompanies stromal cell proliferations. Immunohistochemical stains for histiocytes, such as lysozyme, KP-1, or HAM 56, are useful for identifying these cells.

Clinical Queries and Reporting

Low-grade stromal cell proliferations are difficult to classify with precision, since the interface with myometrium is not represented in biopsy material. Consequently, when the sections demonstrate an apparent low-grade stromal tumor, it is necessary to clearly indicate the differential diagnosis. In perimenopausal or postmenopausal women, a total abdominal hysterectomy should be performed in order to establish the diagnosis. In young women a conservative approach can be undertaken. If the uterus is not enlarged, repeat curettage and simultaneous hysteroscopy can be done. In addition, an MRI scan should be performed to rule out the presence of intramural involvement. If all of these tests are negative, care-

ful follow-up and a repeat curettage in 3 to 6 months is appropriate. Continued long-term follow-up for many years is necessary, since low-grade stromal sarcomas may recur after symptom-free intervals of up to 20 years.

In cases of high-grade stromal sarcoma where the tumor cells are poorly differentiated, the separation of stromal sarcoma from other forms of sarcoma may be extremely difficult in small samples of tissue. Establishing the presence of high-grade sarcoma is sufficient to guide further therapy, however, and the subclassification of the neoplasm has little clinical relevance.

Smooth Muscle Tumors

Leiomyoma

Smooth muscle tumors are rarely encountered in endometrial biopsy and curettage specimens. Those sampled usually are benign leiomyomas. Tissue from a submucosal leiomyoma ("submucous fibroid") or a pedunculated intracavitary leiomyoma occasionally is obtained. These specimens show fragments of smooth muscle, although the tissue usually is too fragmented to allow definitive diagnosis of a leiomyoma. In premenopausal women, leiomyomas can affect endometrial development. Endometrium overlying a leiomyoma may show focal hypoplasia or atrophy, being thin with sparse glands that are underdeveloped and small compared to surrounding tissue (Fig. 11.15).[55] Endometrium adjacent to leiomyomas also can become distorted.[55] The glands may lose their perpendicular orientation relative to the surface epithelium. These focal distortions of endometrial growth can yield a pattern of irregular maturation, with fragments of normally developed proliferative or secretory endometrium adjacent to fragments with irregular or poorly developed glands. Such morphologic abnormalities of the glands generally are nonspecific, however, and are not sufficient to establish the diagnosis of a submucous leiomyoma. Often the endometrial tissue from biopsy material shows either no demonstrable effects from the leiomyomas or nonspecific glandular and stromal breakdown, and in these cases it is not possible to diagnose leiomyomas from a biopsy or curettage specimen.

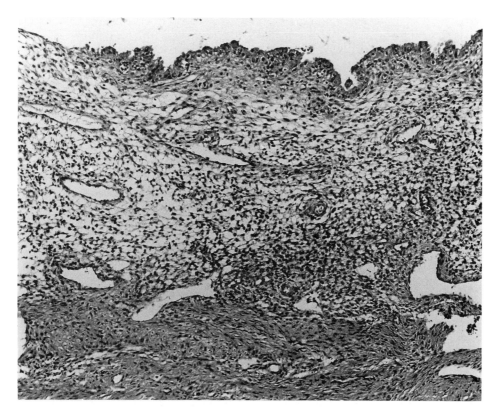

FIGURE 11.15. Endometrium overlying a leiomyoma. A fragment of endometrium is markedly thinned and atrophic, with a thin underlying layer of smooth muscle. Other fragments showed a secretory phase pattern. These findings are suggestive of a leiomyoma but require clinical correlation. In this case subsequent hysterectomy showed submucosal leiomyomas.

Variants of Leiomyoma

There are a number of variants of benign leiomyoma characterized either by increased mitotic activity or by deviation from the typical pattern of interlacing spindle cells, including cellular leiomyoma, leiomyoma with bizarre nuclei (atypical leiomyoma), epithelioid leiomyoma, and mitotically active leiomyoma.[1,16,41,56–63] As previously indicated, it is very unusual to encounter these tumors in biopsies or curettings.

Bizarre, cellular, and epithelioid leiomyomas have mitotic rates of four or less per 10 HPFs.[41,56,61,62] Generally the mitotic rate is very low, averaging less than one mitosis per 10 HPFs. Mitotically active leiomyomas have high mitotic rates, up to 15 mitoses per 10 HPFs, but lack cytologic atypia.[59,60,64] These tumors often are submucosal.[59] In the rare event that any of these lesions are sampled by curette, they are fragmented and only partially removed (Fig. 11.16). Sampling is therefore inadequate and precludes an accurate diagnosis. It is impossible to be certain that the tumor would not have a higher mitotic rate in the portion that is not removed or that more marked nuclear atypia is not present elsewhere. Also, other features, such as size of the lesion and interface of the tumor with normal myometrium, cannot be assessed.

Tumorlets

Small, circumscribed mesenchymal proliferations called tumorlets occasionally may be found in endometrial curettings. One such lesion is the plexiform tumorlet, a rare small epithelioid leiomyoma that usually occurs in the myometrium but that can involve the endometrium.[28,65] Often

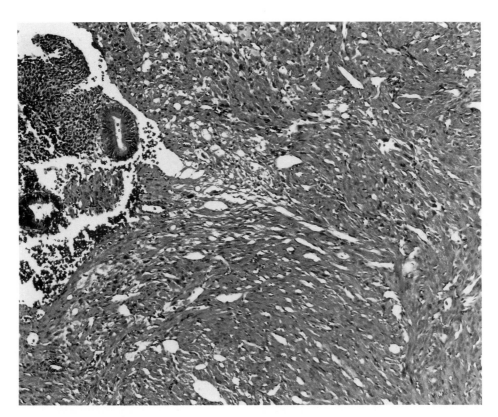

FIGURE 11.16. Portion of bizarre leiomyoma in curettings. A fragment of smooth muscle with moderate nuclear pleomorphism is admixed with fragments of endometrium. Despite the nuclear atypia, the smooth muscle lacked mitotic activity. Nonetheless, hysterectomy was necessary to exclude a leiomyosarcoma, and the uterus showed a small submucosal bizarre leiomyoma.

these are multifocal. In the endometrium they typically occur near the endometrial–myometrial interface and show transitions to normal endometrial stroma. These lesions form circumscribed microscopic nodules and are composed of small, oval to polygonal cells in an organoid arrangement, typically forming small anastomosing trabeculae or cords with an intervening hyaline matrix.

In another pattern of tumorlet or small leiomyoma that may be seen in curettings, the cells have a more spindled appearance (Fig. 11.17). In these small proliferations, the cells interlace in a less well-defined plexiform pattern, and although they are circumscribed, the cells at the periphery blend into surrounding endometrial stroma. Sometimes they encompass glands. Their intimate relationship to endometrial stroma is another example of how stromal and smooth muscle

cells can coexist with transitional cells that bridge the morphology of these two cell types.

Tumorlets, unlike other leiomyoma variants, are sufficiently small that they can be confidently recognized in curettings. When they occur in the endometrium, they often are completely removed by curettage. They have no known clinical significance and are only noteworthy for their unusual pattern. They should be recognized to prevent misclassification of a more serious lesion.

Leiomyosarcoma

Leiomyosarcoma typically occurs in patients over the age of 40. Usually the neoplasm is confined to the myometrium, but it may involve the endometrial cavity and be sampled by a curette. Leiomyosarcomas show features of high-grade sarcoma, with closely spaced hyperchromatic nuclei show-

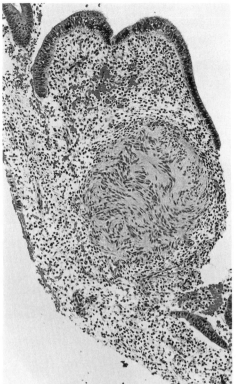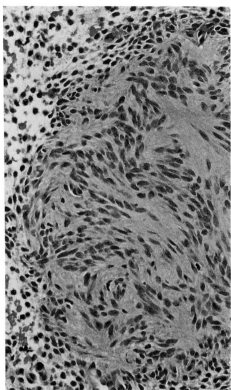

FIGURE 11.17. Tumorlet. *Left*: The lesion forms a small, circumscribed nodule within the endometrial stromal that is composed of an organoid, plexiform-like arrangement of ovoid cells. *Right*: At higher magnification the tumorlet shows strands of small benign cells with intervening hyaline zones. The lesion blends imperceptibly into surrounding endometrial stroma. Lesions such as this are invariably benign and of no clinical significance.

ing pleomorphism, a high mitotic rate, and abnormal mitotic figures.[1,16,41,66] Tumor necrosis usually is present, too. The mitotic rate should be greater than five per 10 HPFs and often is well over 10 per 10 HPFs; the cellularity and nuclear atypia combined with the mitotic index are used in making the diagnosis. The cells grow in interlacing fascicles with abundant eosinophilic fibrillary cytoplasm and elongate nuclei with blunt ends. Epithelioid variants occur in which the cells are polygonal rather than spindle shaped.[41]

Immunohistochemical evaluation of leiomyosarcoma shows diffuse cytoplasmic reactivity for actin, muscle-specific actin, and desmin, but because of the overlap of the immunophenotype with stromal sarcoma, morphologic analysis is generally the best method of classifying this neoplasm.

Clinical Queries and Reporting

Smooth muscle tumors other than ordinary leiomyomas are so unusual in endometrial samples that they require a comment regarding their appearance and possible malignant potential. Unless the tumor is obviously malignant, it probably will be necessary to describe the lesion and wait for the hysterectomy to determine the biologic potential of the tumor. Even in hysterectomy specimens, where thorough sampling is possible, an occasional tumor remains borderline, and some have proposed the term "smooth muscle tumors of uncertain malignant potential"[41,60,67] or "smooth muscle tumor of low malignant potential"[61] for equivocal lesions.

High-grade leiomyosarcoma usually is readily recognized. Often precise classification of the sarcoma may be difficult from a biopsy specimen, but in general, recognition of high-grade sarcoma is sufficient for clinical management. A brief microscopic description with a mitotic count helps to clarify the diagnosis.

Rare Neoplasms

Lymphoma and Leukemia

Lymphoma or leukemic infiltration of the endometrium is a highly unusual finding in biopsy material.[68,69] When this does occur, it commonly is found in a patient with known disseminated disease. Primary involvement is rare, and lymphoma is more common than leukemia. Most of the lymphomas that involve the corpus are diffuse

large cell type or follicular of the small-cleaved cell, large cell, or mixed type.[69] Other types of lymphoma are rare. Diffuse small cell and mixed small and large cell patterns, undifferentiated lymphoma of Burkitt and non-Burkitt type, and Hodgkin disease all have been reported, however. Leukemic infiltrates most commonly are due to myelogenous leukemia and may present as granulocytic sarcoma.[69]

Involvement of the endometrium by lymphoma or leukemia results in extensive infiltration of the stroma with atypical lymphoid cells that may envelop a few residual glands (Fig. 11.18). The process should be distinguished from severe endometritis, which may show scattered lymphoid follicles, transformed lymphocytes, and immunoblasts.[69,70] The mixed inflammatory infiltrate of endometritis and the frequent presence of a

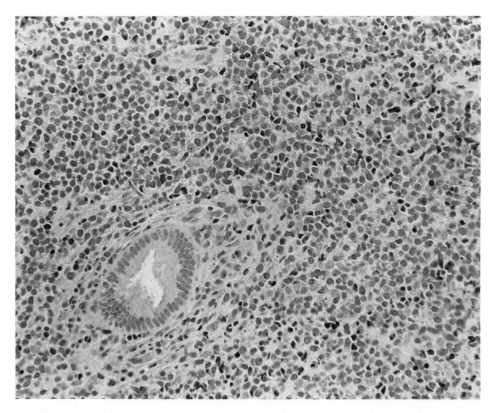

FIGURE 11.18. Lymphoma. Diffuse large cell lymphoma infiltrates the endometrium and encompasses a residual benign gland. The patient presented with abnormal bleeding and had no known disease prior to endometrial biopsy. Shortly after endometrial sampling, however, she presented with symptoms of extrauterine disease. The diffuse infiltrate of large, malignant lymphoid cells contrasts with the mixed inflammatory infiltrate, including plasma cells, seen in chronic endometritis.

neutrophilic infiltrate in the glands and surface epithelium can be helpful features for separating inflammation from a lymphoid neoplasm.

Sheets of malignant lymphoid cells in the endometrium also may mimic a high-grade carcinoma or a stromal tumor. Immunohistochemical stains for leukocyte common antigen and other lymphoid markers as well as keratin and vimentin can help in establishing the correct diagnosis.

Miscellaneous Tumors

It is extremely unusual to encounter pure mesenchymal tumors other than stromal and smooth muscle neoplasms in endometrial biopsies and curettings. An occasional case of a heterologous sarcoma, such as chondrosarcoma, osteosarcoma, or pleomorphic rhabdomyosarcoma, has been reported in the uterine cavity.[71-75] Some of these neoplasms may represent MMMTs in which the carcinomatous component is indistinct or the stromal component has overgrown the carcinomatous elements. All of these neoplasms represent high-grade sarcomas that show aggressive behavior similar to MMMTs. High-grade sarcoma that resembles malignant fibrous histiocytoma or fibrosarcoma is best classified as a variant of high-grade endometrial stromal sarcoma. Other sarcomas, such as alveolar soft part sarcoma and malignant rhabdoid tumor, also have been reported, with most cases occurring in the fourth or fifth decades.[76-79] Hemangiopericytoma is a diagnosis that should be used with great caution; most of the reported cases of so-called hemangiopericytoma of the uterus actually represent endometrial stromal sarcoma. Uterine hemangiopericytoma is vanishingly rare, if it exists at all.

Benign mesenchymal tumors also are extremely rare. Occasional lipomas and heman-

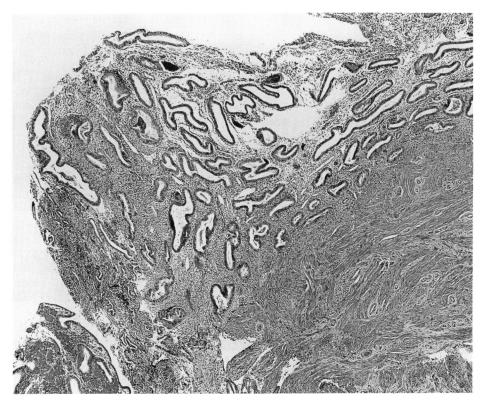

FIGURE 11.19. Tissue from uterine septum. Biopsy of endometrium from a septum confirmed by hysteroscopy. The tissue shows poorly developed secretory endometrium overlying smooth muscle. The histologic findings are not diagnostic by themselves and require clinical correlation.

giomas have been encountered, but they are so unusual that other, more common primary processes should be excluded before diagnosing these rare lesions in a biopsy specimen. For example, adipose tissue in an endometrial biopsy usually represents omental fat indicating a uterine perforation rather than a lipomatous tumor or focal fatty change of the endometrium. In these instances the clinician should be contacted immediately. Likewise, lesions with prominent vascularity usually represent a low-grade stromal tumor or vascular ectasia at the surface of a polyp rather than hemangioma.

Other primary tumors of the corpus that may be encountered in endometrial biopsies or curettings are extremely unusual. These oddities include yolk sac tumor,[80,81] teratoma,[82,83] primitive neuroectodermal tumor,[84,85] glioma,[22] paraganglioma,[86-88] and Wilms tumor.[89] Adenomatoid tumors of the myometrium only rarely involve the endometrium but may be diagnosed in endometrial samples.[90]

Other Lesions and Tumorlike Conditions

On occasion, an endometrial sample may contain fragments of bone or cartilage that represent residual fetal parts from an earlier abortion.[91] Usually the specimen consists of scattered fragments of ossified material without specific relation to the other fragments of endometrial tissue present. These foci may be accompanied by an inflammatory response. Calcification also can occur in a variety of other circumstances.[92-98] Sometimes the calcification is extensive, leading to ossification.[95-97] A few cases of psammoma body formation in association with exogenous hormone use have been reported.[93,98] Rarely, gland contents or stroma may show microscopic areas of dystrophic calcification that have no apparent significance.

Sampling of a uterine septum in a premenopausal patient may yield fragments of poorly developed endometrium with underlying smooth muscle (Fig. 11.19). These changes resemble the changes encountered adjacent to submucosal leiomyomas, and the differential diagnosis requires clinical correlation.

References

1. Zaloudek CJ, Norris HJ: Mesenchymal tumors of the uterus. In: Blaustein's Pathology of the Female Genital Tract. 4th ed. Kurman RJ, ed. New York: Springer-Verlag, 1994;487–528.

2. Clement PB: Tumorlike lesions of the uterine corpus. In: Tumors and Tumorlike Lesions of the Uterine Corpus and Cervix. Clement PB, Young RH, eds. New York: Churchill Livingstone, 1993; 137–179.

3. Clement PB, Scully RE: Tumors with mixed epithelial and mesenchymal elements. In: Tumors and Tumorlike Lesions of the Uterine Corpus and Cervix. Clement PB, Young RH, eds. New York: Churchill Livingstone, 1993;329–370.

4. DiSaia PJ, Creasman WT: Clinical Gynecologic Oncology. 4th ed. St. Louis: Mosby-Year Book, 1993.

5. Goff BA, Rice LW, Fleischhacker D, Muntz HG, Falkenberry SS, et al: Uterine leiomyosarcoma and endometrial stromal sarcoma: Lymph node metastases and sites of recurrence. Gynecol Oncol 1993; 50:105–109.

6. Leibsohn S, d'Ablaing G, Mishell DR, Jr, Schlaerth JB: Leiomyosarcoma in a series of hysterectomies performed for presumed uterine leiomyomas. Am J Obstet Gynecol 1990;162: 968–976.

7. Kahanpaa KV, Wahlstrom T, Grohn P, Heinonen E, Nieminen U, et al: Sarcomas of the uterus: A clinicopathologic study of 119 patients. Obstet Gynecol 1986;67:417–424.

7a. Ali S, Wells M; Mixed Mullerian tumors of the uterine corpus: A review. Int J Gynecol Cancer 1993;3:1–11.

8. Debrito PA, Silverberg SG, Orenstein JM: Carcinosarcoma (malignant mixed mullerian (mesodermal) tumor) of the female genital tract—Immunohistochemical and ultrastructural analysis of 28 cases. Hum Pathol 1993;24:132–142.

9. Silverberg SG, Major FJ, Blessing JA, Fetter B, Askin FB, et al: Carcinosarcoma (malignant mixed mesodermal tumor) of the uterus. A Gynecologic Oncology Group pathologic study of 203 cases. Int J Gynecol Pathol 1990;9:1–19.

10. Bitterman P, Chun B, Kurman RJ: The significance of epithelial differentiation in mixed mesodermal tumors of the uterus. A clinicopathologic and immunohistochemical study. Am J Surg Pathol 1990;14:317–328.

11. George E, Manivel JC, Dehner LP, Wick MR: Malignant mixed mullerian tumors: An immunohistochemical study of 47 cases, with histogenetic considerations and clinical correlation. Hum Pathol 1991;22:215–223.

12. Meis JM, Lawrence WD: The immunohistochemical profile of malignant mixed mullerian tumor. Overlap with endometrial adenocarcinoma. Am J Clin Pathol 1990;94:1–7.

13. Colombi RP: Sarcomatoid carcinomas of the female genital tract (malignant mixed mullerian tumors). Semin Diagn Pathol 1993;10:169–175.

14. Geisinger KR, Dabbs DJ, Marshall RB: Malignant mixed mullerian tumors. An ultrastructural and immunohistochemical analysis with histogenetic considerations. Cancer 1987;59:1781–1790.

15. Auerbach HE, Livolsi VA, Merino MJ: Malignant mixed mullerian tumors of the uterus. An immunohistochemical study. Int J Gynecol Pathol 1988;7:123–130.

16. Silverberg SG, Kurman RJ: Tumors of the uterine corpus and gestational trophoblastic disease. Atlas of Tumor Pathology, 3rd series, Fascicle 3. Washington, DC: Armed Forces Institute of Pathology, 1992.

17. Dinh TV, Slavin RE, Bhagavan BS, Hannigan EV, Tiamson EM, et al: Mixed mullerian tumors of the uterus. A clinicopathologic study. Obstet Gynecol 1989;74:388–392.

18. Norris HJ, Roth E, Taylor HB: Mesenchymal tumors of the uterus. II. A clinical and pathologic study of 31 mixed mesodermal tumors. Obstet Gynecol 1966;28:57–63.

19. Norris HJ, Taylor HB: Mesenchymal tumors of the uterus. III. A clinical and pathologic study of 31 carcinosarcomas. Cancer 1966;19:1459–1465.

20. Gagne H, Tetu B, Blondeau L, Raymond PE, Blais R: Morphologic prognostic factors of malignant mixed mullerian tumor of the uterus: A clinicopathologic study of 58 cases. Mod Pathol 1989;2:433–438.

21. Schweizer W, Demopoulos R, Beller U, Dubin H: Prognostic factors for malignant mixed mullerian tumors of the uterus. Int J Gynecol Pathol 1990;9:129–136.

22. Young RH, Kleinman GM, Scully RE: Glioma of the uterus. Report of a case with comments on histogenesis. Am J Surg Pathol 1981;5:695–699.

23. Gersell DJ, Duncan DA, Fulling KH: Malignant mixed mullerian tumor of the uterus with neuroectodermal differentiation. Int J Gynecol Pathol 1989;8:169–178.

24. Azumi N, Czernobilsky B: Immunohistochemistry. In: Blaustein's Pathology of the Female Genital Tract. 4th ed. Kurman RJ, ed. New York: Springer-Verlag, 1994;1131–1159.

25. Felix JC, Sherrod AE, Taylor CR: Gynecologic and testicular neoplasms. In: Immunomicroscopy: A Diagnostic Tool for the Surgical Pathologist. 2nd ed. Taylor CR, Cote RJ, eds. Philadelphia: W.B. Saunders, 1994;236–255.

26. Clement PB, Scully RE: Mullerian adenosarcoma of the uterus: A clinicopathological analysis of 100 cases with a review of the literature. Hum Pathol 1990;21:363–381.

27. Clement PB, Scully RE: Mullerian adenosarcoma of the uterus: A clinicopathologic analysis of ten cases of a distinctive type of Mullerian mixed tumor. Cancer 1974;34:1138–1149.

28. Zaloudek CJ, Norris HJ: Adenofibroma and adenosarcoma of the uterus. A clinicopathologic study of 35 cases. Cancer 1981;48:354–366.

29. Kaku T, Silverberg SG, Major FJ, Miller A, Fetter B, et al: Adenosarcoma of the uterus: A Gynecologic Oncology Group clinicopathologic study of 31 cases. Int J Gynecol Pathol 1992;11:75–88.

30. Abell MR: Papillary adenofibroma of the uterine cervix. Am J Obstet Gynecol 1971;110:990–993.

31. Vellios F, Ng AB, Reagan JW: Papillary adenofibroma of the uterus. A benign mesodermal mixed tumor of mullerian origin. Am J Clin Pathol 1973;60:543–551.

32. Bocklage T, Lee KR, Belinson JL: Uterine mullerian adenosarcoma following adenomyoma in a woman on tamoxifen therapy. Gynecol Oncol 1992;44:104–109.

33. Kerner H, Lichtig C: Mullerian adenosarcoma presenting as cervical polyps—A report of seven cases and review of the literature. Obstet Gynecol 1993;81:655–659.

34. Clement PB: Mullerian adenosarcomas of the uterus with sarcomatous overgrowth. A clinicopathological analysis of 10 cases. Am J Surg Pathol 1989;13:28–38.

35. Clement PB, Scully RE: Mullerian adenosarcomas of the uterus with sex cord-like elements. Am J Clin Pathol 1989;91:664–672.

36. Tavassoli FA, Norris HJ: Mesenchymal tumors of the uterus. VII. A clinicopathologic study of 60 endometrial stromal nodules. Histopathology 1981;5:1–10.

37. Chang KL, Crabtree GS, Lim-Tan SK, Kempson RL, Hendrickson MR: Primary uterine endometrial stromal neoplasms. A clinicopathologic study of 117 cases. Am J Surg Pathol 1990;14:415–438.

38. Hart WR, Yoonessi M: Endometrial stromatosis of the uterus. Obstet Gynecol 1977;49:393–403.

39. Norris HJ, Taylor HB: Mesenchymal tumors of the uterus. I. A clinical and pathological study of 53 endometrial stromal tumors. Cancer 1966;19:755–766.

40. Yoonessi M, Hart WR: Endometrial stromal sarcomas. Cancer 1977;40:898–906.

41. Clement PB: Pure mesenchymal tumors. In: Tumors and Tumorlike Lesions of the Uterine Corpus and Cervix. Clement PB, Young RH, eds. New York: Churchill Livingstone, 1993;265–328.

42. Fekete PS, Vellios F: The clinical and histologic spectrum of endometrial stromal neoplasms: A report of 41 cases. Int J Gynecol Pathol 1984;3:198–212.

43. Evans HL: Endometrial stromal sarcoma and poorly differentiated endometrial sarcoma. Cancer 1982;50:2170–2182.

44. Piver MS, Rutledge FN, Copeland L, Webster K, Blumenson L, et al: Uterine endolymphatic stromal myosis: A collaborative study. Obstet Gynecol 1984;64:173–178.

45. Mansi JL, Ramachandra S, Wiltshaw E, Fisher C: Endometrial stromal sarcomas. Gynecol Oncol 1990;36:113–118.

46. Larson B, Silfversward C, Nilsson B, Pettersson F: Endometrial stromal sarcoma of the uterus. A clinical and histopathologic study. The Radiumhemmet series 1936–1981. Eur J Obstet Gynecol Reprod Biol 1990;35:239–249.

47. Gloor E, Schnyder P, Cikes M, et al: Endolymphatic stromal myosis: Surgical and hormonal treatment of extensive abdominal recurrence 20 years after hysterectomy. Cancer 1982;50:1888.

48. Thatcher SS, Woodruff JD: Uterine stromatosis: A report of 33 cases. Obstet Gynecol 1982;59:428.

49. Farhood AI, Abrams J: Immunohistochemistry of endometrial stromal sarcoma. Hum Pathol 1991; 22:224–230.

50. Lillemoe TJ, Perrone T, Norris HJ, Dehner LP: Myogenous phenotype of epithelial-like areas in endometrial stromal sarcomas. Arch Pathol Lab Med 1991;115:215–219.

51. Clement PB, Scully RE: Uterine tumors resembling ovarian sex-cord tumors. A clinicopathologic analysis of fourteen cases. Am J Clin Pathol 1976;66:512–525.

52. McCluggage WG, Shah V, Walsh MY, Toner PG: Uterine tumour resembling ovarian sex cord tumour—Evidence for smooth muscle differentiation. Histopathology 1993;23:83–85.

53. Clement PB, Scully RE: Endometrial stromal sarcomas of the uterus with extensive endometrioid glandular differentiation: A report of three cases that caused problems in differential diagnosis. Int J Gynecol Pathol 1992;11:163–173.

54. Franquemont DW, Frierson HF, Mills SE: An immunohistochemical study of normal endometrial stroma and endometrial stromal neoplasms—Evidence for smooth muscle differentiation. Am J Surg Pathol 1991;15:861–870.

55. Deligdish L, Loewenthal M: Endometrial changes associated with myomata of the uterus. J Clin Pathol 1970;23:676–680.

56. Kempson RL, Hendrickson MR: Pure mesenchymal neoplasms of the uterine corpus: Selected problems. Semin Diagn Pathol 1988;5:172–198.

57. Clement PB: Pathology of the uterine corpus. Hum Pathol 1991;22:776–791.

58. Evans HL, Chawla SP, Simpson C, et al: Smooth muscle tumors of the uterus other than ordinary leiomyoma. A study of 46 cases, with emphasis on diagnostic criteria and prognostic factors. Cancer 1988;62:2239–2247.

59. Prayson RA, Hart WR: Mitotically active leiomyomas of the uterus. Am J Clin Pathol 1992;97:14–20.

60. O'Connor DM, Norris HJ: Mitotically active leiomyomas of the uterus. Hum Pathol 1990;21:223–227.

61. Hendrickson MR, Kempson RL: The uterine corpus. In: Diagnostic Surgical Pathology. 2nd ed. Sternberg SS, ed. New York: Raven Press, 1994; 2091–2193.

62. Kurman RJ, Norris HJ: Mesenchymal tumors of the uterus. VI. Epithelioid smooth muscle tumors including leiomyoblastoma and clear cell leiomyoma. Cancer 1976;37:1853–1865.

63. Mazur MT, Kraus FT: Histogenesis of morphologic variations in tumors of the uterine wall. Am J Surg Pathol 1980;4:59–74.

64. Perrone T, Dehner LP: Prognostically favorable "mitotically active" smooth-muscle tumors of the uterus. A clinicopathologic study of 10 cases. Am J Surg Pathol 1988;12:1–8.

65. Kaminski PF, Tavassoli FA: Plexiform tumorlet: A clinical and pathologic study of 15 cases with ultrastructural observations. Int J Gynecol Pathol 1984;3:124–134.

66. Taylor HB, Norris HJ: Mesenchymal tumors of the uterus. IV. Diagnosis and prognosis of leiomyosarcomas. Arch Pathol 1966;82:40–44.

67. Kempson RL, Hendrickson MR: Pure mesenchymal neoplasms of the uterine corpus: Selected problems. Semin Diagn Pathol 1988;5:172–198.

68. Harris N, Scully R: Malignant lymphoma and granulocytic sarcoma of the uterus and vagina. A clinicopathologic analysis of 27 cases. Cancer 1984;53:2530–2545.

69. Ferry JA, Young RH: Malignant lymphoma, pseudolymphoma, and hematopoietic disorders of the female genital tract. Pathol Annu 1991;26:227–263.

70. Young RH, Harris NL, Scully RE: Lymphoma-like lesions of the lower female genital tract. A report of 16 cases. Int J Gynecol Pathol 1985;4:289–299.

71. Vakiani M, Mawad J, Talerman A: Heterologous

sarcomas of the uterus. Int J Gynecol Pathol 1982;1:211–219.

72. Podczaski E, Sees J, Kaminski P, Sorosky J, Larson JE, et al: Rhabdomyosarcoma of the uterus in a postmenopausal patient. Gynecol Oncol 1990;37: 439–442.

73. Hart WR, Craig JR: Rhabdomyosarcoma of the uterus. Am J Clin Pathol 1978;70:217–223.

74. De Young B, Bitterman P, Lack EE: Primary osteosarcoma of the uterus: Report of a case with immunohistochemical study. Mod Pathol 1992; 5:212–215.

75. Clement PB: Chondrosarcoma of the uterus: Report of a case and review of the literature. Hum Pathol 1978;6:726–727.

76. Guillou L, Lamoureux E, Masse S, Costa J: Alveolar soft-part sarcoma of the uterine corpus: Histological, immunocytochemical and ultrastructural study of a case. Virchows Arch [A] Pathol Anat 1991;418:467–471.

77. Cho KR, Rosenchein NB, Epstein JI: Malignant rhabdoid tumor of the uterus. Int J Gynecol Pathol 1989;8:381–387.

78. Gray GJ, Glick A, Kurtin P, Jones H: Alveolar soft part sarcoma of the uterus. Hum Pathol 1986; 17:297–300.

79. Nolan N, Gaffney E: Alveolar soft part sarcoma of the uterus. Histopathology 1990;16:97–99.

80. Joseph MG, Fellows FG, Hearn SA: Primary endodermal sinus tumor of the endometrium. A clinicopathologic, immunocytochemical, and ultrastructural study. Cancer 1990; 63:297–302.

81. Ohta M, Sakakibara K, Mizuno K, Kano T, Matsuzawa K, et al: Successful treatment of primary endodermal sinus tumor of the endometrium. Gynecol Oncol 1988;31:357–364.

82. Clement PB: Miscellaneous primary neoplasms and metastatic neoplasms. In: Tumors and Tumorlike Lesions of the Uterine Corpus and Cervix. Clement PB, Young RH, eds. New York: Churchill Livingstone, 1993;371–418.

83. Martin E, Scholes J, Richart R, Fenoglio C: Benign cystic teratoma of the uterus. Am J Obstet Gynecol 1979;135:429–431.

84. Daya D, Lukka H, Clement PB: Primitive neuroectodermal tumors of the uterus—A report of four cases. Hum Pathol 1992;23:1120–1129.

85. Hendrickson MR, Scheithauer BW: Primitive neuroectodermal tumor of the endometrium: Report of two cases, one with electron microscopic observations. Int J Gynecol Pathol 1986;5:249–259.

86. Beham A, Schmid C, Fletcher CDM, Aubock L, Pickel H: Malignant paraganglioma of the uterus. Virchows Arch [A] 1992;420:453–457.

87. Tavassoli F: Melanotic paraganglioma of the uterus. Cancer 1986;58:942–948.

88. Young TW, Thrasher TV: Nonchromaffin paraganglioma of the uterus. Arch Pathol Lab Med 1982;106:608–609.

89. Bittencourt AL, Britto JF, Fonseca LE, Jr: Wilms' tumor of the uterus: The first report of the literature. Cancer 1981;47:2496–2499.

90. Carlier MT, Dardick I, Lagace AF, Sreeram V: Adenomatoid tumor of the uterus: Presentation in endometrial curettings. Int J Gynecol Pathol 1986;5:69–74.

91. Kurman RJ, Mazur MT: Benign diseases of the endometrium. In: Blaustein's Pathology of the Female Genital Tract. 4th ed. Kurman RJ, ed. New York: Springer-Verlag, 1994;367–409.

92. Alpert LC, Haufrect EJ, Schwartz MR: Uterine lithiasis. Am J Surg Pathol 1990;14:1071–1075.

93. Herbold DR, Magrane DM: Calcifications of the benign endometrium. Arch Pathol Lab Med 1986; 110:666–669.

94. Untawale VG, Gabriel JB, Chauhan PM: Calcific endometritis. Am J Obstet Gynecol 1982;144: 482–483.

95. Ceccacci L, Clancy G: Endometrial ossification: Report of an additional case. Am J Obstet Gynecol 1981;141:;103–104.

96. Bhatia NN, Hoshiko MG: Uterine osseous metaplasia. Obstet Gynecol 1982;60:256–259.

97. Waxman M, Moussouris HF: Endometrial ossification following an abortion. Am J Obstet Gynecol 1978;130:587–588.

98. Valicenti JF, Priester SK: Psammoma bodies of benign endometrial origin in cervicovaginal cytology. Acta Cytol 1977;21:550–552.

12
Methods of Endometrial Evaluation

Endometrial Sampling Techniques

There are several methods of sampling the endometrium. The "gold standard" is dilatation and curettage (D&C), which requires dilatation of the cervix to allow insertion of a curette into the endometrial cavity.[1-5] This technique allows for the most thorough sampling of the endometrium but requires anesthesia for cervical dilatation. The curette is drawn across the anterior and posterior endometrial surfaces, scraping the tissue free. D&C also readily allows for a fractional curettage, with sampling of both the endometrial and the endocervical mucosa. Fractional sampling is especially useful for evaluating possible endocervical pathology, such as extension of endometrial adenocarcinoma to the endocervix.[6] D&C is most commonly used in situations in which more extensive sampling of the endometrium is needed to exclude significant pathology or to remove as much endometrium as possible in patients with severe abnormal endometrial bleeding.[1-5,7-11]

Complications of D&C can include hemorrhage, infection, or perforation, although each of these appears to occur at a rate of between 4 and 6 per 1,000 procedures.[1] Since many patients who undergo D&C do not come to hysterectomy, the overall sensitivity and specificity of this technique have been difficult to determine. One study found that D&C performed immediately before hysterectomy often sampled less than half of the cavity, suggesting that this procedure may fail to fully document significant endometrial pathology.[12] Curettage before hysterectomy for leiomyomas also has little value, rarely identifying a significant lesion.[13] Several investigators also have found discrepancies between the grade of endometrial carcinoma in curettings as compared to hysterectomy specimens.[9,11,14-16]

Strictly applied, the term "endometrial biopsy" refers to a limited sampling procedure that does not require endocervical dilatation prior to sampling. Endometrial biopsy is relatively painless and does not require the anesthetic used for D&C; it is usually an office-based procedure.[3-5,17] These samples are taken either with a small sharp curette, such as the Novak or Randall curette, or with a device that uses suction to aspirate the tissue, such as the Pipelle endometrial aspirator (Unimar, Wilton, CT) or the Z-Sampler (Zinnatti Surgical Instruments, Chatsworth, CA). Limited sampling techniques are especially useful for obtaining smaller specimens for endometrial dating in infertility patients or for evaluating the response of endometrial tissue to steroid hormone therapy of various types. Hyperplasia and neoplasia can be accurately diagnosed by the endometrial biopsy, however, and it is possible to perform limited fractional sampling of endocervical as well as endometrial tissue using some biopsy devices. Because these various biopsy procedures can be done in the office rather than the operating room and because they yield sufficient specimens for diagnosis in most cases, they are cost-effective methods for endometrial evaluation.[1,2,17]

The Pipelle and related devices have received widespread clinical usage because they are simple to use, cost effective, and reliable for giving adequate tissue samples in most cases. The Pipelle-type device uses a hand-held piston to generate negative pressure and aspirate tissue through a narrow cannula inserted into the endometrial cavity. Comparisons of the Pipelle sampling device with other, more traditional, sampling mechanisms show no significant difference in the overall quality of tissue taken for evaluation,[18-29] although some studies find that the Pipelle technique samples much less of the endometrial surface than other biopsy devices.[27] The Pipelle instrument does change the pattern of tissue fragmentation, however, yielding cylinders of tissue with small portions of endometrium mixed with fresh blood clot.

Other aspiration devices, such as the Vabra aspirator (Berkeley Medevices, Berkeley, CA) or the Tis-u-trap (Milex Products, Chicago, IL), use a mechanical vacuum to extract tissue into a tissue trap collection apparatus.[1,17-19,27,30] The cannula for these devices is thin, ranging from 3 to 4 mm, so general anesthesia is not required. This technique tends to result in extensive fragmentation of the tissue, but the overall quality is comparable to that of a D&C specimen for diagnosis. They also have the advantage of sampling much of the endometrium.

An aspiration technique called suction curettage is used in evacuating early (first trimester) abortion specimens. The procedure requires cervical dilatation and is often done under local anesthesia (paracervical block), since general anesthesia increases the risk of perforation, visceral injury, and hemorrhage during extraction of the aborted gestation.[31,32] In very early pregnancy, however, endometrial aspiration, which is often termed "menstrual extraction," can be done using a small plastic cannula without anesthesia or dilatation. After the first trimester, but generally before the 20th week, abortion can be performed by dilatation and evacuation (D&E), a technique that employs gradual cervical dilatation using an osmotic dilator (*Laminaria japonica*).[31,32]

Noninvasive Methods of Endometrial Evaluation

Hysteroscopy

Hysteroscopy with fiberoptic illumination is widely used for visualizing the endometrium and allowing directed biopsy or excision of lesions.[3,33-38] Hysteroscopy, especially with a large-diameter hysteroscope, may require local or general anesthesia, and in some patients cervical dilatation is necessary. The technique is usually performed by distending the endometrial cavity to allow visualization, a procedure termed "panoramic hysteroscopy."[3,39] Often the distending medium is dextran, although other substances, such as carbon dioxide gas, may be used. A nondistending technique known as "contact hysteroscopy," which does not require a distending medium, also has been developed. In this technique the surface to be viewed is touched, and lesions are identified by their contour, color, vascular pattern, and spatial relationships.[3,40]

Hysteroscopy has the advantage of giving directed biopsy specimens, in contrast to the blind biopsy offered by other procedures. It is useful for evaluation of women with abnormal uterine bleeding. It can reveal polyps or small submucosal leiomyomas and enhances clinicopathologic correlations. The technique is useful before and after D&C to make certain that lesions such as polyps or adhesions are removed by the curettage. In addition, hysteroscopy can help in evaluation of women with repetitive abortions who may have a congenital abnormality, such as a septum. This procedure also can be used to determine the extent and possible cervical extension of endometrial carcinoma. The technique of hysteroscopically directed transcervical resection of the endometrium can be used as a therapy for dysfunctional uterine bleeding, obliterating the endometrium.[38,41]

Ultrasound

Transvaginal ultrasound is another adjunctive technique for examining the endometrium.[42–52] Sonography with a transvaginal probe evaluates the thickness and morphology of the endometrium. The technique permits measurement of the thickness of the combined anterior and posterior endometrium, which is referred to as the endometrial "stripe." This parameter can assist in determining pathologic and physiologic changes in the endometrium.[43,52] In postmenopausal patients a thin endometrial stripe of less than 4 or 5 mm indicates that a significant pathologic lesion of the endometrium is unlikely,[44,46,48,51,53,54] whereas a stripe thicker than 5 mm suggests the presence of polyps, hyperplasia, or carcinoma. In addition, this procedure can help to determine the presence or absence of myometrial invasion by endometrial carcinoma. Ultrasonography also is useful for determining the degree of development of the endometrium in the secretory phase by determining its thickness and texture.[42,43,45,47,49,55] This technique cannot replace biopsy for accurate evaluation of endometrial morphology, however.[50]

Both transvaginal and transabdominal ultrasound are useful for assessing the possible presence of an ectopic pregnancy. When ectopic pregnancy is suspected, sonography can determine whether a gestation is in utero or tubal.[56] Both methods of ultrasound also are used in the diagnosis of gestational trophoblastic disease, especially hydatidiform mole.[57–59]

Magnetic Resonance Imaging

Magnetic resonance imaging (MRI) provides a clear view of the uterine anatomy that is especially useful in the evaluation of tumors.[3,60–63] MRI demonstrates the endometrial–myometrial interface or "junctional zone," so it can be used to assess myometrial invasion by endometrial carcinoma. It also can demonstrate myometrial invasion in gestational trophoblastic disease.[64] On occasion this technique is useful for careful follow-up or assessment of other forms of uterine neoplasia, such as stromal tumors or leiomyomas. MRI is time-consuming and expensive, however, and it is not practical for routine evaluation of non-neoplastic conditions.

Histologic Techniques

Gross examination of endometrial tissue is generally not reliable for selecting tissue for microscopy. Consequently, in most cases the whole tissue specimen should be submitted. For abortion specimens containing abundant tissue, three cassettes are sufficient to verify the presence of placental tissue (chorionic villi or trophoblast). If gross examination shows placental tissue, however, one cassette will be sufficient if the study is intended only to document the presence of an intrauterine gestation. An exception is examination of hydatidiform mole. A minimum of eight tissue blocks should be submitted to ensure adequate assessment of the chorionic villi, including the degree of trophoblastic hyperplasia and atypia.

Proper technique is requisite to ensure adequate histologic evaluation. Biopsy tissue that suffers from suboptimal fixation, processing, or sectioning will have artifacts that hinder microscopic evaluation. Fixation of endometrial tissue often is difficult because of the large amount of blood that is admixed with the tissue fragments. Some pathologists advocate special fixatives such as Bouin's for endometrial biopsies, since they offer (Bouin's and other fixatives) excellent cytologic detail,[65] but formalin is the most widely available and accepted fixative and, in our opinion, is the fixative of choice. Acid-containing fixatives such as Bouin's degrade DNA, limiting any type of molecular analysis of the tissues.

Before processing, tissue fragments should be separated from as much blood as possible. Well-fixed tissue can be placed in a tea strainer and briefly rinsed with water to remove some blood before placing into a cassette. Wrapping the tissue in thin, porous paper (tissue wrap or lens paper) or placing tissue in a porous "biopsy bag" in the cassette prevents loss of small tissue fragments. Experience has shown that sponges used to hold small specimens in cassettes cause artifacts and distort the three-dimensional configuration of the tissue.[66] During processing, immersion in alcohol–formalin removes some of the blood, which aids in subsequent sectioning. Modern tissue processors using vacuum provide optimal dehydration and penetration of paraffin into tissue. In our experience, ethanol is a better dehydrating agent than denatured alcohol. To achieve optimum processing, it is best to change reagents in the processor daily.

Endometrial biopsies and curettings are among the more difficult tissues to section, because they are highly fragmented and bloody. The paraffin-embedded tissue tends to be dry, resulting in shatter and a "venetian blind" effect. Warming the block in warm water and then applying ice to the surface of the block facilitates even sectioning, with decreased fragmentation and shatter. Specimens should be cut at 4 to 6 μm.

The paraffin blocks should be cut at multiple levels (two or three) in most cases. Multiple levels, or step sections, are especially important for smaller samples embedded in one or two cassettes. Step sections provide the most comprehensive study of the tissue, allowing the pathologist to assess the three-dimensional aspects of the tissue, and are especially useful for endometrial samples, because the tissue tends to be highly fragmented and haphazardly oriented. Furthermore, levels on the block can uncover occasional subtle abnormalities that would not be noticed if only a single section was reviewed. For example, levels may clarify the presence of a polyp or they may reveal that an apparent polypoid structure simply represents tangential sectioning of normal endometrium. Levels also help to determine whether apparently disordered glands represent a true abnormality or are simply an artifact of the procedure. Even endometrial biopsies for histologic dating in infertility patients benefit from multiple levels; frequently the histologic date is correctly adjusted by identifying more advanced secretory changes in step sections.

Routine hematoxylin and eosin (H&E) stains generally suffice for the diagnosis of most specimens. Other histochemical stains are rarely necessary. The use of the periodic acid–Schiff (PAS) stain to demonstrate glycogen in the early secretory phase has no advantage over careful examination of routine H&E sections for subnuclear vacuoles. Biopsies showing granulomatous inflammation should be stained for acid-fast and fungal organisms. Tissue Gram stains are not useful for evaluation of most cases of endometritis. Stains for epithelial mucin, such as mucicarmine and alcian blue, are useful for establishing the diagnosis of adenocarcinoma in a poorly differentiated malignant tumor. Mucin stains have little utility for determining endometrial versus endocervical primary sites, however, since tumors at either site show variable amounts of cytoplasmic and luminal mucin (Chapter 10).

Frozen Section

Frozen sections can be useful in the evaluation of occasional cases. Usually, however, frozen sections cause significant artifacts in endometrial tissue, since the tissue often is edematous and contains considerable blood. These tissues have very different consistency and water content compared to other specimens, such as lymph nodes or breast tissue. Consequently, laboratories that routinely use frozen section for the latter tend to have greater difficulty obtaining sections from endometrial samples.

On occasion a frozen section is requested just prior to hysterectomy in a perimenopausal or postmenopausal woman with abnormal uterine bleeding to determine whether carcinoma is present. This technique is helpful if the tissue is clearly benign or clearly malignant. The subtleties of glandular patterns, which are crucial in distinguishing atypical hyperplasia from well-differentiated adenocarcinoma, can be substantially obscured by artifacts caused by the frozen section technique, however. Often a better method of assessing the endometrium preoperatively is to obtain an office-based biopsy. Formalin-fixed specimens can be rapidly processed and reported, offering greater diagnostic accuracy.

One other occasional application of frozen section is in the evaluation of the patient with a possible ectopic pregnancy. Frozen section can help establish the presence or absence of intrauterine trophoblastic tissue in selected cases. Usually, however, measurement of serum progesterone, serum beta-human chorionic gonadotropin (beta-hCG) measurements, and transvaginal ultrasound can be used to assess the possible presence of an ectopic gestation before resorting to curettage.[67] When curettings are obtained, an attempt should be made to visualize villi by flotation of the specimen in saline before resorting to frozen section.

Immunohistochemistry

Accurate interpretation of most endometrial biopsies depends primarily on evaluation of well-fixed and carefully prepared H&E sections. In an occasional case, however, optimal assessment of an abnormality is aided by immunohistochemical stains.[68,69] Immunohistochemistry generally is most helpful either to assess trophoblastic tissue or to evaluate a neoplasm. Despite the large number of antibodies available, only a few are useful adjuncts for the diagnosis of most endometrial lesions. The applications of immunohistochemistry for specific diagnoses also are discussed in the relevant chapters. The following is a brief summary of instances where immunohistochemistry can assist in the diagnosis.

For trophoblastic tissue, one of the most useful immunostains is keratin. Since trophoblastic cells are epithelial, any type of trophoblast (cytotrophoblast, intermediate trophoblast, or syncytiotrophoblast) is immunoreactive to keratin unless fixation and preservation have masked the presence of the filaments. Consequently, a keratin stain can be very useful for demonstrating trophoblastic cells, especially intermediate trophoblast, in specimens in which chorionic villi and trophoblastic cells are not clearly evident. An example would be identification of trophoblast in assessing the possible presence of an ectopic pregnancy.[70–74] In these cases the infiltrate of intermediate trophoblast at the placental implantation site can be very difficult to distinguish from decidua (Chapter 3). In addition to keratin, the placental hormones hCG and human placental lactogen (hPL) are produced by syncytiotrophoblast and intermediate trophoblast. Immunostains for these proteins, especially hPL, which is present in intermediate trophoblast at the placental implantation site, can be helpful in ruling out an ectopic pregnancy.[70,71,73–76]

Demonstration of hCG and hPL also is useful in establishing the diagnosis of choriocarcinoma and placental site trophoblastic tumor (PSTT) when routine H&E sections fail to clearly demonstrate the diagnostic histologic features of these neoplasms (Chapter 4).[75,77,78] One other trophoblastic protein, human placental alkaline phosphatase (PLAP), has utility in separating complete from partial hydatidiform mole.[79] In complete moles, the syncytiotrophoblast covering the villi contains much more hCG than PLAP, whereas in partial moles the reverse is found.

In early pregnancy the endometrial glands are immunoreactive for S-100 protein, and this staining disappears after the 12th week of gestation.[80,81] Normal proliferative and secretory endometrium and hyperplastic and neoplastic glands do not stain for S-100 protein. No antibodies assist in distinguishing atypical hyperplasia from well-differentiated adenocarcinoma.

In the evaluation of neoplasia, immunohistochemical stains may assist in the differential diagnosis of endometrial and endocervical primary adenocarcinoma. Endometrial carcinoma generally is immunoreactive for vimentin, while endocervical carcinoma is not.[68,82,83] Conversely, the cells of endocervical adenocarcinoma often contain carcinoembryonic antigen (CEA), which is not present in endometrial carcinoma (Chapter 10).[68,83–85] However, neither vimentin nor CEA is a completely specific marker for primary site.

Keratin immunostains also can help to determine whether a solid proliferation of cells represents an epithelial tumor or a lesion of mesenchymal or lymphoid cells. If the lesion represents a malignant mixed mesodermal tumor (MMMT) (carcinosarcoma), keratin staining also is extremely useful for highlighting the biphasic nature of the tumor, with the keratin-positive epithelial component standing out against the background of nonreactive sarcomatous cells (Chapter 11).[86–91] Epithelial membrane antigen (EMA) also stains epithelial components. The sarcomatous spindle cell component may stain focally with keratin and EMA, but this staining is limited and less intense than the reactivity of the clearly carcinomatous component.[86–92]

In assessing a possible MMMT, other markers can be useful for establishing the presence of sarcomatous elements, although the subtype of sarcoma has no influence on the prognosis of the lesion. The sarcomatous component typically is reactive for vimentin and actin, and if the sarcomatous component includes leiomyosarcoma or rhabdomyosarcoma, muscle-specific actin and desmin reactivity also is found.[86,87,90–92] Myoglobin also stains rhabdomyoblasts.[89,90] Occasionally other stains are useful. A tumor with glial differentiation will stain for S-100 protein or glial fibrillary acidic protein. Cartilaginous tissue is immunoreactive for S-100 protein. Although immunohistochemical stains are useful adjuncts for tumor diagnosis, correlation of histologic features with immunoreactivity is essential for proper classification of cell types.

Muscle filaments, including actin and desmin, are present in both smooth muscle and stromal tumors, so immunostains have little utility in distinguishing between these tumors.[93–95] These tumors also may show immunoreactivity for keratin, although the staining usually is focal, so positive staining for keratin needs to be carefully assessed, especially for the number and intensity of positive cells. In contrast to keratin, EMA is much more specific as an epithelial marker in our experience. It is not present in stromal or smooth muscle tumors.

Other applications of immunohistochemistry are relatively infrequent. On occasion the endometrium will contain metastatic tumor from an unknown primary site, and immunohistochemical evaluation can help determine the type of tumor present.[96] An immunostain for S-100 protein can help identify metastatic melanoma. Metastatic carcinoma from the gastrointestinal tract typically is immunoreactive for CEA, while primary endometrial cancer usually is not. Lymphoma and leukemia can be characterized using a number of lymphoid markers.[97] Antibodies for herpesvirus and cytomegalovirus can help establish the presence of these viral infections.

References

1. Grimes DA: Diagnostic dilation and curettage. A reappraisal. Am J Obstet Gynecol 1982;142:1–6.
2. Smith J, Schulman H: Current dilation and curettage. A need for revision. Am J Obstet Gynecol 1985;65:516–518.
3. Droegemueller W: Diagnostic procedures. In: Comprehensive Gynecology. 2nd ed. Herbst AL, Mishell DR, Jr, Stenchever MA, Droegemueller W, eds. St. Louis: Mosby-Year Book, 1992;213–251.
4. Swartz DP, Butler WJ: Normal and abnormal uterine bleeding. In: Te Linde's Operative Gynecology. 7th ed. Thompson JD, Rock JA, eds. Philadelphia: J.B. Lippincott Co., 1992;297–316.
5. Friedman F, Brodman ML: Endometrial sampling techniques. In: The Uterus: Pathology, Diagnosis and Management. Altchek A, Deligdish L, eds. New York: Springer-Verlag, 1991;155–162.
6. Caron C, Tetu B, Laberge P, Bellemare G, Raymond P-E: Endocervical involvement by endometrial carcinoma on fractional curettage: A clinicopathological study of 37 cases. Mod Pathol 1991;4:644–647.
7. Nickelsen C: Diagnostic and curative value of uterine curettage. Acta Obstet Gynecol Scand 1980;65:693–697.
8. Schlaerth JB, Morrow CP, Rodriguez M: Diagnostic and therapeutic curettage in gestational trophoblastic disease. Am J Obstet Gynecol 1990;162:1465–1471.
9. Daniel AG, Peters WA, III: Accuracy of office and operating room curettage in the grading of endometrial carcinoma. Obstet Gynecol 1988;71:612–614.
10. Berkowitz RS, Desai U, Goldstein DP, Driscoll SG, Marean AR, et al: Pretreatment curettage—A predictor of chemotherapy response in gestational trophoblastic disease. Gynecol Oncol 1980;10:39–43.
11. Cowles TA, Magrina JF, Masterson BJ, Capen CV: Comparison of clinical and surgical staging in patients with endometrial carcinoma. Obstet Gynecol 1985;66:413–416.
12. Stock RJ, Kanbour L: A pre-hysterectomy curettage. Obstet Gynecol 1975;45:537–560.
13. Moller LMA, Berget A: Prehysterectomy curettage in women with uterine fibromyomata is not worthwhile. Acta Obstet Gynecol Scand 1993; 72:374–376.
14. Soothill PW, Alcock CJ, MacKenzie IZ: Discrepancy between curettage and hysterectomy histology in patients with stage I uterine malignancy. Br J Obstet Gynaecol 1989;96:478–481.
15. Piver MS, Lele SB, Barlow JJ, Blumenson L: Para-aortic lymph node evaluation in stage I endometrial cancer. Obstet Gynecol 1982;59:97–100.
16. Sant Cassia LJ, Weppelmann B, Shingleton, H, Soong SJ, Hatch K, et al: Management of early endometrial carcinoma. Gynecol Oncol 1989; 35:362–366.

17. Feldman S, Berkowitz RS, Tosteson ANA: Cost-effectiveness of strategies to evaluate postmeno-pausal bleeding. Obstet Gynecol 1993;81:968–975.

18. Koonings PP, Moyer DL, Grimes DA: A random-ized clinical trial comparing Pipelle and Tis-u-trap for endometrial biopsy. Obstet Gynecol 1990; 75:293–295.

19. Kaunitz AM, Masciello A, Ostrowski M, Rovira EZ: Comparison of endometrial biopsy with the endometrial Pipelle and Vabra aspirator. J Re-prod Med 1988;33:427–431.

20. Hill GA, Herbert CM, III, Parker RA, Wentz AC: Comparison of late luteal phase endometrial biop-sies using the Novak curette or Pipelle endometrial suction curette. Obstet Gynecol 1989;73:443–446.

21. Eddowes HA, Read MD, Codling BW: Pipelle—A more acceptable technique for outpatient endome-trial biopsy. Br J Obstet Gynaecol 1990; 97:961–962.

22. Stovall TG, Photopulos GJ, Poston WM, Ling FW, Sandles LG: Pipelle endometrial sampling in pa-tients with known endometrial carcinoma. Obstet Gynecol 1991;77:954–956.

23. Silver MM, Miles P, Rosa C: Comparison of Novak and Pipelle endometrial biopsy instruments. Obstet Gynecol 1991;78:828–830.

24. Stovall TG, Ling FW, Morgan PL: A prospective, randomized comparison of the Pipelle endome-trial sampling device with the Novak curette. Am J Obstet Gynecol 1991;165:1287–1290.

25. Fothergill DJ, Brown VA, Hill AS: Histological sampling of the endometrium—A comparison be-tween formal curettage and the Pipelle sampler. Br J Obstet Gynaecol 1992;99:779–780.

26. Ferry J, Farnsworth A, Webster M, Wren B: The efficacy of the Pipelle endometrial biopsy in detecting endometrial carcinoma. Aust N Z J Obstet Gynaecol 1993;33:76–78.

27. Rodriguez GC, Yaqub N, King ME: A comparison of the Pipelle device and the Vabra aspirator as measured by endometrial denudation in hysterec-tomy specimens: The Pipelle device samples sig-nificantly less of the endometrial surface than the Vabra aspirator. Am J Obstet Gynecol 1993; 168:55–59.

28. Check JH, Chase TS, Nowroozi K, Wu CH, Chern R: Clinical evaluation of the Pipelle endometrial suction curette for timed endometrial biopsy. J Reprod Med 1989;34:218–220.

29. Henig I, Chan P, Treadway PR, Maw BM, Gullett AJ, et al: Evaluation of the Pipelle curette for endo-metrial biopsy. J Reprod Med 1989;34: 786–789.

30. Einerth Y: Vacuum curettage by the Vabra method. A simple procedure for endometrial diag-nosis. Acta Obstet Gynecol Scand 1982;61: 373–376.

31. Stubblefield PM: Conception control: Contracep-tion, sterilization, and pregnancy termination. In: Gynecology: Principles and Practice. 4th ed. Kist-ner RW, ed. Chicago: Year Book Medical Pub-lishers, 1986;583–621.

32. Grimes DA: Surgical management of abortion. In: Te Linde's Operative Gynecology. 7th ed. Thompson JD, Rock JA, eds. Philadelphia: J.B. Lippincott Co., 1992;317–342.

33. Loffer FD: Hysteroscopy with selective endome-trial sampling compared with D&C for abnormal uterine bleeding. The value of a negative hystero-scopic view. Obstet Gynecol 1989;73: 16–20.

34. Friedler S, Margalioth EJ, Kafka I, Yaffe H: Inci-dence of post-abortion intra-uterine adhesions evaluated by hysteroscopy. A prospective study. Hum Reprod 1993;8:442–444.

35. Mencaglia L, Perino A, Hamou J: Hysteroscopy in perimenopausal and postmenopausal women with abnormal uterine bleeding. J Reprod Med 1987 32:577–582.

36. Fraser IS: Hysteroscopy and laparoscopy in women with menorrhagia. Am J Obstet Gynecol 1990;162:1264–1269.

37. Wortman M, Daggett A: Hysteroscopic manage-ment of intractable uterine bleeding—A review of 103 cases. J Reprod Med 1993;38:505–510.

38. Hellen EA, Coghill SB, Shaxted EJ: The histo-pathology of transcervical resection of the endo-metrium—An analysis of 200 cases. Histopathol-ogy 1993;22:361–365.

39. Valle RF: Technique of panoramic hysteroscopy. In: Diagnostic and Operative Hysteroscopy: A Text and Atlas. Baggish MS, Barbot J, Valle RF, eds. Chicago: Year Book Medical Publishers, 1989;94–101.

40. Baggish MS: Contact hysteroscopy. In: Diagnostic and Operative Hysteroscopy: A Text and Atlas. Baggish MS, Barbot J, Valle RF, eds. Chicago: Year Book Medical Publishers, 1989;102–113.

41. Daniell JF, Kurtz BR, Ke RW: Hysteroscopic en-dometrial ablation using the rollerball electrode. Obstet Gynecol 1992;80:329–332.

42. Rogers PAW, Polson D, Murphy CR, Hosie M, Susil B, et al: Correlation of endometrial histol-ogy, morphometry, and ultrasound appearance after different stimulation protocols for in vitro fertilization. Fertil Steril 1991;55:583–587.

43. Fleischer AC, Gordon AN, Entman SS, Kepple DM: Transvaginal scanning of the endometrium. J Clin Ultrasound 1990;18:337–349.

44. Nasri MN, Coast GJ: Correlation of ultrasound findings and endometrial histopathology in postmenopausal women. Br J Obstet Gynaecol 1989; 96:1333–1338.

45. Khalifa E, Brzyski RG, Oehninger S, Acosta AA, Muasher SJ: Sonographic appearance of the endometrium—The predictive value for the outcome of in vitro fertilization in stimulated cycles. Hum Reprod 1992;7:677–680.

46. Dorum A, Kristensen GB, Langebrekke A, Sornes T, Skaar O: Evaluation of endometrial thickness measured by endovaginal ultrasound in women with postmenopausal bleeding. Acta Obstet Gynecol Scand 1993;72:116–119.

47. Dickey RP, Olar TT, Curole DN, Taylor SN, Rye PH: Endometrial pattern and thickness associated with pregnancy outcome after assisted reproduction technologies. Hum Reprod 1992; 7:418–421.

48. Sheth S, Hamper UM, Kurman RJ: Thickened endometrium in the postmenopausal woman—sonographic-pathologic correlation. Radiology 1993; 87:135–139.

49. Dickey RP, Olar TT, Taylor SN, Curole DN, Matulich EM: Relationship of endometrial thickness and pattern to fecundity in ovulation induction cycles—Effect of clomiphene citrate alone and with human menopausal gonadotropin. Fertil Steril 1993;59:756–760.

50. Doherty CM, Silver B, Binor Z, Molo MW, Radwanska E: Transvaginal ultrasound and the assessment of luteal phase endometrium. Am J Obstet Gynecol 1993;168:1702–1709.

51. Smith P, Bakos O, Heimer G, Ulmsten U: Transvaginal ultrasound for identifying endometrial abnormality. Acta Obstet Gynecol Scand 1991;70: 591–594.

52. Fleischer AC, Gordon AN, Entman SS, Keple DM: Transvaginal sonography of the endometrium: Current and potential clinical applications. In: The Principles and Practice of Ultrasonography in Obstetrics and Gynecology. 4th ed. Fleischer AC, Romero R, Manning FA, Jeanty P, James AE, Jr, eds. Norwalk: Appleton and Lange, 1991;583–596.

53. Varner RE, Sparks JM, Cameron CD, Roberts LL, Soong S: Transvaginal sonography of the endometrium in postmenopausal women. Obstet Gynecol 1991;78:195–199.

54. Goldchmit R, Katz Z, Blickstein I, Caspi B, Dgani R: The accuracy of endometrial Pipelle sampling with and without sonographic measurement of endometrial thickness. Obstet Gynecol 1993;82: 727–730.

55. Grunfeld L, Walker B, Bergh PA, Sandler B, Hoff-

mann G, et al: High-resolution endovaginal ultrasonography of the endometrium: A noninvasive test for endometrial adequacy. Obstet Gynecol 1991;78:200–204.

56. Fleischer AC, Cartwright PS, Pennell RG, Sacks GA: Sonography of ectopic pregnancy with transabdominal and transvaginal scanning. In: The Principles and Practice of Ultrasonography in Obstetrics and Gynecology. 4th ed. Fleischer AC, Romero R, Manning FA, Jeanty P, James AE, Jr, eds. Norwalk: Appleton and Lange, 1991;57–76.

57. Fleischer AC, Gordon AN: Sonography of trophoblastic diseases. In: The Principles and Practice of Ultrasonography in Obstetrics and Gynecology. 4th ed. Fleischer AC, Romero R, Manning FA, Jeanty P, James AE, Jr, eds. Norwalk: Appleton and Lange, 1991;501–508.

58. Romero R, Horgan JG, Kohorn EI, Kadar N, Taylor KJW, et al: New criteria for the diagnosis of gestational trophoblastic disease. Obstet Gynecol 1985;66:553–558.

59. Berkowitz RS, Birnholz J, Goldstein DP, Bernstein MR: Pelvic ultrasonography and the management of gestational trophoblastic disease. Gynecol Oncol 1983;15:403–412.

60. Lange RC, Buberg AC, McCarthy SM: An evaluation of MRI contrast in the uterus using synthetic imaging. Magn Reson Med 1991;17: 27-284.

61. Brown HK, Stoll BS, Nicosia SV, Florica JV, Hambley PS, et al: Uterine junctional zone: Correlation between histologic findings and MR imaging. Radiology 1991;179:409-413.

62. Scoutt LM, Flynn SD, Luthringer DJ, McCauley TR, McCarthy SM: Junctional zone of the uterus: Correlation of MR imaging and histologic examination of hysterectomy specimens. Radiology 1991;179:403-407.

63. Brown JJ, Thurnher S, Hricak H: MR imaging of the uterus: Low-signal-intensity abnormalities of the endometrium and endometrial cavity. Magn Reson Imaging 1990;8:309-313.

64. Barton JW, McCarthy SM, Kohorn EI, Scoutt LM, Lange RC: Pelvic MR imaging findings in gestational trophoblastic disease, incomplete abortion, and ectopic pregnancy: Are they specific? Radiology 1993;186:163–168.

65. Buckley CH, Fox H: Biopsy Pathology of the Endometrium. New York: Raven Press, 1989.

66. Kepes JJ, Oswald O: Tissue artefacts caused by sponge in embedding cassettes. Am J Surg Pathol 1991;15:810–812.

67. Carson SA, Buster JE: Ectopic pregnancy. N Engl J Med 1993;329:1174–1181.

68. Azumi N, Czernobilsky B: Immunohistochemistry.

In: Blaustein's Pathology of the Female Genital Tract. 4th ed. Kurman RJ, ed. New York: Springer-Verlag, 1994;1131–1159.

69. Felix JC, Sherrod AE, Taylor CR: Gynecologic and testicular neoplasms. In: Immunomicroscopy: A Diagnostic Tool for the Surgical Pathologist. 2nd ed. Taylor CR, Cote RJ, eds. Philadelphia: W.B. Saunders Co., 1994;236–255.

70. O'Connor DM, Kurman RJ: Intermediate trophoblast in uterine curettings in the diagnosis of ectopic pregnancy. Obstet Gynecol 1988;72:665–670.

71. Kaspar HG, To T, Dinh TV: Clinical use of immunoperoxidase markers in excluding ectopic gestation. Obstet Gynecol 1991;78:433–437.

72. Daya D, Sabet L: The use of cytokeratin as a sensitive and reliable marker for trophoblastic tissue. Am J Clin Pathol 1991;95:137–141.

73. Yeh IT, O'Connor DM, Durman RJ: Intermediate trophoblast: Further immunocytochemical characterization. Mod Pathol 1990;3:282–287.

74. Sorensen FB, Marcussen N, Daugaard HO, Kristiansen JD, Moller J, et al: Immunohistological demonstration of intermediate trophoblast in the diagnosis of uterine versus ectopic pregnancy—A retrospective survey and results of a prospective trial. Br J Obstet Gynaecol 1991; 98:463–469.

75. Kurman RJ, Main CS, Chen HC: Intermediate trophoblast: A distinctive form of trophoblast with specific morphological, biochemical and functional features. Placenta 1984;5:349–370.

76. Angel E, Davis JR, Nagle RB: Immunohistochemical demonstration of placental hormones in the diagnosis of uterine versus ectopic pregnancy. Am J Clin Pathol 1985;84:705–709.

77. Kurman RJ, Young RH, Norris HJ, Main CS, Lawrence WD, et al: Immunocytochemical localization of placental lactogen and chorionic gonadotropin in the normal placenta and trophoblastic tumors, with emphasis on intermediate trophoblast and the placental site trophoblastic tumor. Int J Gynecol Pathol 1984;3:101–121.

78. Young RE, Kurman RJ, Scully RE: Proliferations and tumors of intermediate trophoblast of the placental site. Semin Diagn Pathol 1988; 5:223–237.

79. Brescia RJ, Kurman RJ, Main CS, Surti U, Szulman AE: Immunocytochemical localization of chorionic gonadotropin, placental lactogen, and placental alkaline phosphatase in the diagnosis of complete and partial hydatidiform moles. Int J Gynecol Pathol 1987;6:213–229.

80. Nakamura Y, Moritsuka Y, Ohta Y, Itoh S, Haratake A, et al: S-100 protein in glands within decidua and cervical glands during early pregnancy. Hum Pathol 1989;20:1204–1209.

81. Agarwal S, Singh UR: Immunoreactivity with S100 protein as an indicator of pregnancy. Indian J Med Res 1992;96:24–26.

82. Dabbs DJ, Geisinger KR, Norris HT: Intermediate filaments in endometrial and endocervical carcinomas. The diagnostic utility of vimentin patterns. Am J Surg Pathol 1986;10:568–576.

83. Tamimi HK, Gown AM, Kimdeobald J, Figge DC, Greer BE, et al: The utility of immunocytochemistry in invasive adenocarcinoma of the cervix. Am J Obstet Gynecol 1992;166:1655–1662.

84. Cohen C, Shulman G, Budgeon LR: Endocervical and endometrial adenocarcinoma: An immunoperoxidase and histochemical study. Am J Surg Pathol 1982;6:151–157.

85. Maes G, Fleuren GJ, Bara J, Nap M: The distribution of mucins, carcinoembryonic antigen, and mucus-associated antigens in endocervical and endometrial adenocarcinomas. Int J Gynecol Pathol 1988;7:112–122.

86. Debrito PA, Silverberg SG, Orenstein JM: Carcinosarcoma (malignant mixed mullerian (mesodermal) tumor) of the female genital tract—Immunohistochemical and ultrastructural analysis of 28 cases. Hum Pathol 1993;24:132–142.

87. George E, Manivel JC, Dehner LP, Wick MR: Malignant mixed mullerian tumors: An immunohistochemical study of 47 cases, with histogenetic considerations and clinical correlation. Hum Pathol 1991;22:215–223.

88. Geisinger KR, Dabbs DJ, Marshall RB: Malignant mixed mullerian tumors. An ultrastructural and immunohistochemical analysis with histogenetic considerations. Cancer 1987;59:1781–1790.

89. Auerbach HE, Livolsi VA, Merino MJ: Malignant mixed mullerian tumors of the uterus. An immunohistochemical study. Int J Gynecol Pathol 1988;7:123–130.

90. Meis JM, Lawrence WD: The immunohistochemical profile of malignant mixed mullerian tumor. Overlap with endometrial adenocarcinoma. Am J Clin Pathol 1990;94:1–7.

91. Costa MJ, Khan R, Judd R: Carcinosarcoma (malignant mixed mullerian [mesodermal] tumor) of the uterus and ovary. Correlation of clinical, pathologic, and immunohistochemical features in 29 cases. Arch Pathol Lab Med 1991;115:583–590.

92. Bitterman P, Chun B, Kurman RJ: The significance of epithelial differentiation in mixed mesodermal tumors of the uterus. A clinicopathologic and immunohistochemical study. Am J Surg Pathol 1990;14:317–328.

93. Farhood AI, Abrams J: Immunohistochemistry of endometrial stromal sarcoma. Hum Pathol 1991;22:224–230.

94. Franquemont DW, Frierson HF, Mills SE: An immunohistochemical study of normal endometrial stroma and endometrial stromal neoplasms —Evidence for smooth muscle differentiation. Am J Surg Pathol 1991;15:861–870.

95. Lillemoe TJ, Perrone T, Norris HJ, Dehner LP: Myogenous phenotype of epithelial-like areas in endometrial stromal sarcomas. Arch Pathol Lab Med 1991;115:215–219.

96. Barr NJ, Taylor CR: Approach to the "unknown primary"—Anaplastic tumors. In: Immunomicroscopy: A Diagnostic Tool for the Surgical Pathologist. 2nd ed. Taylor CR, Cote RJ, eds. Philadelphia: W.B. Saunders Co., 1994; 368–400.

97. Taylor CR: Lymphoma/hematopathology: The antibodies. In: Immunomicroscopy: A diagnostic Tool for the Surgical Pathologist. 2nd ed. Taylor CR, Cote RJ, eds. Philadelphia: W.B. Saunders, 1994;71–106.

Index

ISBN 0-387-94230-0